Cosmetic Injectables in Practice
Dermal Fillers and Botulinum Toxin

Cosmetic Injectables in Practice
Dermal Fillers and Botulinum Toxin

Editors

Rashmi Sarkar MD MNAMS
Professor
Department of Dermatology
Maulana Azad Medical College and Associated
Lok Nayak Jai Prakash Narayan Hospital
New Delhi, India

Vivek Nair MD FAAD (USA) FISD (USA)
Consultant Dermatologist and Dermatosurgeon
Dr Nair's Skin Clinic and Hair Transplant Center
Gurugram, Haryana, India

Associate Editor

Gillian Ruth Britto MD AAAM
Dermatologist, Derma Care Center
Al-Salam International Hospital, Kuwait

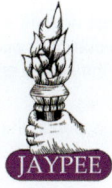

JAYPEE BROTHERS MEDICAL PUBLISHERS
The Health Sciences Publisher
New Delhi | London

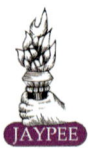 **Jaypee Brothers Medical Publishers (P) Ltd**

Headquarters
Jaypee Brothers Medical Publishers (P) Ltd
4838/24, Ansari Road, Daryaganj
New Delhi 110 002, India
Phone: +91-11-43574357
Fax: +91-11-43574314
Email: jaypee@jaypeebrothers.com

Overseas Office
J.P. Medical Ltd
83 Victoria Street, London
SW1H 0HW (UK)
Phone: +44 20 3170 8910
Fax: +44 (0)20 3008 6180
Email: info@jpmedpub.com

Website: www.jaypeebrothers.com
Website: www.jaypeedigital.com

© 2020, Jaypee Brothers Medical Publishers

The views and opinions expressed in this book are solely those of the original contributor(s)/author(s) and do not necessarily represent those of editor(s) of the book.

All rights reserved. No part of this publication may be reproduced, stored or transmitted in any form or by any means, electronic, mechanical, photocopying, recording or otherwise, without the prior permission in writing of the publishers.

All brand names and product names used in this book are trade names, service marks, trademarks or registered trademarks of their respective owners. The publisher is not associated with any product or vendor mentioned in this book.

Medical knowledge and practice change constantly. This book is designed to provide accurate, authoritative information about the subject matter in question. However, readers are advised to check the most current information available on procedures included and check information from the manufacturer of each product to be administered, to verify the recommended dose, formula, method and duration of administration, adverse effects and contraindications. It is the responsibility of the practitioner to take all appropriate safety precautions. Neither the publisher nor the author(s)/editor(s) assume any liability for any injury and/or damage to persons or property arising from or related to use of material in this book.

This book is sold on the understanding that the publisher is not engaged in providing professional medical services. If such advice or services are required, the services of a competent medical professional should be sought.

Every effort has been made where necessary to contact holders of copyright to obtain permission to reproduce copyright material. If any have been inadvertently overlooked, the publisher will be pleased to make the necessary arrangements at the first opportunity. The **CD/DVD-ROM** (if any) provided in the sealed envelope with this book is complimentary and free of cost. **Not meant for sale.**

Inquiries for bulk sales may be solicited at: jaypee@jaypeebrothers.com

Cosmetic Injectables in Practice-Dermal Fillers and Botulinum Toxin

First Edition: **2020**

ISBN 978-93-89188-37-0

Printed at Replika Press Pvt. Ltd.

Dedicated to
*My late parents, Dr Asim Kumar Sarkar and Mrs Chhobi Sarkar
for your constant blessings and strength.*
—**Rashmi Sarkar**

My daughters, Anaisha and Zoya. Thank you for choosing us.
—**Vivek Nair**

Contributors

Abhay Talathi DNB MD FCPS DDVL
Consultant Dermatologist and Cosmetologist
SkinSpace Clinic
Mumbai, Maharashtra, India

Ayushi Khandelwal MD
Associate Dermatologist
MS Skin Clinic
Bengaluru, Karnataka, India

Banani Choudhury MD DNB MNAMS
Consultant
Department of Dermatology
Jaslok Hospital and Research Center
Mumbai, Maharashtra, India

Bhavesh K Swarnakar MBBS DVD DNB MNAMS
Dermatologist and Esthetician
Swarnkar Superspeciality Center
Indore, Madhya Pradesh, India

Deepak Jhakar MD
Senior Resident
Department of Dermatology
Municipal Corporation Medical College and
Hindurao Hospital
New Delhi, India

Deepak Vedamurthy MD FHM
Associate, Division of Hospital Medicine
Christiana Care Health System
Newark, Delaware, USA

Gillian Ruth Britto MD AAAM
Dermatologist, Derma Care Center
Al-Salam International Hospital
Kuwait

Gulhima Arora DNB MNAMS
Consultant Dermatologist
Department of Dermatology
Mehektagul Dermaclinic
New Delhi, India

Hema Pant MD
Medical Director
Sculpt Aesthetics and Cosmetic Clinic
New Delhi, India

Indu Ballani MD
Visiting Consultant
BL Kapoor Hospital
New Delhi, India

Ishad Aggarwal MD
Consultant Dermatologist
Wizderm Skin Clinic
Kolkata, West Bengal, India

Ishmeet Kaur MD
Assistant Professor
NDMC and Hindu Rao Hospital
New Delhi, India

Jaishree Sharad MBBS DDV FAAD Fellowship in
Cosmetic Dermatology
Fellowship in Lasers
Director
Skinfiniti Aesthetic Skin and Laser Clinic
Mumbai, Maharashtra, India

Komal Sharma MD
Fellow in Dermatology
Medanta—The Medicity
Gurugram, Haryana, India

Kritu Bhandari MD
Medical Director
Orijine—Skin, Hair and Wellness
Pune, Maharashtra, India

Kuldeep Singh MBBS MS (Surg) MCh (Plastic Surg)
Senior Consultant
Department of Aesthetic, Plastic and
Reconstructive Surgery
Indraprastha Apollo Hospitals
New Delhi, India

Latika Arya MD
Consultant Dermatologist, Laser and
Esthetic Physician
LA Skin and Aesthetic Clinic
New Delhi, India

Madhuri Agarwal MBBS MD DDV
Founder and Medical Director
Yavana Aesthetics Clinic
Mumbai, Maharashtra, India

Malavika Kohli MD DVD DNB
Director, Skin Secrets
Jaslok Hospital and Research Center
Breach Candy Hospital Trust
Mumbai, Maharashtra, India

Manogna Vellala MD DVL
Civil Assistant Surgeon
Institute of Preventive Medicine
Hyderabad, Telangana, India

Maya Vedamurthy MD MAMS FRCP (Edin)
Consultant Dermatologist
RSV Skin and Laser Research Center
Apollo Hospitals
Chennai, Tamil Nadu, India

MK Shetty MD
Consultant Dermatologist and
Esthetic Laser Physician
Dr Shetty's Center for Aesthetic Medicine
Vikram Hospital; Carefit Group of Clinics
Bengaluru, Karnataka, India

Mukta Sachdeva MD DPD (UK) Dip Derm (UK) DD
(UK) Fellow in Cos Derm (USA)
Head and Consultant
Manipal Hospital
Bengaluru, Karnataka, India

Nidhi Sharma MD
Consultant Dermatologist
Dermdoctors Clinic
Amritsar, Punjab, India

Pallavi Ailawadi MD DNB
Consultant Dermatologist
Skinacea Clinic
Faridabad, Haryana, India

Rajat Kandhari MBBS MD MSc
Consultant Dermatologist
Dr Kandhari's Skin and Dental Clinic
Veya Aesthetics
New Delhi, India

Rashmi Sarkar MD MNAMS
Professor
Department of Dermatology
Maulana Azad Medical College and Associated
Lok Nayak Jai Prakash Narayan Hospital
New Delhi, India

Richa Ojha Sharma MD FAAD
Consultant Dermatologist
Twacha Skin Clinics, New Delhi
Medical Director
MaxDermCare Skin and Lasers Pvt. Ltd.
New Delhi, India

Rungsima Wanitphakdeedecha MD MA MSc
Associate Professor
Department of Dermatology
Faculty of Medicine, Siriraj Hospital, Mahidol
University
Bangkok, Thailand

Sandeep Arora MD
Professor and Head
Department of Dermatology
Command Hospital Air Force
Bengaluru, Karnataka, India

Sheilly Kapoor MD
Consultant Dermatologist
Medanta—The Medicity
Gurugram, Haryana, India

Shilpa Garg DNB
Consultant Dermatologist
Department of Dermatology
Sir Ganga Ram Hospital
New Delhi, India

Sonali Langar MD
Post Graduate Diploma in Aesthetics
American Academy of Aesthetic Medicine
Consultant Dermatologist
Apollo Hospital
Skin Remedies Clinic and Laser Centre
Noida, Uttar Pradesh, India

Sudha Vani Damarla MD
Associate Professor
Department of Dermatology
Osmania Medical College
Hyderabad, Telangana, India

Swati Mutha MBBS DDV
Associate Dermatologist
Dr Malavika Kohli and Associates
ACI-Cumballa Hill Hospital
Mumbai, Maharashtra, India

Tanvi Gupta Arora MD DNB
Consultant Dermatologist
Skintillate Skin, Hair and Laser Clinic
New Delhi, India

Vanravi Vachatimanont MD MSc BMedSci BSc
Dermatologic Surgeon and Esthetic Practitioner
Innovative SKin and Laser surgerY (iSKY) Center
Bangkok, Thailand

Varsha Vaidyanathan MD DNB
Senior Resident
Department of Dermatology
North DMC Medical College and Hindurao Hospital
New Delhi, India

Vivek Nair MD FAAD (USA) FISD (USA)
Consultant Dermatologist and Dermatosurgeon
Dr Nair's Skin Clinic and Hair Transplant Center
Gurugram, Haryana, India

Weeranut Phothong MD
Assistant Professor
Department of Dermatology
Faculty of Medicine Siriraj Hospital, Mahidol University
Bangkok, Thailand

Woraphong Manuskiatti MD
Professor
Department of Dermatology
Faculty of Medicine Siriraj Hospital,
Mahidol University, Bangkok, Thailand

Preface

Somewhere around 3 years back, I was approached by M/s Jaypee Brothers Medical Publishers (P) Ltd, New Delhi, India to edit a book on Cosmetic Injectables-Dermal Fillers and Botulinum toxin, which should be useful for the Asian readers as well as the rest of the world. Honestly, this was not really in my comfort zone, but I am always in for new adventures. I spoke to three more co-editors, those who are successful injectors to help me in this venture. However, life is unpredictable and two of them dropped out along the way. Dr Vivek Nair, my younger colleague and student, remained on board, and we decided to take this ahead, in spite of the odds.

A lot happened in these 2–3 years in our lives. I could feel once again that I was at professional crossroads and would perhaps have to take uncomfortable decisions. I lost my dear mother who was my strength, a wonderful professional colleague and good friend. The editorial team also changed thrice! And wanting to be true to the subject, I started learning injectables whenever and wherever I could and I feel I could at least learn some important techniques. And importantly, a dermatologist mostly following medical dermatology can also learn. It was our mission to make an easily comprehensible book on botulinum toxin and fillers available to practitioners and dermatology students, so they inject properly and safely.

I would like to thank our authors, national and international, for writing wonderful chapters and providing expert tips. A big word of thanks to Vivek Nair for his patience and expertise on this book. And thank you, Dr Gillian Ruth Britto for helping us as an Assistant Editor and Dr Latika Arya for giving us valuable insights into this project and helping us with the table of contents.

I would like to thank Shri Jitendar P Vij (Group Chairman), Mr Ankit Vij (Managing Director), Ms Chetna Malhotra Vohra (Associate Director–Content Strategy), Dr Rajul Jain (Development Editor) and the staff of M/s Jaypee Brothers Medical Publishers (P) Ltd, New Delhi, India, in helping me out with this difficult project. Thanks Srikanta and Abhik for being understanding. And to the readers, happy reading and safe injecting!

Rashmi Sarkar

Preface

When I started injecting in 2010 there were very few of us actively practicing cosmetic dermatology. Since then the numbers of dermatologists interested in injectables have grown in leaps and bounds. It is heartening to see that most injectors today have sound knowledge of the fundamentals around the use of fillers and botulinum toxin; quite unlike the situation when we started. This book fulfills the need of a handy reference tool for injecting different areas of the face. Expert injectors from all over the country have given their valuable personal experience for the most common indications treated. Under Dr Rashmi Sarkar's guidance, editing this book has been a learning experience for me, and we hope that the readers will find it useful. I would like to thank her for giving me this opportunity and for helping to keep me connected with academia despite being in private practice for over a decade. The love and support of my family is the bedrock which makes all else possible.

Vivek Nair

Contents

Introduction and History of Dermal Fillers and Botulinum Toxin — xix
Pallavi Ailawadi, Rashmi Sarkar

SECTION 1: DERMAL FILLERS

1. **Classification of Fillers** — 3
   Rashmi Sarkar, Gillian Ruth Britto

2. **Science and Properties of Hyaluronic Acid Fillers** — 9
   Maya Vedamurthy, Deepak Vedamurthy

3. **Guide for Selection and Use of Fillers** — 16
   Richa Ojha Sharma, Rashmi Sarkar

4. **Facial Anatomy for Dermal Fillers** — 23
   Kuldeep Singh

5. **Facial Assessment** — 50
   Malavika Kohli, Banani Choudhury

6. **Patient Selection and Esthetic Consult** — 66
   Latika Arya

7. **Pre-requisites for Filler Treatment** — 70
   Rashmi Sarkar, Vivek Nair

8. **Anesthesia** — 72
   Tanvi Gupta Arora

9. **Filler Injection Techniques** — 75
   Richa Ojha Sharma

10. **Fillers for Upper Face—Forehead and Temporal Region** — 79
    Vanravi Vachatimanont, Rungsima Wanitphakdeedecha

11. **Fillers for Upper Face—Temples** — 85
    Gulhima Arora, Sandeep Arora

12. **Fillers for Upper Face—Eyebrow** — 90
    MK Shetty

13. **Fillers for Upper Face—Upper Eyelid** — 94
    Indu Ballani

14. **Fillers for Midface—Tear Trough and Infraorbital Areas**   98
    Rajat Kandhari, Deepak Jhakar

15. **Fillers for Midface—Cheeks**   107
    Madhuri Agarwal

16. **Fillers for Midface—Tear-Trough and Nose**   112
    Vanravi Vachatimanont, Rungsima Wanitphakdeedecha

17. **Fillers for Midface—Nasolabial Folds**   118
    Vivek Nair

18. **Fillers for Lower Face—Marionette Lines**   123
    Richa Ojha Sharma

19. **Fillers for Lower Face—Chin**   128
    Gillian Ruth Britto, Rashmi Sarkar

20. **Fillers for Lower Face—Jawline**   133
    Hema Pant, Gillian Ruth Britto, Vivek Nair

21. **Fillers for Lower Face—Lip Augmentation**   137
    Gillian Ruth Britto

22. **Fillers for Nonfacial Areas and Scars**   149
    Madhuri Agarwal

23. **Complications of Fillers and their Treatment**   154
    Mukta Sachdeva, Ayushi Khandelwal

24. **Combination Therapies with Fillers**   160
    Ishad Aggarwal

25. **Fractional Laser-assisted Botulinum Toxin Delivery**   171
    Weeranut Phothong, Woraphong Manuskiatti

SECTION 2: BOTULINUM TOXIN

26. **Neurotoxin Preparations**   179
    Abhay Talathi

27. **Frown Lines**   182
    Varsha Vaidyanathan, Shilpa Garg, Rashmi Sarkar

28. **Forehead Lines**   186
    Richa Ojha Sharma, Rashmi Sarkar

29. **Crow's Feet and Lower Eyelid**   191
    Nidhi Sharma

30. **Brow Lift with Botulinum Toxin**   197
    Jaishree Sharad

31.	**Bunny Lines** Sonali Langar	202
32.	**Nose** Indu Ballani	208
33.	**Smoker's Lines (Lip Lines)** Gulhima Arora, Sandeep Arora	213
34.	**Gummy Smile—Botulinum Toxin** Malavika Kohli, Swati Mutha	218
35.	**Botulinum Toxin for Marionette Lines** Ishad Aggarwal	225
36.	**Dimpled Chin** Rajat Kandhari, Kritu Bhandari	229
37.	**Botulinum Toxin in Platysmal Bands** Sudha Vani Damarla, Manogna Vellala	234
38.	**Nefertiti Lift** Bhavesh K Swarnkar	237
39.	**Botulinum Toxin in Masseteric Hypertrophy** Sudha Vani Damarla, Manogna Vellala	241
40.	**Complications of Botulinum Toxin and their Management** Sheilly Kapoor, Komal Sharma	245
41.	**Botulinum Toxin in Men** Rajat Kandhari	253
42.	**Microdosing in Botulinum Toxin** Rajat Kandhari, Ishmeet Kaur	259
43.	**Neurotoxin Resistance** Vivek Nair, Rashmi Sarkar	267

Index   *273*

Introduction and History of Dermal Fillers and Botulinum Toxin

Pallavi Ailawadi, Rashmi Sarkar

Beauty is defined as "the quality of being pleasing, especially to look at". Apart from this dictionary meaning, there are various definitions of beauty, both subjective and objective, albeit on a philosophical level, with multidimensional perspectives. However, since time immemorial, high emphasis has been put on physical appearance, and the things or people thought of as beautiful, tend to be appreciated more by society.

Through history, beauty standards have been defined by youthful appearance, smooth blemish-free and taut skin, delicate features with symmetrical face, long hair, slender and petite body in women, whereas men were supposed to have sharp features, broad chiseled face with muscular tall body frame. The desire to maintain the youthful appearance has been seen through the oldest civilizations and continues till date. Even in those times, they created scented oils, perfumes, and elixirs in a desire for eternal youth. On the other hand, the modern scientists have created botulinum toxin (BoNT), fillers, light, and laser devices in order to fulfill the same purpose.

SKIN AGING

As life expectancy has increased over time and people are living longer, the issues associated with aging, more so—reversal of aging, have become a major area of interest and research.

The skin is incredibly durable, but like all other organs, it also undergoes aging and is rather, the most visible indicator of passing time.

Skin aging is a complex process, affected by combination of endogenous (genetics, cellular metabolism, hormone, and metabolic processes) and exogenous (sun exposure, pollution, smoking, radiation, chemicals, and toxins) factors.[1] These factors lead to cumulative structural and physiological degradation and progressive changes in each skin layer. The aged skin becomes thin, atrophic, rough, dry, and wrinkled and these changes are more marked in the photoaged skin. Gradual loss of skin elasticity leads to sagging. A marked loss of fibrillin and collagen type VII contributes to wrinkles by weakening dermoepidermal junction **(Fig. 1)**. The overall collagen content, glycosaminoglycans, and hyaluronic acid (HA) decrease, reduces skin turgor.[2]

Also, other factors like gravity, muscle action, loss of volume, reduction and redistribution of superficial and deep fat pockets, and loss of bony support contribute to facial aging and lead to sagging, changes in shape and contour.

ANTIAGING IN DERMATOLOGY

This is one of the fastest growing subspecialties in dermatology and is a huge market in itself.

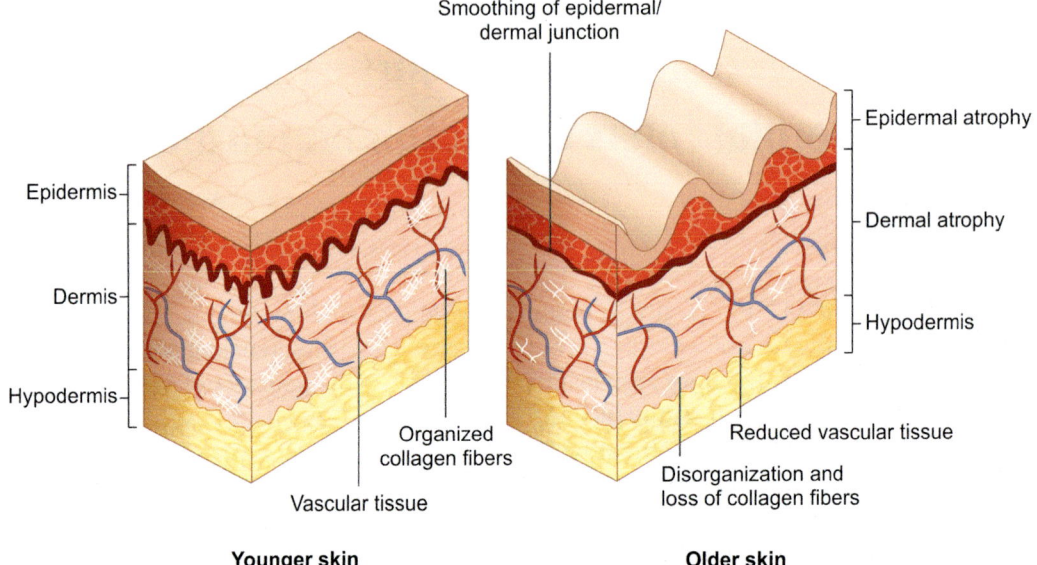

Fig. 1: Depiction of ageing of skin.

The latest statistics from The American Society for Aesthetic Plastic Surgery report Botox injections as the number one aesthetic procedure performed since 1999, with over 1,801,033 procedures done in 2018 itself, followed by 810,240 HA fillers and more than one billion dollars were spent on injectable procedures in the same year.[3] The pharmaceutical industry has responded massively with breakthrough research and has flooded the market with various antiaging modalities.

Multiple skin antiaging strategies are used these days, including nonsurgical ones like—BoNT, fillers, chemical peels, microdermabrasion, microneedling, light and laser-based devices, radiofrequency, ultrasound, and surgical methods. Each of these treatments has its own indications and a patient may require single or sometimes a combination of these to achieve the desired result. In this textbook, we shall be mainly focusing on role of BoNT and fillers in dermatology.

BOTULINUM TOXIN

Clostridium botulinum is a rod-shaped, gram-positive anaerobic bacterium which produces BoNT, having seven different subtypes (A, B, C, D, E, F, G).[4] Types A, B, and E are commonly implicated in human botulism, while type A is most commonly used for cosmetic injections.

The Origins of Botox

In the late 1700s, an unknown disease led to many deaths in Europe, caused by human ingestion of a toxin present in contaminated foods, primarily smoked blood sausages. In 1820, Justinus Kerner **(Fig. 2)**, a German physician, gave the first description of clinical botulism based on clinical observations of "sausage poisoning". In 1870, Muller coined the name botulism, *botulus*, Latin word for sausage. Later, in 1895, Émile van Ermengem, a bacteriologist described *Clostridium botulinum* as the bacterial source of the toxin. In 1928, scientists at the University of California, San Francisco, first isolated the

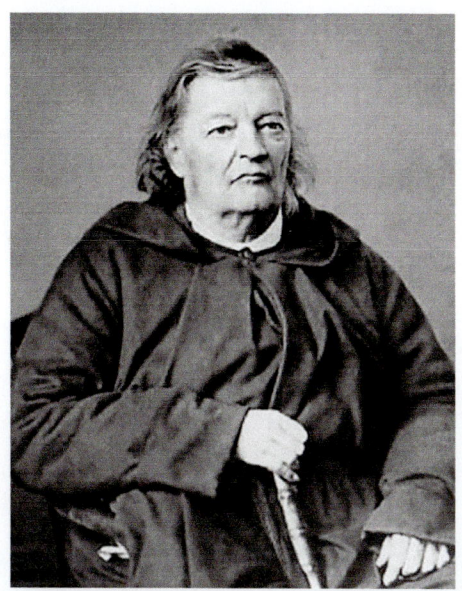

Fig. 2: Justinus Kerner (1786-1862).

appearance of moderate-to-severe glabellar lines. Subsequently, it has been approved for various medical and cosmetic uses.

Mechanism of Action

The BoNT is synthesized as a 150 kD single chain molecule and then cleaved to form two active chains bound with a disulfide bridge. The light chain acts as zinc endopeptidase with proteolytic activity, while the heavy chain provides cholinergic specificity and binds to presynaptic receptors. BoNT binds presynaptically on cholinergic nerve terminals and decreases the release of acetylcholine into the neuromuscular junction and thus prevents signal transmission, causing neuromuscular blockade. All seven subtypes of the toxin have same end result but their intracellular target proteins and potencies vary substantially. While subtypes A and E cleave synaptosome-associated protein (SNAP-25), subtypes B, D, and F cleave a vesicle-associated membrane protein (VAMP), synaptobrevin, and BoNT-C acts by cleaving syntaxin, all of these being components of the SNARE complex **(Fig. 3)**.

stable precipitate of BoNT. However, it took another 20 years for the toxin to be finally isolated in pure crystalline form by Dr Edward Schantz. Over the next few years, scientists established the exact mechanism of action of BoNT, neuromuscular blockade.[5] During world war II, American officers had planned for BoNT to be packed in capsules and used as biological weapon on Japanese soldiers, but the plan was aborted.

In 1970s, animal experiments on the use of BoNT to treat strabismus gave good results and human studies began in early 1980s, ultimately leading to US Food and Drug Administration (FDA) approval for use of BoNT-A (BOTOX®) for treatment of strabismus (1989).[5]

In a serendipitous discovery, ophthalmologists Jean and Alastair Carruthers observed that blepharospasm patients treated with periorbital Botox injections also enjoyed diminished facial glabellar lines, thereby initiating the cosmetic use of the toxin.[6] In 2002, following clinical trials, FDA approved Botox for temporarily improving the

The basic premise of action of BoNT is chemodenervation, leading to muscle paresis when injected in striate muscle. This leads to decreased wrinkling on dynamic movements of the face and decreased muscle spasms in dystonias. When injected into the exocrine glands, it leads to decreased glandular function, thereby reducing sweating in axillary hyperhidrosis. Other effects on spinal stretch reflex, muscle spindle, and reduced substance P and glutamate, make it useful in some chronic pain disorders. The onset of action takes 3-7 days from the time of injection and effect wears off in 4-6 months. Recovery occurs through proximal axonal sprouting and muscle reinnervation by formation of new neuromuscular junctions.[4]

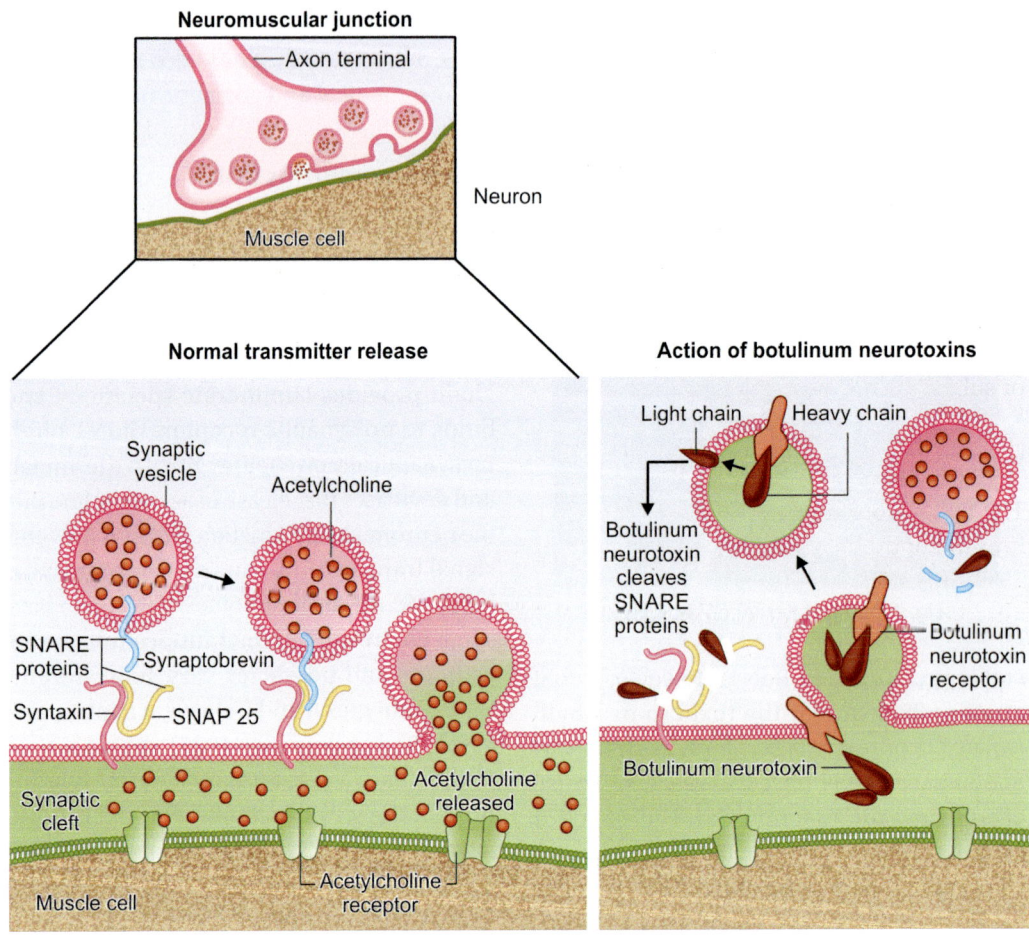

Fig. 3: Mechanism of action of botulinum toxin at the neuromuscular junction.

Current Role

Once a lethal food poison and later exploited in biological warfare, BoNT is currently one of the most versatile drugs for treatment of human diseases in ophthalmology, dermatology, and neurology.

It has been integrated into popular culture as a cosmetic enhancement tool, not just for antiaging, but also for facial shaping and contouring. BoNT-A is a mainstay in aesthetics and therapeutics, while BoNT-B has also demonstrated efficacy in aesthetics and cervical dystonia. Only BoNT-A and BoNT-B are available as approved drugs; other serotypes have shown results but have been used only in experimental settings.

Though FDA has approved Botox® (Allergan Inc) for temporary improvement of mild-to-moderate glabellar lines (2002), lateral canthal lines (2013), axillary hyperhidrosis (2004), forehead lines (2017), current aesthetic uses also include perioral lines, eyebrow lifts, widening of eyes, gummy smile, platysmal bands, horizontal neck lines, and masseter as well as palmar hyperhidrosis. Different preparations of BoNT-A are available in the market, manufactured by different companies, having variable potencies, dilution characteristics and dosages, and it is important to know the differences while using them.

FILLERS

Injectable dermal fillers are available in various forms in the market and are used for soft-tissue augmentation to enhance or replace volume that is lost in any part of skin or subcutaneous fat.

The Origin of Fillers

The first reported use of a material injected into the body for cosmetic purposes was in 1899, by Robert Gersuny (**Fig. 4**), who injected liquid paraffin to create testicular prosthesis in patients with tuberculous epididymitis. Overtime, it became treatment of choice for nasal augmentation but lost favor due to serious complications like embolization, migration, and granuloma formation (paraffinoma). Subsequently, similar injectables such as vegetable oil, mineral oil, lanolin, and beeswax were used, but abandoned due to undesirable complications.[7]

In the early 1900s, autologous fat grafts were used for correction of depressed facial defects and scar. These were relatively safe but the results and longevity were unpredictable. In 1960s, liquid silicone injections were used for soft tissue augmentation, however, frequent complications ruled out further use. The quest for the perfect injectable has been a fascinating journey and has taken an interesting course with multiple new agents formulated in last 40 years. In 1981, bovine dermal collagen was first approved by FDA as a xenogenic substance for dermal injection. However, there was a need for fillers that did not require a prior skin test and would last longer. In 2003, FDA approved new fillers for temporary soft-tissue augmentation, the HA fillers, which remain the most widely used filler material even today.[7] Subsequently, longer-lasting synthetic fillers like calcium hydroxylapatite and poly-L-lactic acid became quite popular.

Mechanism of Action

The process of aging does not occur uniformly in all areas of face and the differential impact of gravity, reduction and resorption of fat pockets and loss of bony skeletal support lead to changes in facial shape and contour. Further, subcutaneous fat of the face is not a single layer but is compartmentalized and these show variable aging over time and differ according to individual patient anatomy. Hence, it is imperative to correct these compartments separately for correcting the aging face. Fillers are used for volume correction, providing support to the tissue and filling up the rhytides. Some of the new fillers also induce production of collagen and thus the effects last longer, even after resorption of the substance. Fillers can be classified as temporary, semipermanent, or permanent depending on the longevity of the substance in tissue. They can also be classified by the composition of product—collagen (bovine, porcine, and human), HA, poly-L-lactic acid, calcium hydroxylapatite, polyacrylamide gels, and polymethyl methacrylates.[8] Over 30 fillers have been approved by FDA over last two decades. The type of product, area and volume of injection depend on indication of use and amount of correction required. HA fillers are the most commonly used temporary fillers for cosmetic purposes.

Current Role

Dermal fillers have revolutionized the field of cosmetic dermatology and form an effective tool in nonsurgical treatment of aging face as well as skin rejuvenation, either as stand-alone treatment or combination. Injectable dermal fillers are classified as medical implant device and FDA has approved various fillers for different indications. The absorbable or temporary fillers have been approved for filling up wrinkles and acne scars, lip, cheek and hand augmentation, correcting lipoatrophy in human immunodeficiency virus (HIV) patients and a nonabsorbable or permanent filler only for correction of nasolabial folds.[9] However, they have also been used for several other indications like facial shaping and contouring, eyebrow lift, filling up scars from several diseases, and volume augmentation of other body sites.

Since aesthetic treatments are mainly elective, the safety profile of procedures should be high and risk-benefit ratio should be balanced. The products used in fillers are relatively safe and most of the adverse effects happen due to improper patient or product selection, injection technique, and patient factors. Nevertheless, it is imperative for the treating doctor to know about the product, constituents, particles per mg, cross-linking, additives like lignocaine, and shelf life. There are multiple such products available in the market and it is essential to have a sound knowledge and choose the filler correctly as per the indication. The ideal filler should be safe, effective, easy to use, biocompatible, nontoxic and noninflammatory, as well as have a long life.

REFERENCES

1. Cevenini E, Invidia L, Lescai F, et al. Human models of aging and longevity. Expert Opin Biol Ther. 2008;8(9):1393-405.
2. Fisher GJ. The pathophysiology of photoaging of the skin. Cutis. 2005;75(Suppl 2):5-8.
3. American Society for Aesthetic Plastic Surgery. [online] Available from: https://www.surgery.org/sites/default/files/ASAPS-Stats2018_0.pdf. [Last accessed on June, 2019].
4. Dressler D, Saberi FA, Barbosa ER. Botulinum toxin: mechanisms of action. Arq Neuropsiquiatr. 2005;63(1):180-5.
5. Ting PT, Freiman A. The story of *Clostridium botulinum*: from food poisoning to Botox. Clin Med (Lond). 2004;4(3):258-61.
6. Carruthers JD, Carruthers JA. Treatment of glabellar frown lines with *C. botulinum*-A exotoxin. J Dermatol Surg Oncol. 1992;18:(1)17-21.
7. Kontis TC, Rivkin A. The history of injectable facial fillers. Facial Plast Surg. 2009;25(2):67-72.
8. Gilbert E, Hui A, Waldorf HA. The basic science of dermal fillers: past and present Part I: background and mechanisms of action. J Drugs Dermatol. 2012;11(9):1059-68.
9. US Food and Drug Administration. Dermal fillers (soft tissue fillers). [online] Available from: (https://www.fda.gov/medical-devices/cosmetic-devices/dermal-fillers-soft-tissue-fillers. [Last accessed on June, 2019].

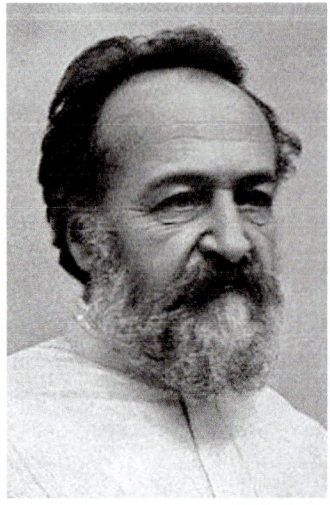

Fig. 4: Robert Gersuny (1844-1924).

SECTION 1

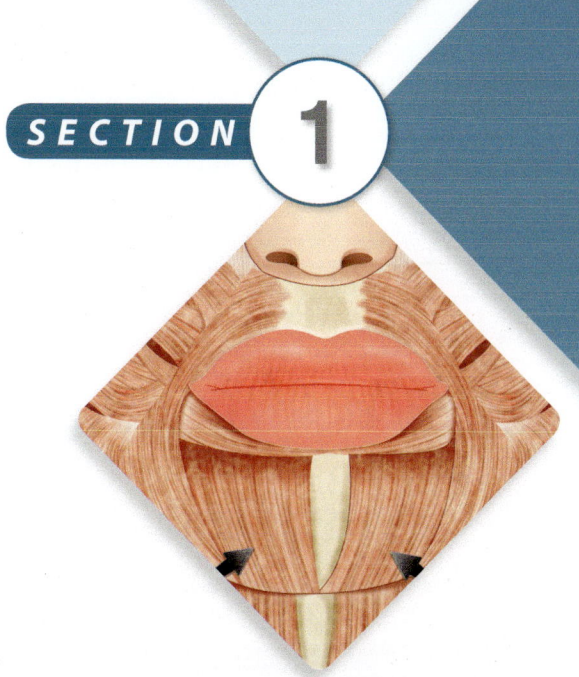

DERMAL FILLERS

SECTION OUTLINE

1. Classification of Fillers
2. Science and Properties of Hyaluronic Acid Fillers
3. Guide for Selection and Use of Fillers
4. Facial Anatomy for Dermal Fillers
5. Facial Assessment
6. Patient Selection and Esthetic Consult
7. Pre-requisites for Filler Treatment
8. Anesthesia
9. Filler Injection Techniques
10. Fillers for Upper Face—Forehead and Temporal Region
11. Fillers for Upper Face—Temples
12. Fillers for Upper Face—Eyebrow
13. Fillers for Upper Face—Upper Eyelid
14. Fillers for Midface—Tear Trough and Infraorbital Areas
15. Fillers for Midface—Cheeks
16. Fillers for Midface—Tear-Trough and Nose
17. Fillers for Midface—Nasolabial Folds
18. Fillers for Lower Face—Marionette Lines
19. Fillers for Lower Face—Chin
20. Fillers for Lower Face—Jawline
21. Fillers for Lower Face—Lip Augmentation
22. Fillers for Nonfacial Areas and Scars
23. Complications of Fillers and their Treatment
24. Combination Therapies with Fillers
25. Fractional Laser-assisted Botulinum Toxin Delivery

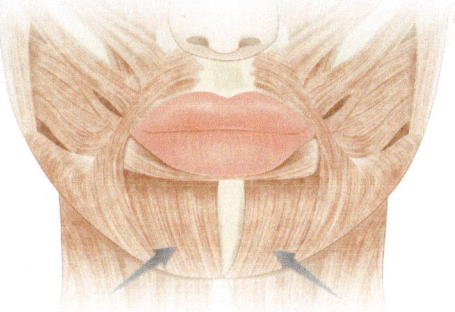

Classification of Fillers

Rashmi Sarkar, Gillian Ruth Britto

INTRODUCTION

Esthetic enhancement has been a desire since ancient times of people from various cultures. There are several methods available to improve the facial appearance such as topical and systemic agents, surgical intervention, energy-based devices (like radiofrequency, high intensity focused ultrasound, intense pulse light) and injectables like botulinum toxin and fillers. Fillers by far are the simplest and effective method to get instant results, both for the patient and the treating physician.[1] Paraffin was the first injectable substance that was used as dermal filler but its complication of embolization and granuloma formation abandoned its use as dermal filler. However, fillers have been the most popular method since the 1980s when bovine collagen was injected to treat facial lines and creases and to restore volume deficits. It was the first Food and Drug Administration (FDA) approved facial filler and it has been used for almost 30 years.[2] It was originally used to treat viral pox scars, acne scars, lipoatrophy, and soft tissue augmentation. Since the augmentation effect lasts only for 6 months and due to its side effects, physicians were on the lookout for more sustainable and effective fillers. An ideal filler has not yet been discovered; however, hyaluronic acid (HA)-based fillers have helped revolutionize the filler market with a number of ideal products available to patients.

CLASSIFICATION OF DERMAL FILLERS

Classification of dermal fillers is based on the following ***(Table 1):***[3]

- *Based on the origin*: Natural/synthetic.
- *Based on the source*: Autograft/allograft/heterograft.
- *Based on effect*: Temporary/semi-permanent/permanent.
- *Content*: Collagen/fat/hyaluronic acid/silicone/peptides.

Based on the Origin

Natural

This group of fillers was the bovine derived collagen products, namely Zyderm® and Zyplast® collagen. The collagen material was derived from a closed herd of cattle and purified for human use. Zyderm® I was first approved by the FDA in 1981 and recommended for injection into the superficial papillary dermis, and was approved for the treatment of superficial lines and wrinkles, as well as shallow acne scars. Zyderm® II, FDA approved in 1983 to treat postacne and traumatic scars on the face, although it worked well for lines and wrinkles. Zyplast® was best injected into the mid-deep dermis and its recommended use was for deep lines and folds.[4]

Table 1: Classification of dermal fillers.[3]

Dermal fillers	Examples
Based on origin	
Natural	Zyderm, fibrel, restylane, Juvederm
Synthetic	ArteFill® (PMMA), Bellafill (PMMA), Aquamid (Polyacrylamide hydrogel), Alcamid (Polyalkylimide) Silicone (Silikon 1000, Bioplastique, Pro fill), calcium hydroxylapatite (Radiesse), poly-L-lactic acid (PLLA) (Sculptra/New fill)
Based on source	
Autograft	Fat, dermal graft, isolagen (Autologous collagen)
Allograft	Fascian (cadaver), cymetra (cadaver)
Xenograft	Zyderm, zyplast, fibroquel, endoplast-50 (Bovine collagen)
Based on effect	
Temporary	Zyderm, fibrel, cymetra, fibroquel, endoplast-50 restylane, Juvederm, autologous fat, frozen fat
Semi-permanent	Autologous fat, CaHA (Radiesse), PLLA (Sculptra)
Permanent	Artefill® (PMMA), expanded polytetrafluoroethylene (EPTFE), adatoSil 5000, silicone (Silikon 1000, Biocell ultra vital)
Based on content	
Collagen	Zyderm, zyplast, fibroquel, CosmoDerm, CosmoPlast
Fat	Autologous fat, Frozen fat
Hyaluronic acid (HA)	Hylaform, restylane, Juvederm, prevelle, esthelis, belotero, captique, puragen, elevess, teosyal
Silicone	Silikon 1000, biocell ultra vital, bioplastique
Peptides	SYN®

(PMMA: polymethyl methacrylate)

Since Zyderm®/Zyplast® had hypersensitivity concerns, human-derived collagen products were developed, namely CosmoDerm® and CosmoPlast®. These fillers are made from cultured human fibroblasts and were FDA approved in 2003 for facial Esthetic procedures. They do not require intradermal testing, which was a major drawback with bovine collagen.[4] These products had longevity of approximately 3 months.

Synthetic

Poly-L-lactic acid (PLLA): Injectable PLLA is biocompatible, biodegradable, biostimulatory, synthetic filler that must be injected into the reticular dermis or subcutaneous fat. PLLA, marketed as Sculptra®, was FDA approved in 2009 as soft tissue augmentation filler.[5,6] It stimulates neocollagenesis through fibroblast activation.[7] Histological studies show increase in type 1 collagen over 8–30 months after the injection.[8,9] It is degraded by nonenzymatic hydrolysis into carbon dioxide and water over 9–24 months. However, due to neocollagenesis the augmentation effect lasts for about 24 months.[10] Side effects of Sculptra include immediate effects of swelling, bruising, inflammation, and pruritus which lasts for a few days.[11] Long-term effects include foreign body granuloma formation and extremely rare effect of anaphylactic reaction has been noted.

Calcium hydroxylapatite: Calcium hydroxylapatite (CaHA) is a biocompatible, biodegradable, resorbable, and biostimulatory filler that contains microspheres which can stimulate the endogenous production of collagen.[12] Histopathologically, they appear bluish and round or oval in shape and packed together, 25–40 μm and surrounded by fibrin fibers and mild cellular infiltrate. These microspheres are degraded by enzymatic process and disappear clinically by 9–12 months.[13] It has been used in cases of lipoatrophy of HIV, hand rejuvenation, and lip augmentation. There are reports of nodule formation after lip injections. Migration to a distant location from the injection site, a foreign body granulomatous reaction, seen as blue-gray microspheres in the extracellular matrix or within multinucleated giant cells has also been reported.[14]

Polymethyl methacrylate: Polymethyl methacrylate (PMMA) is rigid, transparent and colorless, thermoplastic permanent skin filler with low cost, easy accessibility, and potential to achieve lasting results. It has been used as an injectable filler to treat hollows and reduce rhytids. ArteFill® became the first and only permanent injectable wrinkle filler to receive FDA approval in 2006. ArteFill® is a third-generation polymeric microsphere-based filler, following its predecessor Artecoll®. It has been approved for the treatment of nasolabial folds. ArteFill® consists of PMMA microspheres (20% by volume), 30–50 μm in diameter, suspended in 3.5% bovine collagen solution (80% by volume), and 0.3% lidocaine. The collagen carrier is absorbed within 1 month after injection and completely replaced by the patient's own connective tissue within 3 months.[15]

First-generation polymerized PMMA microspheres (Arteplast) are purified with diameter greater than 20 μm, which may produce foreign body granulomas, larger microsphere (second generation Artecoll) of 30–50 μm resist phagocytosis; however, it was demonstrated that giant cell reaction still occurs with larger particles.[16,17] Complications of PMMA injection were classified as nodular masses, inflammation, allergies, and skin hypopigmentation.[18]

Polyacrylamide hydrogel: Aquamid is a biocompatible and nonabsorbable hydrogel consisting of 97.5% water and 2.5% cross-linked polyacrylamide gel (PAAG). The gel is manufactured through polymerization of the acrylamide monomers and N,N'-methylenbisacrylamide.[19] PAAG is available in more than 40 countries worldwide (Europe, Asia, the Middle East, and Latin America) and awaiting FDA approval. After injection, the implant is encapsulated and surrounded by fibroblasts and microphages, theoretically preventing migration. It is used for treating various rhytides (deep rhytides and folds), facial contouring, and correction of HIV lipoatrophy. It usually lasts for about 1 year after injection.[20] There have been reported cases of inflammation, nodule and granuloma formation, and delayed hypersensitivity reactions of Aquamid injections.[21]

Polyvinylpyrrolidone-silicone suspension: It is a permanent filler comprised of particles of polymerized silicone elastomer, 100–600 μm in size, dispersed in a carrier of polyvinylpyrrolidone. It has been used for lip augmentation and the correction of facial rhytids. It is injected into the subcutaneous plane and this avoids any phagocytosis due to its large particle size. Cases of foreign body granuloma formation, swelling, and induration have been reported.[22,23]

Polyalkylimide gel: Polyalkylimide gel is a permanent hydrophilic translucent gel filler composed of a hydrophilic biopolymer with 96% sterile water and 45% polyalkylimide polymer (Alcamid®), and different from polyacrylamide. It has been used for lipoatrophy of HIV, skeletal deformities such as pectus excavatum. Complications noted with this filler include swelling, bruising, and nodule formation.[24-26]

Based on the Source

Autograft

Fat, dermal graft: Fat grafts are taken from the lower abdomen and inner thigh especially in younger patients. When processed with proper centrifugation they can reliably produce purified fat, concentrated growth factors, and adipose-derived stem cells.[27]

Allograft

Allograft includes fascia (cadaver).

Heterograft

Heterografts include fibroquel which is bovine derived.[3]

Based on Effect

Temporary fillers are fillers which last for >12 months, such as HA fillers. Semi-permanent fillers last for 1–2 years and permanent fillers more than 2 years **(Table 2)**.[3]

Based on Content

Hyaluronic acid based fillers are one of the most popular and widely used materials in esthetic procedures. HA was first discovered by two American scientists, Carl Meyer and John Palmer. This polymer also known as Hyaluronan, is the most abundant *glycosaminoglycans* found in the human dermis. It is a ubiquitous component of all membrane connected tissue. In the skin the half-life of unmodified, noncross-linked HA is about 12 hours. Therefore to increase longevity when injected into the skin HA is cross-linked. Currently there are a large number of dermal fillers available to the physician based on various cross-linked HA technologies. Some

Table 2: Classification of dermal fillers based on duration.[3]

Temporary (Biodegradable) <1 year	Semi-permanent (Biodegradable) 1–2 years	Permanent (Nonbiodegradable) >2 years
Collagen	Calcium hydroxyapatite (CaHA) (Radiesse)	Polymethyl methacrylate (PMMA) (ArteFill®, Artecoll, Arteplast)
Collagen-human (Cosmoderm 1,2, Cosmoplast)		Polyacrylamide gel (PAAG) (Aquamid)
Collagen-Bovine (Zyderm 1,2, Zyplast)	Poly-L-lactic acid (PLLA) (Sculptra)	Polyalkylimide (Alcamid)
Hyaluronic acid-avian (Hylaform)		Silicone (Polydimethylsiloxane oil)
Hyaluronic acid-bacterial (Restylane, Juvederm)	Hydroxyethylmethacrylate (HEMA) (Dermaline/Derma deep)	

of these technologies include VYCROSS (Allergan Inc.), NASHA (Galderma Pharma), CPM (Merz Pharmaceuticals) and OXIFREE technology (Kylane laboratories).[6] The main differentiators for HA fillers are: Source of HA; concentration of HA in each syringe being utilized; the particulate size of the HA; whether the HA is cross-linked; the type of cross-linking agent used in the HA; whether the HA is monophasic or biphasic; and whether there is an anesthetic in the HA syringe.[4]

REFERENCES

1. Smith KC. Reversible vs. nonreversible fillers in facial aesthetics: concerns and considerations. Dermatology Online J. 2008;14(8):3.
2. Chacon AH. Fillers in dermatology: from past to present. Cutis. 2015;96(5):E17-9.
3. Karthik R, Mohan N. Dermal fillers. International Journal of Oral Health Dentistry. 2017;3(1):6-9.
4. Use of hyaluronic acid fillers for the treatment of the aging face. Clinical Interv Aging. 2007;2(3):369-76.
5. Schierle CF, Casas LA. Nonsurgical rejuvenation of the aging face with injectable poly-L-lactic acid for storation of soft tissue volume. Aesthet Surg J. 2011;31(1):95-109.
6. Ladewig K, Abberton K, Andrea J O'Connor. Designing in vivo bioreactors for soft tissue engineering. J Biomater Tissue Engineering. 2012;2:1-13.
7. Lam SM, Azizzadeh B, Graivier M. Injectable poly-L-lactic acid (Sculptra): technical considerations in soft-tissue contouring. Plast Reconstr Surg. 2006;118(Suppl 3):S55-63.
8. Vleggaar D. Facial volumetric correction with injectable poly-L-lactic acid. Dermatol Surg. 2005;31(11 Pt 2):1511-7.
9. Vleggaar D, Bauer U. Facial enhancement and the European experience with Sculptra (poly-L-lactic acid). J Drugs Dermatol. 2004;3(5):542-7.
10. Vleggaar D. Soft-tissue augmentation and the role of poly-L-lactic acid. Plast Reconstr Surg. 2006;118(Suppl 3):S46-54.
11. Valantin MA, Aubron-Olivier C, Ghosn J, et al. Polylactic acid implants (New-Fill) to correct facial lipoatrophy in HIV-infected patients: results of the open-label study. AIDS. 2003;17(17):2471-7.
12. Marmur ES, Phelps R, Goldberg DJ. Clinical, histologic and electron microscopic findings after injection of a calcium hydroxylapatite filler. J Cosmet Laser Ther. 2004;6(4):223-6.
13. Tzikas TL. Evaluation of the Radiance FN soft tissue filler for facial soft tissue augmentation. Arch Facial Plast Surg. 2004;6(4):234-9.
14. Beer KR. Radiesse nodule of the lips from a distant injection site: report of a case and consideration of etiology and management. J Drugs Dermatol. 2007;6(8):846-7.
15. Lemperle G, Knapp TR, Sadick NS, et al. ArteFill permanent injectable for soft tissue augmentation: I. Mechanism of action and injection techniques. Aesthetic Plast Surg. 2010;34(3):264-72.
16. Lemperle G, Nacul AM, Fortes FB. Can injection of PMMA-microspheres cause hypercalcemia? Clin Cases Miner Bone Metab. 2015;12(1):82-3.
17. Bachmann F, Erdmann R, Hartmann V, et al. Adverse reactions caused by consecutive injections of different fillers in the same facial region: risk assessment based on the results from the Injectable Filler Safety study. J Eur Acad Dermatol Venereol. 2011;25(8):902-12.
18. Limongi RM, Tao J, Borba A, et al. Complications and Management of Polymethylmethacrylate (PMMA) injections to the midface. Aesthet Surg J. 2016;36(2):132-5.
19. Christensen LH, Breiting VB, Aasted A, et al. Long-term effects of polyacrylamide hydrogel on human breast tissue. Plast Reconstr Surg. 2003;111(6):1883-90.
20. von Buelow S, von Heimburg D, Pallua N. Efficacy and safety of polyacrylamide hydrogel for facial soft-tissue augmentation. Plast Reconstr Surg. 2005;116(4):1137-46.
21. Fernández-Cossío S, Casta-ño-Oreja MT. Biocompatibility of two novel dermal fillers: histological evaluation of implants of a hyaluronic acid filler and a polyacrylamide filler. Plast Reconstr Surg. 2006;117(6):1789-96.
22. Ersek RA, Beisang AA 3rd. Bioplastique: a new texture copolymer microparticle promises permanence in soft-tissue augmentation. Plast Reconstr Surg. 1991;87(4):693-702.

23. Rudolph CM, Soyer HP, Schuller-Petrovic S, et al. Foreign body granulomas due to injectable aesthetic microimplants. Am J Surg Pathol. 1999;23(1):113-7.
24. Margolis DM. Treatment for lipoatrophy: facing the real costs. AIDS. 2007;21:1819-20.
25. Karim RB, de Lint CA, van Galen SR, et al. Long-term effect of polyalkylimide gel injections on severity of facial lipoatrophy and quality of life of HIV-positive patients. Aesthetic Plast Surg. 2008;32(6):873-8.
26. Hönig J. Cheek augmentation with Bio-Alcamid in facial lipoatrophy in HIV seropositive patients. J Craniofac Surg. 2008;19(4):1085-8.
27. Pu LLQ. Fat grafting for facial rejuvenation and contouring: a rationalized approach. Ann Plast Surg. 2018;81(6S Suppl 1):S102-8.
28. Molliard SG. Key rheological properties of hyaluronic acid fillers: from tissue integration to product degradation. Plast Aesthet Res. 2018;5:17.

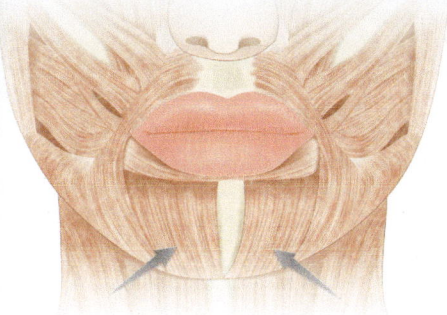

CHAPTER 2

Science and Properties of Hyaluronic Acid Fillers

Maya Vedamurthy, Deepak Vedamurthy

INTRODUCTION

The performance of any hyaluronic acid (HA) filler is based on the science with which it has been formulated. A scientific knowledge of the physical and chemical properties of HA is of utmost importance when choosing a dermal filler product to accomplish expected results and patient satisfaction.

HISTORICAL PERSPECTIVE

Hyaluronic acid was first isolated from the vitreous jelly of cows' eyes by Karl Meyer and his colleague John Paler in 1934.[1] They found the isolated substance to contain two sugar molecules one of which was uronic acid and the other D-N-acetylglucosamine. They proposed the name HA as it was isolated from hyaloid/vitreous (hyalos is the Greek word for glass + uronic acid). Hyaluronic acid was first used commercially in 1942 by Ender Balazs as a substitute for egg white in bakery products.[2]

The first biomedical application was in 1950 when it was used for vitreous substitution in eye surgeries. At first it was isolated from umbilical cords, then rooster combs and later from bacteria.

HYALURONIC ACID MOLECULE

Hyaluronic acid is a linear polysaccharide that exists naturally in all living organisms and is found in the extracellular space in nonsulfated forms. The identical structure of HA in all living species and tissues makes it an ideal substance for use as a biomaterial in medicine.

Chemical Structure

Hyaluronic acid also known as hyaluron has a simple chemical structure—two sugar molecules D-Glucuronic acid and D-N-acetylcysteine connected by glycosidic bonds forming a uniform linear polysaccharide molecule. It has a twisted ribbon structure referred to as the "coiled structure" **(Fig. 1)**.

Distribution of Hyaluronic Acid in the Human Body

Hyaluronic acid is found in highest concentration in connective tissues, epithelial, and neural tissues. About 56% of HA is found in the skin. An average human body weighing 70 kg contains about 15 g of HA, one-third of which is turned over every day.[3]

Functions of Hyaluronic Acid in the Human Body

Hyaluronic acid plays a major role for both mechanical and transport purposes in the body giving volume to the skin, shape to the eyes, and elasticity to the joints.

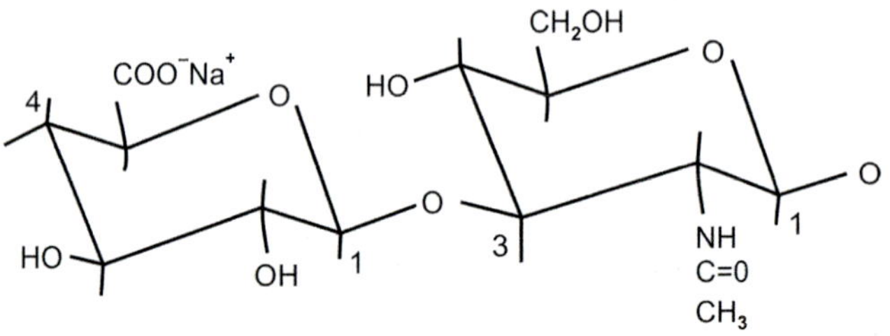

Fig. 1: Chemical structure of hyaluronic acid.

Specific Properties of HA

The HA is made up of sugar units which are hydrophilic in nature. This property and ability to bind water is provided by the HA component of the proteoglycans which can bind multiple times its own weight of water. This property contributes to hydration and restoration of volume loss in tissues. In solution, the HA molecule is present as coils of flexible network of entangled molecules which have the capacity to hold large amounts of water. HAs have a very short life of only few days when injected in humans. The hyaluronidase present naturally in human tissues will degrade the native form of noncross-linked HA into water and carbon dioxide. So, the molecule has to be modified to stay for longer periods in the tissues.[4]

EVOLUTION OF NONANIMAL STABILIZED HYALURONIC ACID

At present, the supply of HAs for medical purposes is either obtained by extraction from animal tissues or produced by biotechnology. The synthesis of HA by certain bacteria is utilized in the production of the raw material for dermal fillers which is then cross linked for stabilization.

PROPERTIES OF HYALURONIC ACID DERMAL FILLERS

There are several properties which determine the performance of the filler substance. For the physician to understand and evaluate dermal fillers, these physical and chemical attributes need to be identified to choose the appropriate product.

PROPERTIES OF HYALURONIC ACID RELEVANT TO DERMAL FILLERS

- Cross-linking
- Concentration
- Gel hardness
- Particle size
- Cohesivity and viscosity
- Tissue integration
- Degradation

Cross-linking

Cross-linking is needed to prevent digestion of the material by the body's own hyaluronidase. Food and Drug Administration (FDA) has approved of three different cross-linkers for this purpose:[5]

1. 1,4-Butanediol diglycidyl ethers (BDDE) used in the Restylane, Belotero and Juvederm range

2. Divinyl sulfone (DVS) used in Prevelle Silk and Hylaform
3. Biscarbodiimide (BCDI) used in Elevess and Puragen.

Practically, these cross-linking molecules are toxic in large amounts, but they are virtually in undetectable quantities in most HA fillers.

The amount of cross-linking is represented as a degree and this has to be within optimal limits to increase the viscosity as well as the longevity of the HA as more cross-linking will make the product less biocompatible and result in a foreign body reaction.

Cross-linking is important to improve biomedical properties while maintaining biocompatibility and biological activity **(Fig. 2)**.[6] HA fillers are classified into two types—monophasic and biphasic.[7] Monophasic HA fillers are also known as solely cross-linked and nonparticulate HA gels, e.g. Juvederm. The monophasic fillers are prepared by mixing the high molecular weight and low molecular weight HAs. The biphasic fillers, e.g. Restylane consist of gel particles of stabilized HA suspended in noncross-linked HA which serves as a lubricant. Studies have shown that monophasic HA filler show a higher degree of swelling than biphasic fillers.[8]

Concentration

The concentration of HA in a dermal filler includes both cross-linked and noncross-linked HA. The degree of correction is determined by the amount of cross-linked HA while the noncross-linked HA serves as a lubricant to help in smooth flow of the product. So the term "effective HA concentration" is used to give an estimate of cross-linked HA minus the noncross-linked HA.

The concentration of HA is important for longevity as well as the swelling properties.

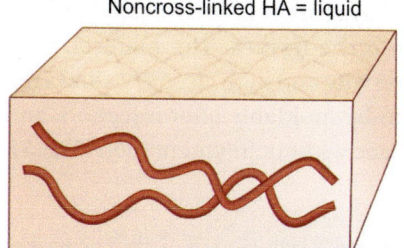
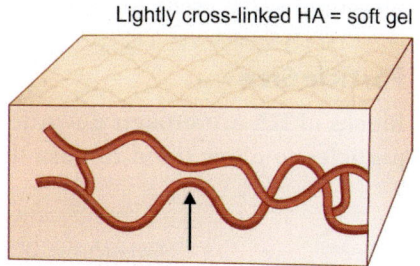
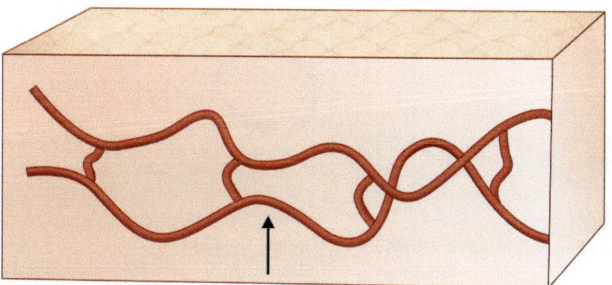

Fig. 2: Types of cross-linking and their mechanical properties.
(HA: hyaluronic acid)

The swelling ratio of the material decreases with the increase in the degree of cross-linking and HA concentration. Highest water uptake indicates a lower cross-linking extent. On the contrary, the more concentrated products in the range of 20–24 mg/mL are below equilibrium hydration and will imbibe more water and cause more tissue swelling.[9]

Gel Hardness

Gel hardness represents the degree of cross-linking between the chains and the total HA concentration. More heavily cross-linked products are stiffer than the less cross-linked products, and this is measured by the elastic modulus G. The higher the G, the more difficult it is to push the product through the needle. But the advantage is that it will be stiffer and harder to displace. Thus, the elastic modulus G represents the ability of the HA filler to resist any dynamic shearing force **(Fig. 3)**.[10] This property or elastic modulus G of a filler is measured by the oscillatory shear stress test.

Particle Size

Blocks of HA are broken down to smaller particles to allow them to pass through a syringe and needle. Particulate gel particles need to conform and bend when pushed through a needle or they will become sheared if pushed through a small orifice with sufficient force. The particle size is important to choose the appropriately sized needle to ensure smooth flow of the product. The particle size is also useful to determine the site of placement of the filler material. Small particle HA (SP-HAL) is a low-density filler with less viscosity and is indicated for the superficial dermis, medium density particles are more viscous and better suited for augmentation of mid dermis, while larger gel particles are high density, longer lasting products suitable for deep dermal injection **(Fig. 4)**.[11,12]

Cohesivity and viscosity

Cohesivity and viscosity is a measure of the capacity of a material not to dissociate because of the affinity of its molecules for one another.

Viscosity is a measure of the capacity of a material to remain at the injected area or spread into the tissues. The material with good cohesivity and high viscosity allows the product to be moldable after injection, and stays in place without fragmentation **(Fig. 5)**.

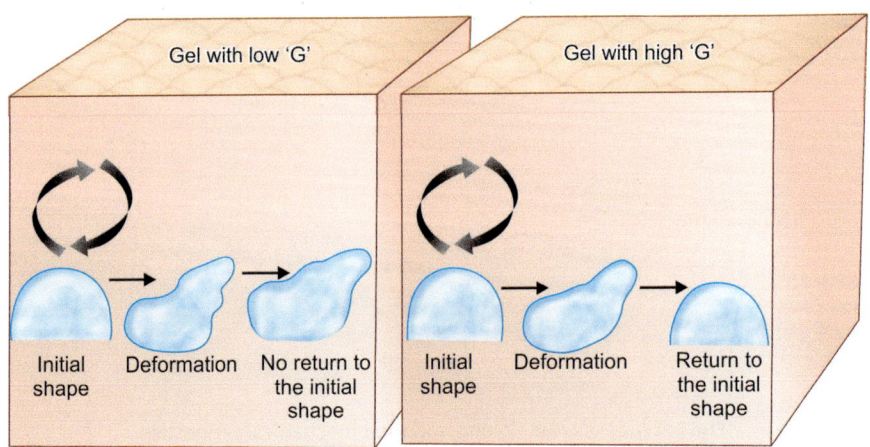

Fig. 3: Impact of elastic modulus G on deformation of the HA gel.

Tissue Integration

This step involves integration of the filler material in the injected area after it is extruded from the syringe. Based on studies, this integration starts within a few hours of injection and continues for up to 2 weeks. This process depends on the rheological properties and cohesivity of the gel and the physicomechanical properties of the recipient tissue.[13]

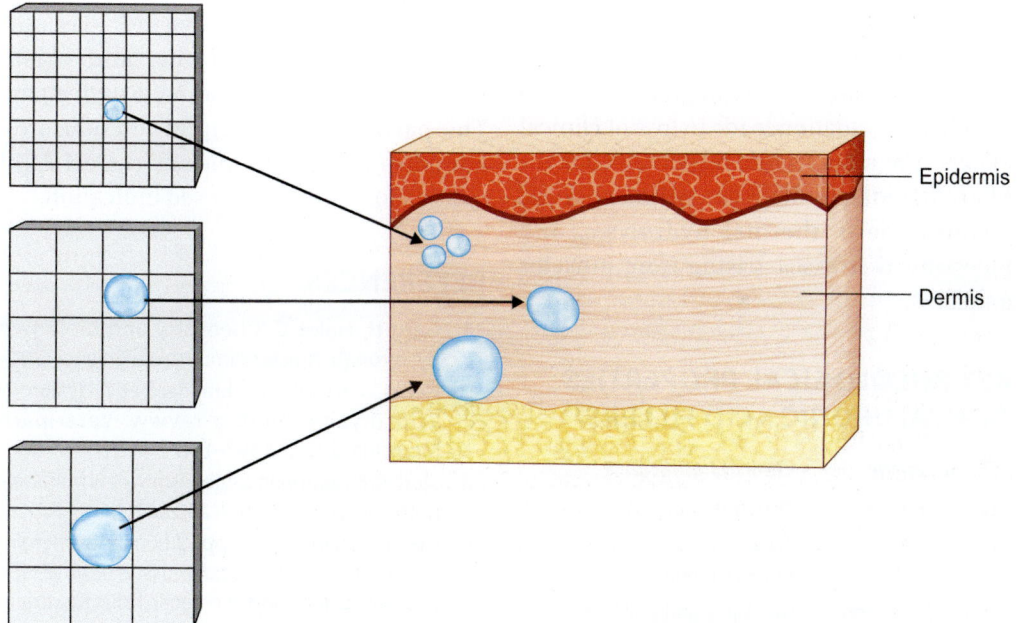

Fig. 4: Placement of particles based on size.

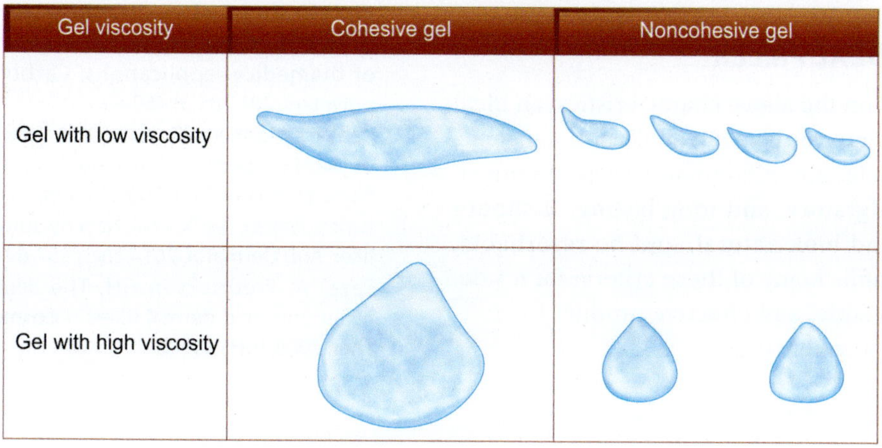

Fig. 5: Impact of the cohesivity and viscosity on shape.

Biodegradation

The unique property of nonanimal, stabilized hyaluronic acid (NASHA) is that it undergoes isovolemic degradation. Normally, biodegradable implants shrink gradually upon degradation, but NASHA maintains the initial volume throughout the degradation phase. When a bridge disappears, water takes its place thus, maintaining the same volume until the implant is fully degraded. *In vivo* HA filler degradation leads to loss of clinical effects. The main factors responsible for HA filler degradation are free radicals, dermal hyaluronidase, thermal hydrolysis, and mechanical stresses arising from muscles and fat.[14]

KEY RHEOLOGICAL PROPERTIES OF HYALURONIC ACID FILLERS[15]

Characteristic	Clinical significance
Gel hardness G	Structure, stiffness
Particle size	Placement depth, extrusion force, degradation
HA concentration	Durability and stability, swelling
Cross-linking	Longevity and viscosity
Cohesivity	"Lifting" capability

AN IDEAL FILLER

Based on the above characteristics, an ideal filler should be biocompatible, non-antigenic, nontoxic, noninflammatory, easy to inject, nonmigratory, and long lasting. It should feel and look natural, and be resorbable. HA fulfills many of these criteria for a safe, predictable, and effective product for soft-tissue augmentation.

CONCLUSION

A thorough knowledge and understanding of the science behind dermal fillers is essential for optimizing treatment outcomes, safety, and patient satisfaction.

The performance of any HA filler is based on the science with which it has been formulated. The four key rheological properties—viscosity, elasticity, extrusion force, and elastic modulus G are very important to understand. The particle size is helpful to choose the administration technique and correct depth of injection for the proposed indication.

REFERENCES

1. Garg H, Hales C. Chemistry and biology of hyaluronan. Amsterdam: Elsevier Science; 2004.
2. Necas J, Bartosikova L, Brauner P, et al. Hyaluronic acid (hyaluronan): a review. Veterinarni Medicina. 2008;53:397-411.
3. Stern R. Hyaluronan catabolism: a new metabolic pathway. Eur J Cell Biol. 2004;83(7):317-25.
4. Fakhari A, Berkland C. Applications and emerging trends of hyaluronic acid in tissue engineering, as a dermal filler and in osteoarthritis treatment. Acta Biomater. 2013 Jul 1;9(7):7081-92.
5. Monheit GD, Coleman KM. Hyaluronic acid fillers. Dermatol Ther. 2006;19(3):141-50.
6. Schanté CE, Zuber G, Herlin C, et al. Chemical modifications of hyaluronic acid for the synthesis of derivatives for a broad range of biomedical applications. Carbohydrate polymers. 2011;85(3):469-89.
7. Kablik J, Monheit GD, Yu L, et al. Comparative physical properties of hyaluronic acid dermal fillers. Dermatol Surg. 2009;35(Suppl 1):302-12.
8. Park S, Park KY, Yeo IK, et al. New hyaluronic acid filler. Ann Dermatol. 2014;26(3):357-62.
9. Tezel A, Fredrickson GH. The science of hyaluronic acid dermal fillers. J Cosmet Laser Ther. 2008;10(1):35-42.

10. Molliard SG, Bétemps JB, Hadjab B, et al. Key rheological properties of hyaluronic acid fillers: from tissue integration to product degradation. Plast Aesthetic Res. 2018;5:17.
11. Rohrich RJ, Ghavami A, Crosby MA. The role of hyaluronic acid fillers (Restylane) in facial cosmetic surgery: review and technical considerations. Plast Reconstr Surg. 2007;120(Suppl 6):41S-54S.
12. Bertucci V, Lynde CB. Current concepts in the use of small-particle hyaluronic acid. Plast Reconstr Surg. 2015;136(Suppl 5):132S-8S.
13. Tran C, Carraux P, Micheels P, et al. In vivo bio-integration of three hyaluronic acid fillers in human skin: a histological study. Dermatology. 2014;228(1):47-54.
14. Stern R, Kogan G, Jedrzejas MJ, et al. The many ways to cleave hyaluronan. Biotechnol Adv. 2007;25(6):537-57.
15. Vedamurthy M. Soft tissue agumentation: Dermal fillers. In: Sharad J, Vedamurthy M (Eds.) Aesthetic Dermatology: Current Perspectives. New Delhi: Jaypee Brothers Medical Publishers; 2019. pp. 192-8.

CHAPTER 3

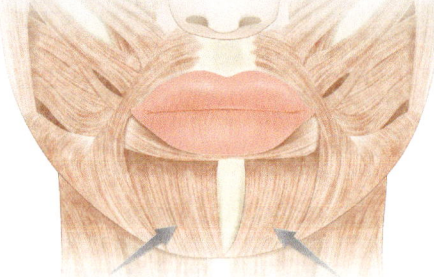

Guide for Selection and Use of Fillers

Richa Ojha Sharma, Rashmi Sarkar

INTRODUCTION

Dermal filling for enhancement of facial features is a science as well as an art. The science part is the understanding of the physics of gel behavior and the art is in the correct utilization and placement of the gel. Although over 50 different brands of dermal fillers are available for use, there is no universal filler which can be used for all indications of face rejuvenation and remodeling. A good understanding of the physics of gels will help us predict with greater accuracy how a filler will behave when injected into a particular area or layer of the skin. Hyaluronic acid (HA) fillers are the ones used most commonly in India, hence this chapter will focus on HA fillers.

Hyaluronic acid fillers are available in different grades and under different names, based on their physical properties. They are differentiated on the basis of HA concentration, amount, degree of cross-linking, particle size, elastic modulus (G′), and extrusion force. These factors influence product selection for different indications. There may be some overlap in the use, but it is not advisable to use fillers interchangeably in all situations.

PHYSICAL PROPERTIES OF GELS

It is to be expected that, when placed inside any layer or plane in the face, a filler gel will undergo various compressive, lateral, and shearing forces. After all, the face is a very complex and dynamic part, subject to intrinsic and extrinsic forces. Knowing the physical, viscoelastic and cohesive properties can help us choose the best filler for a given site.

Cross-Linking

Hyaluronic acid is a glycosaminoglycan disaccharide composed of alternately repeating units of D-glucuronic acid and N-acetyl-D-glucosamine. Free HA polymers have a short half-life. Noncross-linked HA is liquid. Cross-linking of fluid HA converts this liquid into a gel and provides structure and adhesion. This also makes it more resistant to *in vivo* enzymatic degradation resulting in a longer duration of filler effect. Cross-linking of HA units is done using 1,4-Butanediol diglycidyl ether (BDDE), divinyl sulfone, or 2,7,8-diepoxyoctane (DEO).[1] Cross-linking is measured as the percentage of disaccharide units bound to a cross-linking molecule. For example, a 1% cross-linked gel has one cross-linking molecule for every 100 HA monomers. Higher degrees of cross-linking leads to stiffer gels that resist deformation.[2] Lower degree of cross-linking creates a more fluid gel which is also hydrolyzed much faster. A clinical utility of such gels is in creating more hydration and overall rejuvenation in the superficial skin.

For these fillers such as Restylane Vital, IAL, and Princess Rich are injected intradermally.

Particle Size

Cross-linking of HA is quite like making jelly—stirring the gelatin powder in warm water results in a mass of jelly. In order for it to be injectable, this cohesive mass can be "sized" either by homogenization or by passing the gel mass through a series of sieves, making monophasic or biphasic gels respectively.

- Monophasic gels consist of a single "phase" of HAs. They have lower G' values.[3] They are softer and more easily injected than biphasic products. They can be either monodensified, i.e. HA is mixed and cross-linked in a single step (e.g. Juvéderm) or polydensified, i.e. HA goes through two stages of cross-linking (e.g. Belotero).
- Biphasic gels consist of two "phases" of HA—one phase consists of the cross-linked particles the size of which is determined by the grade of the sieve used and the second phase is the free or minimally cross-linked HA, which acts as the vehicle for lubrication and ease of injection. These have a higher G' and are harder to inject (e.g. Restylane).[4,5]

Rheological Properties

Rheology is the study of the flow of materials and their deformability when subjected to various forces.[6]

Rheological parameters are used to describe viscoelastic properties:[6]

- *Elastic modulus [G prime (G')]*: Measures the ability of filler to regain its original shape after being subjected to shear forces. Thus G' hints at the hardness of the product.
- *Viscous Modulus G"*: Measures the *inability* of the gel to recover the original shape after being subjected to shear forces.
- *Complex modulus G**: The total ability of material to withstand deformation. It is defined as the sum of the elastic modulus (G') and viscous modulus (G").

Rheology is influenced by the particle size, HA concentration, and degree of cross-linking.[5]

G' is the most useful parameter for filler selection. A low G' filler will not retain its shape under stress as much as a high G' filler will. One way of illustrating this difference is to compare a low G' gel to chocolate pudding and a high G' gel to a gelatin mold.[7] Thus, a low G' filler will not lead to lifting and volumization to the same degree as a high G' filler will. A high G' filler is therefore best used in areas where lifting is the desired trait, such as cheeks and chin. A low G' filler is better suited where it needs to spread out and in fact lifting is to be avoided such as in tear troughs and lips, and also for fine rhytides. Firm gels with high G' are harder to inject than softer gels. They also cause more inflammation and edema for some days after the injection. Soft gels with low G' are softer to inject and give a more natural appearance when injected superficially.[8]

Cohesivity

The cohesivity of a gel is its tendency to retain its form or shape under stress. Cohesivity increases with both cross-linking degree and HA concentration.[9] Fillers with low cohesivity are used for superficial rhytides as they are easier to mold and integrate better into the skin. On the other hand, high-cohesivity fillers are preferred for lifting and volume building. The 5-point Gavard-Sundaram Cohesivity

Scale[10] measures filler cohesivity and classifies HA fillers into:
- High cohesivity groups (Belotero Balance)
- Medium-high cohesivity (Juvéderm Ultra XC and Ultra Plus XC)
- Low-medium cohesivity (Juvéderm Voluma XC)
- Low cohesivity (Restylane Lyft).

AVAILABLE PRODUCTS

Table 1 lists the properties of some of the HA fillers available.

Juvéderm Ultra, Juvéderm Ultra Plus, and Voluma

Allergan Inc (Irvine, CA) manufactures the Juvéderm and Voluma groups of products. Juvéderm Ultra has the lowest G' (207 Pa) and Juvéderm Ultra Plus has a slightly higher G' (263 Pa). Both are made with proprietary Hylacross technology, which allows high water uptake by the HA gel after injection. For these fillers, undercorrection is advised to avoid a swollen look. Voluma has the highest G' in the Allergan HA basket (398 Pa) and is approved for malar augmentation. Voluma, Volift (G' 340 Pa), and Volbella (G' 271) are manufactured using the proprietary Vycross technology and absorb less water than Juvéderm Ultra or Juvéderm Ultra Plus.[11]

Restylane and Restylane Lyft

The Restylane group of products is made by Galderma (Uppsala, Sweden). Restylane is a firm filler with a moderately high G' and is used for tear troughs and mild nasolabial folds. Restylane Silk is a low G', small particle HA and is US Food and Drug Administration (FDA) approved for lip augmentation and treatment of perioral lines. Due to these properties, it is also used for areas where less lift is needed, such as mild tear troughs.[12] Restylane Lyft (formerly called Perlane) has the highest G' (977 Pa) among the FDA-approved HA products and is best utilized where lift and contouring are needed such as cheek, chin, temple, and nose. Restylane Sub Q, though not

Table 1: G' values and HA concentration of popular HA fillers.

Filler	G' (in Pascals)	HA concentration (mg/mL)
Belotero Balance	128	22.5
Juvéderm Ultra XC	207	24
Juvéderm Ultra Plus XC	263	24
Volbella	271	15
Volift	340	17.5
Voluma	398	20
Yvoire Classic S	251	22
Yvoire Volume	399	22
Yvoire Contour	504	22
Restylane	864	20
Restylane Lyft	977	20
Belotero Volume	NA	26

(G': elastic modulus; HA: hyaluronic acid)

available in India yet, is a very firm gel, having a very high particle size and lifting capacity.

Belotero

The Belotero range of fillers (marketed by Merz Pharmaceuticals GmbH, Frankfurt am Main, Germany) was formerly called as Esthelis, Fortelis, and Modelis (marketed by Anteis SA, Geneva, Switzerland). The Belotero basket has a range of products ranging in increasing order of gel firmness from Belotero Hydro, Soft, Balance, Intense, and Volume. Belotero Balance has a low G′ (128 Pa), which makes it appropriate for treating fine lines and wrinkles. It is approved for mid to deep dermal injections to improve moderate to severe facial wrinkles and folds.[13] The Belotero portfolio also includes other non-FDA approved products—Belotero Volume (a deep volumizer), Belotero Intense (a mid-level volumizer), and Belotero Soft (a superficial volumizer.

Others

A few other brands of fillers marketed in India are following:
- *Princess fillers (produced by Austrian company Croma-Pharma GmbH)*: The Princess range of fillers includes three variants of monophasic HA gel filler with differing cross-linking of HA molecules—Princess Filler for moderate to severe wrinkles, lip contouring and volumizing, Princess Rich for superficial dermis, and Princess Volume for deep wrinkles, and contouring. The HA concentration is 23 mg/mL.
- *Yvoire fillers (LG Life Sciences, Seoul, Korea)*: Yvoire Classic S, Volume, and Contour are available in India. Yvoire Classic S is used for superficial nasolabial folds and lips, while Yvoire Volume is for restoration of cheeks. Yvoire Contour is best used for more robust lifting and contouring of midface and chin.

DURATION OF EFFECT

Studies to determine the duration of clinical improvement after HA injections have shown that Juvéderm products, Restylane products and Belotero Balance, remain in site for at least 6 months and up to 1 year.[14] Voluma has reported longevity of up to 2 years.[15] Persistence of HA fillers in the skin is dependent upon the volume and site of injection, the particle size, manufacturing processes, and host metabolism. Among these, the host metabolism, i.e. the local reaction followed by enzymatic and free-radical degradation of HA is the most important factor in determining filler longevity.[2,8]

SELECTION OF FILLERS FOR DIFFERENT AREAS

Table 2 gives a broad guide of requirements and choice of fillers for different facial zones.

There is no "one size fits all" approach as far as dermal fillers are concerned. An individualized approach is needed after assessing the goals and expectations of treatment. A thorough facial analysis to determine any anatomic uniqueness, possible outcomes to enhance esthetic appeal, and meeting patient expectations is imperative. Broadly, active lines should be targeted with neuromodulator and static lines with HA filler.[16]

Fine Lines

For fine lines of the face we need a nonbulky filler to avoid visible bumps and lumps and

Table 2: Guidelines for filler selection.

Facial zone	Objective	Desirable feature of filler	Rheological properties	Brand recommended
Lips	Intradermal or subdermal placement to restore volume	• Easily moldable • Not bulky	• Low-medium elasticity (G') • Low viscosity for ease of injection • Low cohesivity	Juvéderm Ultra/Ultra Plus, Volbella, Restylane Kysse, Belotero Balance
Midface	Deep dermal or subdermal placement for restoring volume and to achieve projection	• Ability to maintain shape • Resist shear deformation and compression • No displacement	• High elasticity (high G' HA fillers can be injected in the supraperiosteal plane of the malar prominence and low to moderate G' HA can be used more superficially for refinement) • Low viscosity • Medium-high cohesivity	Voluma, Restylane Lyft/Volyme, Belotero Volume
Nasolabial (NL) fold	Supraperiosteal in upper-third of NL fold and intradermal in lower two-third	• Nonbulky • Minimal projection	• Moderate elasticity (G') • Medium cohesivity	Juvéderm Ultra Plus, Restylane Lido/Lyft, Belotero Balance
Lower face	Deep dermal or subdermal placement for restoring volume	• Minimal projection • Easily moldable • Nonpalpable	• Moderate elasticity (G") • Low viscosity • Medium cohesivity	Volift, Restylane Lido, Belotero Intense
Chin and nose	Supraperiosteal placement on dorsal nose and subcutaneous placement for tip correction	• Maximum vertical projection • Minimum lateral spread	• High elasticity (G') • Low viscosity • High cohesivity	Voluma, Restylane Lyft, Belotero Volume
Tear troughs	Supraperiosteal placement to fill troughs and to make lower lid bags less noticeable	• Minimum projection • Nonpalpable	• Moderate elasticity (G') • Low viscosity • Low cohesivity	Volbella (for grade 1 and 2); Ultra plus (for grade 3 and 4), Restylane Lido, Belotero Balance
Fine lines	Intradermal or subdermal placement in crow's feet, perioral lines, fine forehead lines	• Minimum projection • Easily moldable • Nonpalpable • Undercorrection is advised	• Low elasticity (G') • Low viscosity • Low cohesivity	Volbella, Restylane Fynesse, Belotero Soft

(HA: hyaluronic acid)

Fig. 1: Incorrect product choice leading to visible filler in the tear trough region.

also a filler that flows easily between the tight dermal tissue. This translates into a product with a low G' and low cohesivity.

Tear Troughs

Tear troughs can be corrected by carefully placing a filler with moderate G' supraperiosteally. Filler must be chosen carefully to correct this area because of the risk of visibility and palpability of the product **(Fig. 1)**. It is always advisable to undercorrect this area and assess after 2 weeks to touch up if needed.

Midface

To counter aging features and to add esthetic appeal, midface volumization, contouring, and projection are needed. The force exerted by the acts of sleeping on the side, chewing, talking, kissing and animation as well as the shear forces of the skin, muscles and tissue in this area must be resisted by our chosen filler. Rheologically speaking, this means that the filler must have sufficient elastic modulus (G') to withstand shearing and medium to high cohesivity to resist displacement by the compression forces.

Lower Face

The marionette lines, nasolabial folds, and accordion lines are very mobile areas and prone to shearing forces. For these we need fillers that do not project at all and merge well with tissue to move well with the muscles and avoid a lumpy look. For this a filler with moderate G' and low to medium cohesivity is preferred.

Nose and Chin

The nose and chin area is prone to a great deal of tension and pull of the overlying skin and muscle. A filler of choice with high G' and high cohesivity will provide the required projection without spreading laterally.[6]

SUMMARY

- Armed with a thorough knowledge of the science of fillers and careful injection technique an esthetic physician can deliver the best results with fillers.
- Broadly speaking, fillers with high G' and cohesivity are better suited for deeper placement in the subcutaneous tissue or supraperiosteally while those with lower G' and lesser cohesivity are usually better suited for superficial placement.
- However, it must be remembered that a filler with higher G', may not always lift better than a filler with a lower G'. Rather, it is a complex interaction between the G prime, cohesivity, and manufacturing process that determines the lifting capacity of fillers.

REFERENCES

1. Tezel A, Fredrickson GH. The science of hyaluronic acid dermal fillers. J Cosmet Laser Ther. 2008;10:35-42.
2. Bentkover SH. The biology of facial fillers. Facial Plast Surg. 2009;25:73-85.

3. Flynn TC, Sarazin D, Bezzola A, et al. Comparative histology of intradermal implantation of mono and biphasic hyaluronic acid fillers. Dermatol Surg. 2011;37:637-43.
4. Prasetyo AD, Prager W, Rubin MG, et al. Hyaluronic acid fillers with cohesive polydensified matrix for soft-tissue augmentation and rejuvenation: a literature review. Clin Cosmet Investig Dermatol. 2016;9:257-80.
5. Herrmann JL, Hoffmann, Ward CE, et al. Biochemistry, physiology, and tissue interactions of contemporary biodegradable injectable dermal fillers. Dermatol Surg. 2018;44:S19-31.
6. Pierre S, Liew S, Bernardin A. Basics of dermal filler rheology. Dermatol Surg. 2015;41:S120-6.
7. Sundaram H, Voigts B, Beer K, et al. Comparison of the rheological properties of viscosity and elasticity in two categories of soft tissue fillers: calcium hydroxylapatite and hyaluronic acid. Dermatol Surg. 2010;36:1859-65.
8. Kablik J, Monheit GD, Yu L, et al. Comparative physical properties of hyaluronic acid dermal fillers. Dermatol Surg. 2009;35:302-12.
9. Fallacara A, Manfredini S, Durini E, et al. Hyaluronic acid fillers in soft tissue regeneration. Facial Plast Surg. 2017;33:87-96.
10. Sundaram H, Rohrich RJ, Liew S, et al. Cohesivity of hyaluronic acid fillers: development and clinical implications of a novel assay, pilot validation with a five-point grading scale, and evaluation of six U.S. Food and Drug Administration-approved fillers. Plast Reconstr Surg. 2015;136:678-86.
11. Goodman GJ, Swift A, Remington BK. Current concepts in the use of Voluma, Volift, and Volbella. Plast Reconstr Surg. 2015;136:139S-48S.
12. Bertucci VB, Lynde CB. Current concepts in the use of small-particle hyaluronic acid. Plast Reconstr Surg. 2015;136:132S-8S.
13. Sundaram H, Fagien S. Cohesive polydensified matrix hyaluronic acid for fine lines. Plast Reconstr Surg. 2015;136:149S-63S.
14. Goodman GJ, Bekhor P, Rich M, et al. A comparison of the efficacy, safety, and longevity of two different hyaluronic acid dermal fillers in the treatment of severe nasolabial folds: a multicenter, prospective, randomized, controlled, single-blind, within-subject study. Clin Cosmet Investig Dermatol. 2011;4:197-205.
15. Callan P, Goodman GJ, Carlisle I, et al. Efficacy and safety of a hyaluronic acid filler in subjects treated for correction of midface volume deficiency: a 24 month study. Clin Cosmet Investig Dermatol. 2013;6:81-9.
16. Gutowski KA. Hyaluronic acid fillers. Clin Plas Surg. 2016;43:489-96.

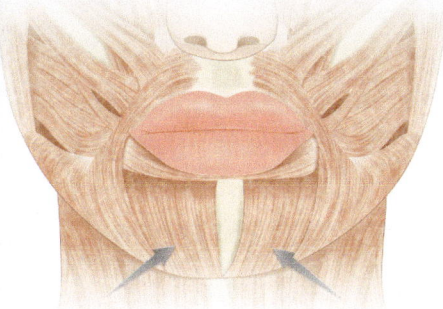

CHAPTER 4

Facial Anatomy for Dermal Fillers

Kuldeep Singh

INTRODUCTION

Knowledge of anatomy of the face is absolutely essential to enable safe and effective injection of fillers which has been evolving over the last three decades. As knowledge has evolved, the techniques of injection have also evolved and have become more predictable, effective, and safer. Anatomy has become clearer because of efforts by researchers through live and cadaver dissections, and also the imaging and staining techniques.[1]

Aging changes in the face include skin texture changes, volume changes in the fat compartments, sagging of the soft tissues, bony resorption, and hyperactive muscles. Whether we want to lift the tissues or restore volume, an accurate knowledge of the structures in the face and the changes in anatomy which happen with time, will help us to be more effective and also safe.

In this chapter, we will be discussing relevant injection anatomy of the face area-wise. The objective is to facilitate a complete understanding of the area to be injected. Each area will be discussed layer-wise so as to understand different planes, tissues, and spaces. Subsequently, the surface landmarks and their relationship to underlying important structures will also be delineated.

FOREHEAD INCLUDING THE BROW

The area of the forehead extends from the frontal hairline to the root of the nose, and sideways from one temporal crest to the other. The layers of the forehead consist of skin, subcutaneous tissue, muscles, galea, the subgaleal space, the periosteum, and bone **(Fig. 1)**.

The skin of the forehead is glabrous and is attached to underlying muscle with fibrous septa.[2] This ensures that the skin remains fairly fixed to underlying muscles and therefore conveys expressions caused by movement

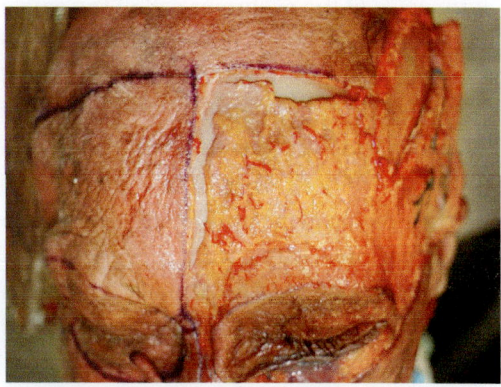

Fig. 1: Layers of soft tissues in the forehead region. Skin has been removed on the left side, and a thin layer of superficial fat overlying the frontalis muscle is seen.

of the muscles to the surface of the skin. In youth, the skin is smooth and rarely shows any lines. But with age, and regular repetitive movements of the forehead muscles strong lines emerge. The pattern of these lines varies in different individuals depending on the pattern of the adherence of the skin via the septa. These lines initially are present during movement (dynamic), but gradually remain present at rest too. The transverse lines on the forehead are due to the underlying frontalis muscle, and the vertical lines in between the eyebrows are due to the underlying corrugator supercilii muscle.

The subcutaneous tissue in the forehead is a thin layer lying on the frontalis muscle. There are two superficial fat compartments in the forehead, the central compartment and the middle fat compartment **(Fig. 1)**. The nerves of the forehead namely the supratrochlear and the supraorbital run on the surface of the frontalis muscle underneath the subcutaneous fat along with the blood vessels. Initially, it was thought that there is no deep fat compartment in the forehead. However, a fat pad exists deep to the frontalis at the level of the eyebrows called the galeal fat pad, which extends upwards for 2–2.5 cm above the supraorbital rim.[3,4] It is covered on its deep surface by the posterior layer of the galea, which invests the frontalis muscle **(Fig. 2)**.

In the region of the eyebrow, another deep fat compartment exists, which lies deep to the orbicularis oculi muscle (orbital part), and is called the retro-orbicularis oculi fat (ROOF) **(Fig. 2)**.

In younger people, most of the brow volume is made up of muscle, whereas in older people most of the brow volume is fat, mostly in the ROOF.

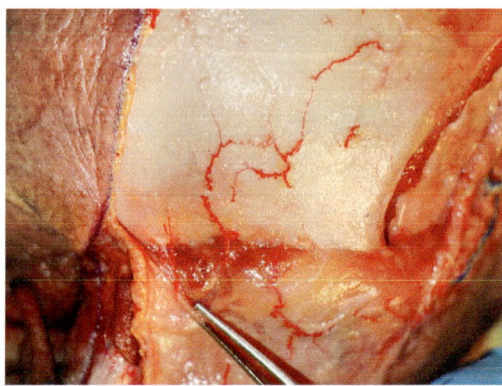

Fig. 2: The frontalis muscle along with galea removed from the forehead showing the supraorbital notch, supratrochlear and supraorbital vessels, the corrugator supercilii muscle. The galea invests the frontalis muscle, and there is a trace of fat on the deep surface of the galea (described by some as the galeal fat pad). The lateral fat seen is the ROOF.

Muscles of the Forehead and Eyebrow Region

Frontalis Muscle

This muscle originates from the galea at the hairline and inserts into the skin in the eyebrow region. The fibers also interlace with the orbicularis and the corrugator supercilii. The two bellies of the frontalis usually do not meet in the midline; however, in some males, they decussate in the midline. The upper part of the muscle pulls the hairline down, while the lower part elevates the eyebrows. It is to be noted that the frontalis muscle is the only elevator of the eyebrows. It is innervated by the temporal branch of the facial nerve **(Figs. 1 and 7)**.

Corrugator Supercilii

This muscle originates from the superomedial part of the orbital rim, and courses transversely to be attached to the skin of the middle of the eyebrow. The corrugator has two bellies,

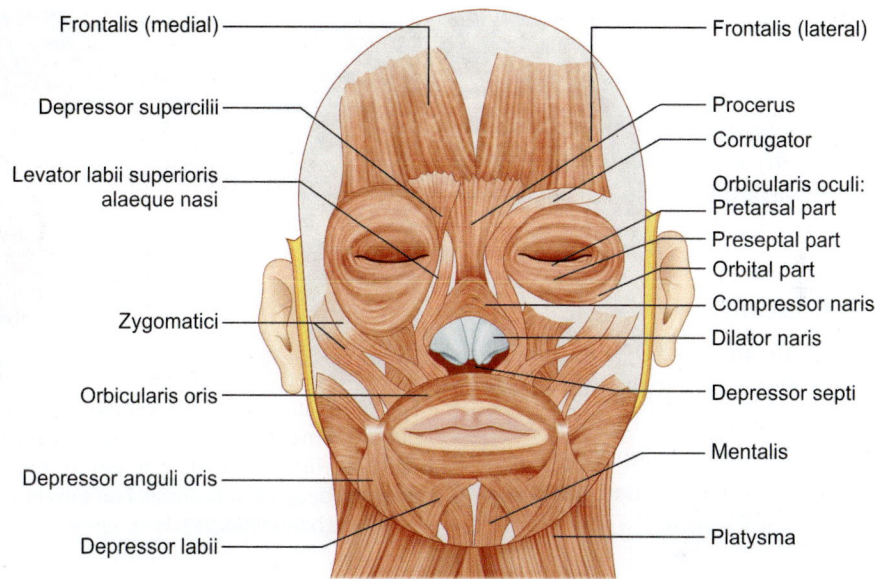

Fig. 3: Muscles of the face.

a transverse belly and an oblique belly. Medially, near its origin, the corrugator is situated deeply close to the bone whereas laterally, near the tail, it is very superficial and subdermal.

The medial part of the corrugator receives its nerve supply from the zygomatic branch and the lateral part from the temporal branch of the facial nerve. Contraction of the corrugator muscle brings the medial ends of the eyebrows together and also depresses the eyebrows. The corrugator crease in the glabellar region is formed over the supratrochlear neurovascular bundle. The supraorbital neurovascular bundle pierces the medial end of the corrugator supercilii before becoming superficial as it ascends into the forehead (**Fig. 3**).

Depressor Supercilii

It is a thin muscle which blends in with the medial fibers of the orbicularis oculi. It arises from the frontal process of the maxilla 2–5 mm below the frontozygomatic suture and inserts into the dermis of the medial brow, and acts as a depressor of the medial brow.

Procerus Muscle

It arises from the lower end of the nasal bones and the upper lateral cartilage. It travels upward and inserts into the skin of the glabella in between the eyebrows. It pulls the nose skin up and the glabellar skin downward, and is responsible for the horizontal crease at the root of the nose. It is believed evolution wise that the procerus is a downward extension of the frontalis muscle (**Fig. 3**). The temporal branch of the facial nerve supplies the procerus.

The scalp in the forehead glides over the underlying pericranium. At the lateral ends these layers are attached to the superior temporal crest and inferiorly at the supraorbital margin with the orbicularis retaining ligament (ORL). These attachments protect the neurovascular structures lying adjacent.

The bony skeleton of the forehead comprises the frontal bone. It is smoothly convex uniformly across its extent in women, but in men has a prominent supraorbital ridge with a more vertical frontal bone above.

Applied Anatomy

Loss of volume in the ROOF contributes to deflation and descent of the tail of the eyebrow.[5] Also, it deepens the upper eyelid sulcus causing the A frame deformity. Injection is placed deep to the orbicularis, and lateral to the supraorbital bundle.[6]

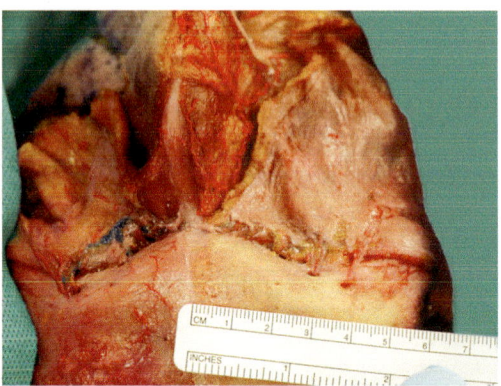

Fig. 4: Supratrochlear and supraorbital neurovascular bundles emerging from their respective foramina, and travelling about 1.5 cm before piercing the galea to become superficial. Frontalis muscle with galea has been reflected

VESSELS AND NERVES OF THE FOREHEAD

The vessels are the paired supratrochlear vessels with the supratrochlear nerve, the supraorbital vessels and nerve, and the anterior (frontal) branch of the superficial temporal arteries.

Supratrochlear artery (branch of the ophthalmic artery) exits the orbit through the supratrochlear foramen at the medial end of the roof of the orbit, on an average of 14 mm from the midline. The medial glabellar fold typically overlies the origin of the vessels.

Supraorbital artery exits the orbit through the foramen of the same name (rarely a notch), which is palpable, and lies about 10 mm lateral to the supratrochlear vessels, or along a line drawn vertically touching the medial limbus. Twenty percent of the time, it is a notch on one side and a foramen on the other.[7]

1 cm after exiting the orbit both the supratrochlear (ST) and supraorbital (SO) vessels pierce the galea and become superficial. They at first pass through the corrugator muscle and then come to lie on the surface of the frontalis muscle, and ascend to the hairline. The vessel diameter ranges from 1 mm to 1.5 mm at the foramen **(Fig. 4)**.

The supraorbital nerve gives off a deep branch which travels laterally and ascends in a supraperiosteal plane about 1.5 cm medial and parallel to the superior temporal crest. It is accompanied by an artery.

Applied Anatomy

Filler injections in the glabellar and brow region should be placed in the dermal or immediate subdermal plane. Deep injections in this region within 2 cm of the supraorbital rim are at a higher risk for intravascular injection, antegrade if slow, and retrograde if injected under pressure. As the viscous filler cannot go distally in a smaller lumen size, it travels proximally till the injection pressure is kept up. Once the pressure is discontinued, it flows distally.

As the glabellar arterial branches are terminal, the entire glabella is a high risk for injection. The SO and ST arteries communicate with branches of the internal carotid artery through the ophthalmic artery and therefore filler material can travel retrograde to the ophthalmic artery and then distally into the central artery of the retina.

Injections into the lateral forehead in the supraperiosteal plane can impinge upon the deep branch of the SO nerve or even embolize the accompanying artery.

Injections in the brow region can be done using a cannula 25 G or greater in the suborbicularis plane, using a lateral to medial approach. Filler injections for contouring the forehead in the upper part are done in the supraperiosteal plane.

TEMPORAL REGION

The temporal region is bound superiorly by the superior temporal septum and inferiorly by the zygomatic arch. The layers of this region from superficial to deep are the skin, subcutaneous tissue, superficial temporal fascia-consisting of two layers, the outer layer and the deep layer, together called the temporoparietal fascia. This is followed by the deep temporal fascia, the temporalis muscle, and the periosteum **(Figs. 6A to C)**. The superficial temporal artery and the frontal branch of the facial nerve travel within the temporoparietal fascia. The frontal branch (or branches) crosses over the zygomatic arch at its midpoint **(Fig. 7)**.

The temporoparietal fascia is separated from the deep temporal fascia by loose areolar tissue. The latter is thickened in the region of the temporal crest and is called the *superior temporal septum*. Also, there is the condensation of the areolar tissue in the middle of the temporal fossa, called the *inferior temporal septum*. Both septum fuse at the anterior end and form the *temporal adhesion* in the region of the tail of the eyebrow **(Fig. 5)**. The temporal ligamentous adhesion (TLA) measures about 20 mm in height and 15 mm in width, and begins 10 mm cephalad to the superior orbital rim.[8]

About 2–3 cm above the zygomatic arch, the deep temporal fascia divides into an outer layer which attaches to the outer surface of the zygomatic arch, and a deeper layer which attaches to the inside edge. In between these

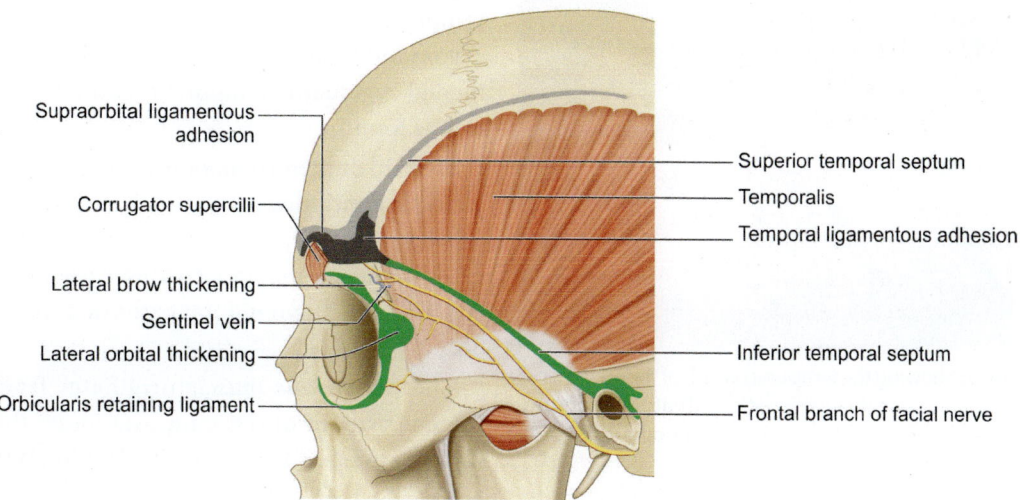

Fig. 5: Ligaments in the periorbital area and the temporal region.

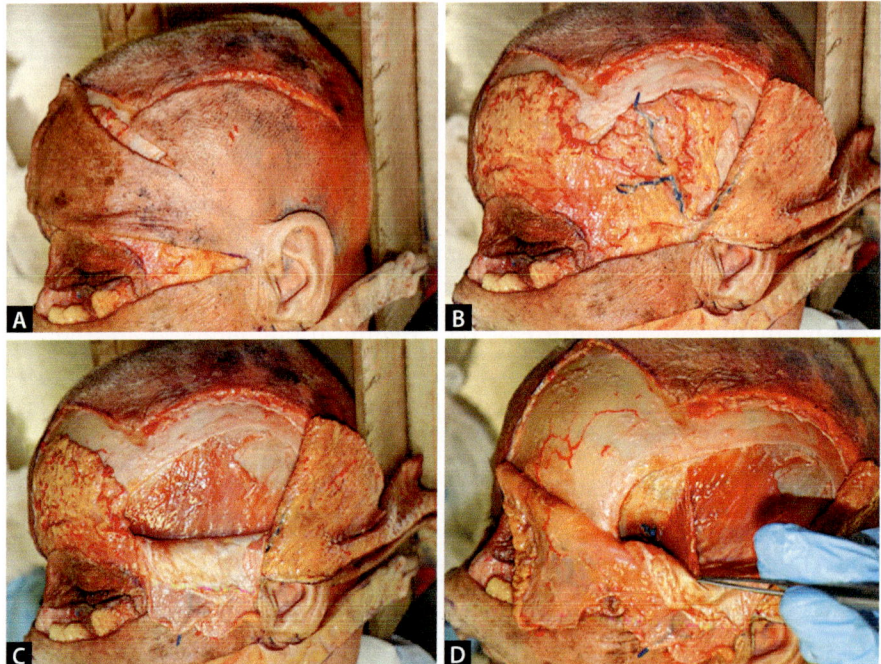

Figs. 6A to D: (A) The temporal region with skin flaps elevated; (B) Exposed temporoparietal fascia showing the superficial temporal artery dividing into its anterior and posterior branches about 5 cm from the tragus, with accompanying veins; (C) Shows reflected deep temporal fascia exposing the temporalis muscle arising from the superior temporal crest and temporal fossa; (D) The reflected anterior edge of the temporalis muscle showing the anterior deep temporal vessels about 2 cm behind the junction of the lateral orbital rim and the superior temporal crest (Swift point is 1 cm above and lateral to avoid the vessels in a temple filler injection).

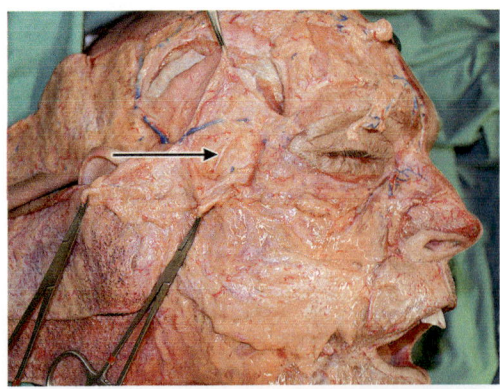

Fig. 7: Showing the temporal branch of the facial nerve crossing over the zygomatic arch at its midpoint, lying in the deep part of the temporoparietal fascia enveloped with fat (black arrow).

two layers, lies a fat pad called the superficial temporal fat pad (also called the supra zygomatic fat pad).[6] Also, in this space the medial zygomaticotemporal (sentinel) vein can be found.

Deep to the deep temporal fascia is a space which is continuous with the infratemporal fossa. Some fat is present in this space and is called the deep temporal fat pad (subzygomatic fat), which is the temporal extension of the buccal pad of fat.

The *temporalis muscle* originates from the periosteum of the temporal fossa, the superior temporal crest and the deep surface of the deep temporal fascia **(Fig. 6C)**, and is inserted into the coronoid process and the anterior surface of the ascending ramus of the mandible. The middle temporal vessels and the deep temporal vessels provide blood supply the muscle. Motor innervation is from the mandibular nerve.

The *superficial temporal artery* is a branch of the external carotid artery, emerges 1 cm anterior and 1 cm superior to the tragus. About 5 cm later, it branches into the anterior (frontal) branch and the posterior (parietal) branch **(Fig. 6B)**. It lies within the temporoparietal fascia.

The frontal branch of the facial nerve runs obliquely from the tragus to the lateral border of the frontalis muscle in the forehead. It crosses the zygomatic arch obliquely at its midpoint, lying under the deeper part of the temporoparietal fascia, just supraperiosteal **(Fig. 7)**. Its surface marking is the Pitanguy line, which runs from point 0.5 cm below the tragus to a point 1.5 cm lateral to the supraorbital rim.

The anterior deep temporal vessels run vertically in the deep part of the temporalis muscle on an average about 1.8 cm posterior to the lateral orbital rim **(Fig. 6D)**.

The anterior and the posterior deep temporal arteries supplying the muscle are branches from the second part of the maxillary artery. They lie between the temporalis muscle and the pericranium **(Fig. 6D)**.

The middle temporal artery arises from the superficial temporal artery immediately above the zygomatic arch and perforates the deep temporal fascia, gives branches to the temporalis muscle, and anastomoses with the deep temporal vessels.

Applied Anatomy

The bone in the temporal region is of varying thickness. One site is particularly thin and is called the *pterion*. This is located 3 cm posterior and 3 cm superior from the lateral canthus. It can also be localized 3 cm posterior to the frontozygomatic suture and 4 cm above the zygomatic arch. Forceful deep injections against the bone in this region can possibly enter the cranial cavity in the region of the pterion.

Injections in the temporal region are usually made deep in the muscle, or in the interface between the muscle and the periosteum. The bony landmarks including the temporal crest, the lateral orbital rim, and the upper border of the zygomatic arch are defined and located before starting injection. Injections are usually made in the anterosuperior quadrant of the temporal region outside the hairline. A point within 1 cm of the lateral orbital rim is considered safe with respect to avoiding the anterior deep temporal vessels.

Swift, DeLorenzi, and Kapoor (2019) have described a safe point 1 cm superior and 1 cm lateral to the tail of the eyebrow **(Fig. 6D)**.[9]

Intravascular injection in this area can enter the anterior deep temporal artery and travel retrograde to the external carotid artery and on releasing pressure embolize into the superficial temporal artery, or any closest branch. Direct injection in the anterior branch of the superficial temporal artery may occur, if one does not look for it and mark it.

Injections in the inferior part of the temporal fossa, just above the zygomatic arch, are avoided as the filler may reach the infratemporal fossa through the space between the deep temporal fascia and the temporalis muscle.

EYELIDS AND ORBIT

This region is also called the periorbital region. It includes the eyebrow, supraorbital rim, infrabrow area, lateral canthal area, the upper and lower eyelids, and the infraorbital area.

The *orbicularis oculi* muscle originates from the nasal part of the frontal bone, the frontal process of maxilla, and the medial canthal tendon and, inserts into the lateral raphe and lateral canthal tendon. It consists of circular fibers extending from the eyelids outward, to cover the orbital septum and then extend across the orbital rim. The infraorbital part extends much farther in the inferolateral part to cover the upper cheek **(Fig. 8)**.[10]

The orbicularis oculi muscle is divided into three parts:
1. The *pretarsal* part which overlies the upper and lower tarsal plates, and is involved in the closure of the eyelids and blinking
2. The *preseptal* part overlies the orbital septum, and
3. The *orbital* part extends over the bony orbit. The orbital fibers in the inferolateral part have been described to have multiple fenestrations by Michaud.[11] Muscle fibers from the medial part extend to cover the lacrimal sac, and are involved in the function of pumping lacrimal fluid downward.

The orbicularis oculi muscle action is to close the eyelids. The superior part is also a depressor of the eyebrow. It is the only cheek elevator.

The infraorbital part of the orbicularis lies between the superficial fat of the cheek viz. the infraorbital fat (IOF) (the malar fat pad), and the deep fat namely the suborbicularis oculi fat (SOOF). In the supraorbital part, the fat of the forehead overlies the orbicularis oculi, and deep to the orbicularis lies the ROOF.

The eyelids have no fat and the orbicularis oculi muscle is intimately adherent to the skin in most areas.

At the orbital rim, the deep surface of the *orbicularis* muscle is attached to the periosteum by a ligament called the ORL. This ligament exists in the upper orbital rim, the lateral orbital rim, and the inferior orbital rim dividing the orbicularis into the septal and orbital parts. In the infraorbital region, the ORL (it is about 2 mm away from the rim

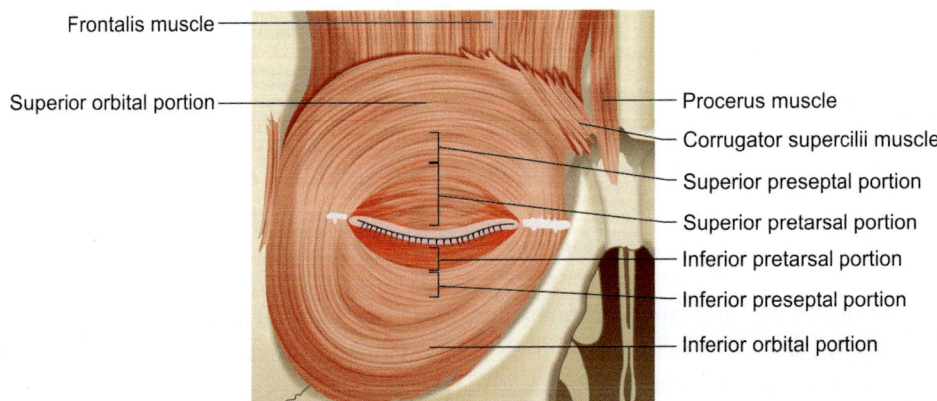

Fig. 8: Orbicularis oculi muscle showing the pretarsal, preseptal and preorbital parts, and its relationship with the corrugator supercilii and frontalis muscles.

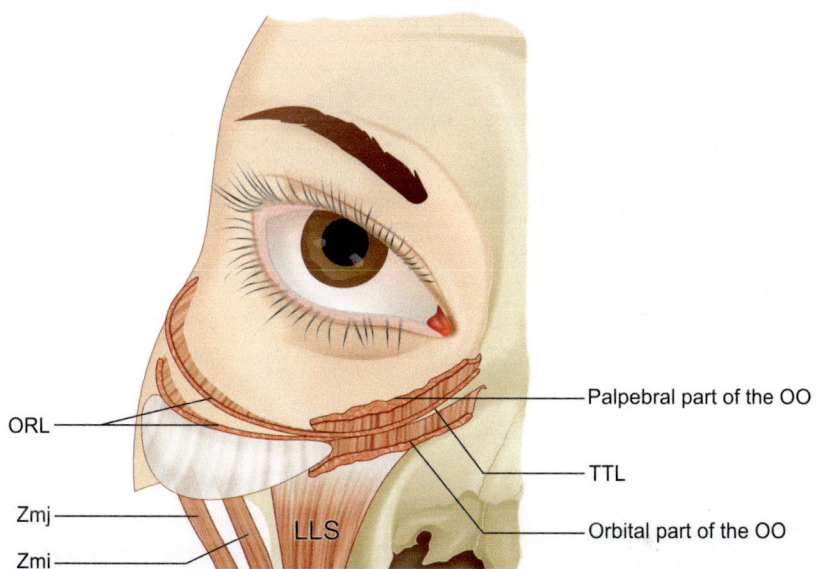

Fig. 9: Orbicularis retaining ligament (ORL) showing 2 lamellae in the lateral infraorbital part and medially single tightly adherent structure. Also showing relationship with prezygomatic space.
(ORL: orbicularis retaining ligament; TTL: tear trough ligament; LLS: levator labii superioris; OO: orbicularis oculi)

here) is split into two lamelli in the lateral part, whereas as it travels medially it fuses, gets more and more tightly adherent to the periosteum, and in the medial most part is called the tear trough ligament (TTL). The orbicularis muscle is also tightly adherent to the periosteum in the medial part **(Figs. 5 and 9)**.

The nerve supply to the orbicularis oculi comes from the frontal branch of the facial nerve in the superolateral part and the zygomatic branch in the inferomedial part.

The corrugator supercilii and the depressor supercilii muscles have been discussed in the section on the forehead.

The SOOF consists of a medial part and a lateral part. The medial part extends from the medial limbus to the lateral canthus, and the lateral part from the lateral canthus to the temporal fat pad. Deep to the SOOF lies the prezygomatic space, and deep to that lies the origin of the zygomaticus major muscle and adjacent periosteum.

The prezygomatic space is bound anteriorly by the SOOF, posteriorly by the body of the zygoma and maxilla, superiorly by the ORL, and inferiorly as well as laterally by the zygomatic ligament. Access to this space (other than by direct puncture) is via a point on the front of the zygoma body in the lateral and upper part **(Fig. 11)**. This gives access (using a cannula) to the SOOF up to the medial canthus, as well as the deep medial cheek fat compartment.

The malar septum is a funnel-like structure which exists in the infraorbital and the lateral orbital region, inferiorly ending on the orbital rim, whereas laterally it is 5 mm away from the rim **(Figs. 12A and B)**. It divides the SOOF into a superficial part and a deep part.[12] The lymphatic drainage of superficial SOOF is already compromised in patients with malar

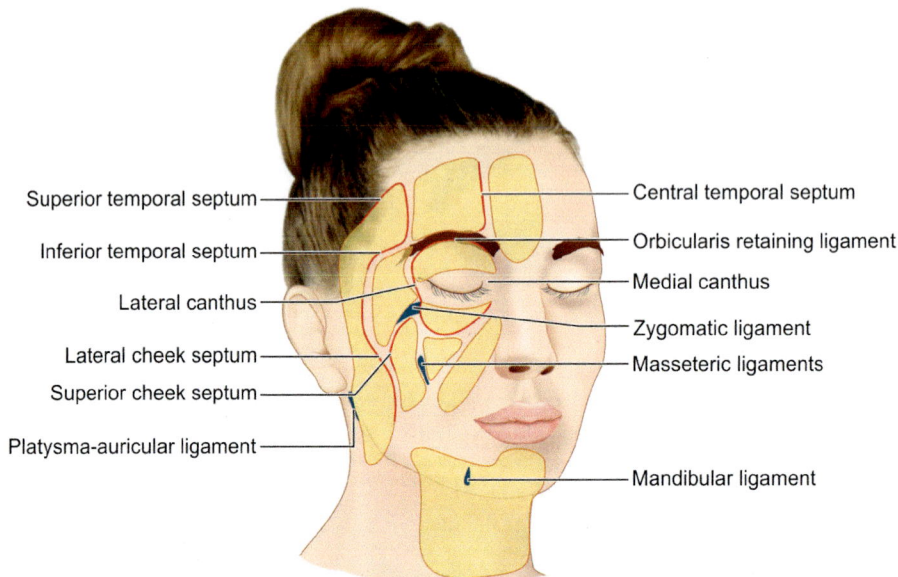

Fig. 10: Fat compartments of the face—showing ligaments and septae demarcating various fat compartments
(*Source*: Prendergast PM. Anatomy of the face and neck. Cosmetic Surgery. Schiffman and Guiseppe (Eds). Springer Verlag 2012)

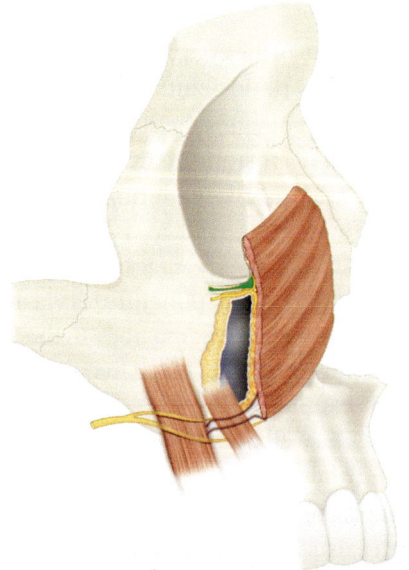

Fig. 11: Prezygomatic space—situated in front of the body of zygoma, superiorly. Bordered by ORL, roof by Preorbital part of the orbicularis oculi muscle, floor by SOOF. The zygomatic ligament forms the lateral part of its floor. Gives access to the SOOF and deep medial cheek fat compartment.

(*Source*: Mendelson B and Wong, C. Anatomy of the ageing face. Aesthetic Surgery of the face. Plastic Suregry. Elsevier 2013)

bags, and any high-volume injection in the deep SOOF will increase edema (malar bags) in the region. Also, superficial injection in a patient with malar bags will worsen them.

Vascular Anatomy

Almost all around the orbit, there is a confluence of arteries and veins between the external carotid and the internal carotid systems. The supratrochlear, supraorbital, lacrimal, infratrochlear, and the dorsal nasal (branches of the ophthalmic artery) arteries anastomose freely with the superficial temporal artery, the transverse facial artery, the infraorbital artery, and the angular artery **(Fig. 13)**.

The superficial temporal artery anastomoses with the supraorbital artery and/or supratrochlear artery. The transverse facial artery and the deep temporal arteries anastomose with the zygomatic branch of the lacrimal artery.

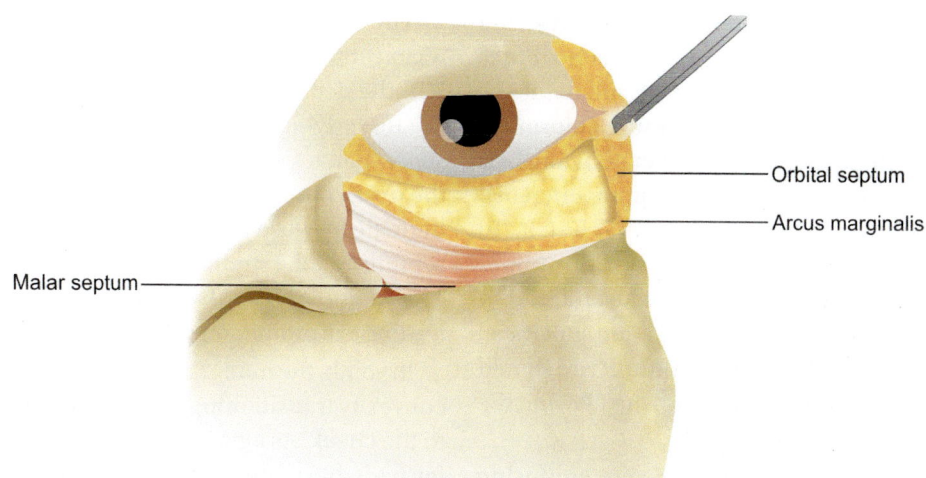

Figs. 12: Structure of the malar septum—(A) cadaver dissection; and (B) diagrammatic representation.
(*Source*: Pessa JE, Garza JR: The malar septum: the anatomical basis of malar mounds and malar edema. Aesthet Plast J. 1997;17(1):11-17)

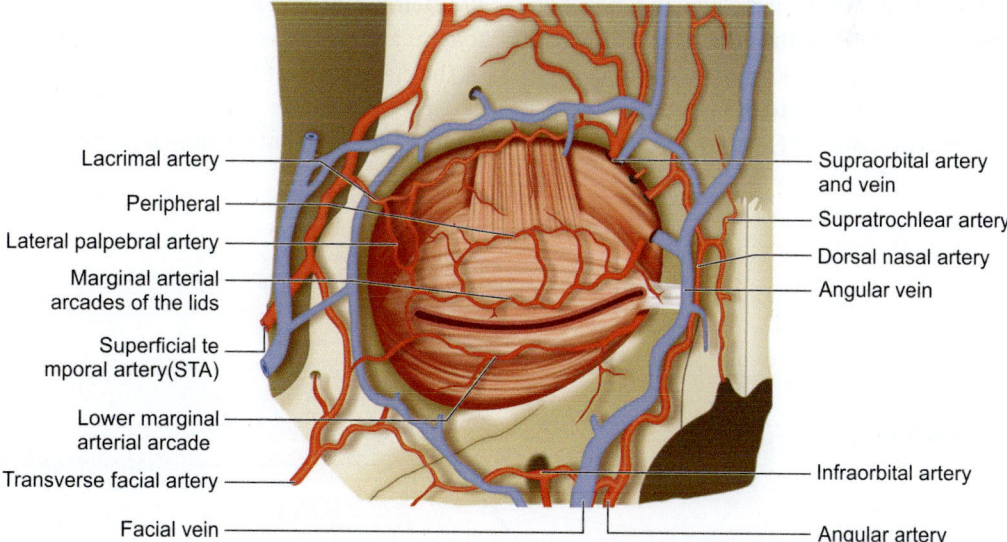

Fig. 13: Periorbital arteries and veins—showing connections between the ECA and the ICA systems, viz. the infraorbital, angular, transverse facial, superficial temporal, supraorbital, supratrochlear, and dorsal nasal arteries.
(ECA: external carotid artery; ICA: internal carotid artery)

Applied Anatomy

The ROOF is the deep fat compartment in the supraorbital region. Here the deep fat is continuous and flows into the preseptal area reaching the levator palpebrae superioris (LPS) muscle unlike the SOOF in the lower eyelid, which is limited by the ORL from communicating with the lower eyelid preseptal space.[13]

Volume loss in the ROOF causes the tail of the eyebrow to descend and contributes to deepening of the superior sulcus of the upper eyelid, called the "a frame deformity". The plane of injection of fillers obviously is deep to the OO muscle, in the suprapericranial plane, lateral to the supraorbital notch. To improve the superior sulcus of the upper eyelid, injection is performed just inferior to the rim, deep to the orbicularis, and superficial to the LPS and the orbital septum. Care should be taken to avoid the septum, the LPS and the upper eyelid fat pads.

The infraorbital area has very confusing anatomical nomenclature. The "tear trough" extends from the medial canthus to the mid-pupillary line, and from the mid-pupillary line to the lateral canthus, it is called the "nasojugal groove". Lateral to the lateral canthus, it is called the "mid-cheek groove". The mid-cheek groove corresponds to the attachment of the zygomatic ligament **(Fig. 14)**.

The fullness/volume of the infraorbital region arises from the underlying muscles, the IOF, the deep fat compartment (SOOF), and the underlying bone. All of these structures show changes with age along with changes in the overlying skin. The lower eyelid fat pads herniate because of attenuation of the orbital septum and the stretched orbicularis muscle. The lateral SOOF also undergoes atrophy leading to a prominent palpebromalar groove.

In youth, the infraorbital region is a smooth convexity transitioning from the lower eyelid to the cheek. As aging progresses, the orbital fat pads herniate causing convexity in the preseptal part of the lower eyelid. Ptosis of the deep cheek fat compartment further exposes the SOOF creating a double convexity. Rohrich, Pessa, and Ristow[14,15] demonstrated that in cadaveric specimens injection of saline in the deep medial cheek fat compartment caused the double convexity to disappear, thereby inferring that the primary determinant

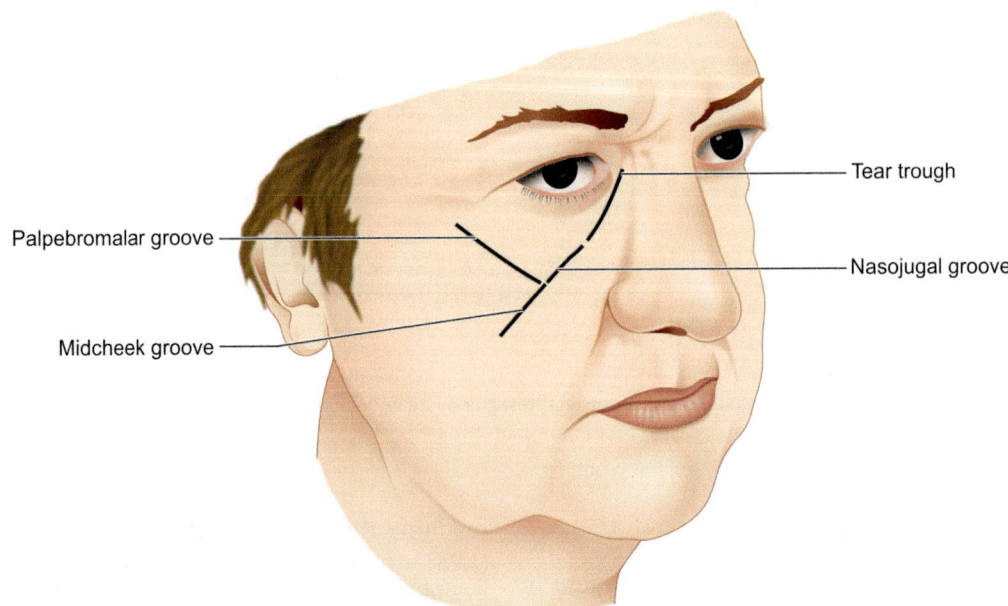

Fig. 14: Face showing 1. Palpebromalar groove, 2. Tear trough 3. Nasojugal groove and 4. The midcheek groove.

of this deformity is likely to be loss of volume in the deep medial cheek fat compartment.

The bony orbit also changes its shape with aging. The orbital aperture increases in size primarily in the superomedial and the inferolateral regions.[16] This leads to some degree of enophthalmos and poor support for the lower eyelid. Also concomitant hyperactivity of the orbicularis oculi leads to a narrowed palpebral fissure.

MIDFACE AND THE PREAURICULAR REGION

The midface extends from the root of the nose to the base of the nose at its junction with the upper lip. Laterally, it is bound by the external ear and also includes the preauricular region. The skeleton of the midface is formed externally by the maxillae, the zygomatic bones, the zygomatic process of the temporal bones (forming the zygomatic arch), and the nasal bones. The piriform (nasal) aperture is formed by the maxilla and the nasal bones. The width of the face is decided by the prominence of the zygomatic eminences (bizygomatic width). The vertical height of the face is decided by the height of the maxilla and the mandible.

The prominent zygomatic eminences give structural support to the midface and control the way the face ages. The central part of the maxilla supports the nasolabial region and the upper lip. An underdeveloped maxilla/absorption of the maxilla is responsible for poor support to the middle third of the face leading to early aging in this area with subsequent crowding of soft tissues in the middle third.

The infraorbital foramen lies beneath a prominent ridge of bone about 5–7 mm below the inferior orbital rim at the junction of the medial one-third with the lateral two-thirds (corresponds to a vertical line dropped from the medial limbus), in a recessed area difficult to reach from above but easily accessible from below. It transmits the infraorbital nerve and vessels.

The zygomaticofacial foramen lies on the summit of the malar eminence (zygomatic eminence) and transmits the zygomaticofacial nerve and vessels.

The soft tissues of the face are divided into a medial mobile area and the lateral relatively immobile area. The medial half does not have a deep fascia, the muscles are all superficial and insert into the skin. In the lateral half, muscles are deep and are covered with the investing layer of the deep fascia. The only superficial muscle in the lateral half is the platysma, and it does not reach higher than the commissure. Internally, a distinct vertical line divides these two halves. The retaining ligaments anchoring the skin to the bone/deep fascia form this line **(Fig. 15)**.[13]

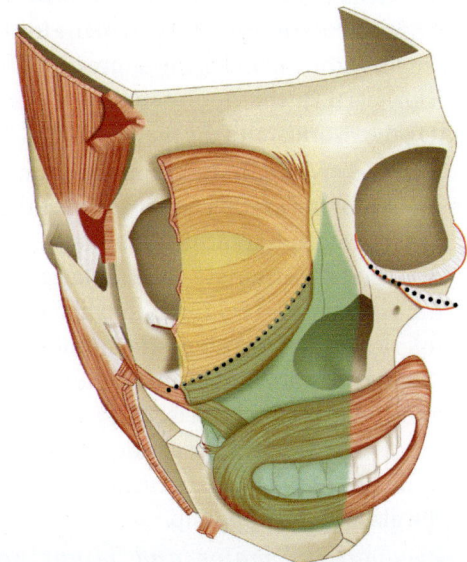

Fig. 15: Regions of the face. The anterior face is mobile, and the lateral part is relatively immobile, and separated from each other by a vertical line of retaining igaments—temporal adhesion, lateral orbital thickening, zygomatic, masseteric and mandibular ligaments.

(*Source*: Mendelson B and Wong, C. Anatomy of the ageing face. Aesthetic Surgery of the face. Plastic Suregry. Elsevier 2013)

The midcheek is the anterior part of the midface. It is triangular, and bound above by the pretarsal part of the lower lid, medially the side of the nose above and nasolabial groove below, and laterally by the lateral cheek at the junction of the zygoma meeting the arch. The soft tissues are composed of three segments overlying specific parts of the midcheek skeleton. The lid-cheek segment lies over the inferior orbital rim, malar segment over the body of the zygoma, and the nasolabial segment over the anterior surface of the maxilla.[13]

MUSCLES OF THE MIDFACE, LIPS, AND LOWER FACE

The muscles of the midface include the levator labii superioris alaeque nasi (LLSAN), levator labii superioris (LLS), the nasalis, the zygomaticus major and minor, the risorius, and the orbicularis oris. Muscles of the lower face include the mentalis, the depressor labii inferioris (DLI), the depressor anguli oris (DAO), the risorius, and the platysma **(Fig. 3)**.

- The *LLSAN* originates from the frontal process of the maxilla and inserts into the lower lateral nasal cartilage and the upper lip. The LLS originates a little lateral to the alaeque nasi from the maxilla at the inferior orbital rim above the infraorbital foramen, and inserts into the upper lip and the orbicularis oris. They are both innervated by the buccal and zygomatic branches of the facial nerve, and elevate the ala and the upper lip.
- *Zygomaticus major and minor* are superficial muscles, which take origin from the body of the zygoma lateral to the origin of the LLS, and insert into the modiolus and adjacent upper lip. Their origin forms the floor of the prezygomatic space, which lies under the medial SOOF. Fibers from the zygomatic and buccal branches supply the muscles on their deep surface. Both these muscles elevate the angle of mouth. The zygomaticus major fuses distally with the orbicularis oris, the superficial musculoaponeurotic system (SMAS), and the buccinator to form the modulus. Proximal to the modiolus, some facial bands from the zygomaticus major attach to the overlying skin. These may explain the dynamic cheek dimples in many individuals.[1]
- The *levator anguli oris (LAO)* arises from the canine fossa of the maxilla and inserts into the upper lip. The nerve supplying it enters the superficial surface, and arises from the zygomatic and buccal branches of the facial nerve.
- The *nasalis* muscle has two components— (1) the transverse nasalis (compressor naris) and (2) the alar nasalis (dilator naris). The compressor arises from the maxilla, above and lateral to the incisive fossa going upward and medially expanding into a thin, flat aponeurosis continuous across the dorsum of the nose with its counterpart on the opposite side **(Fig. 3)**. It compresses the nostrils. The dilator arises from the maxilla from the incisive fossa and inserts into the lower lateral cartilage and dilates the nostrils. Blocking the dilator may cause nasal valve to collapse.
- The *depressor septi* arises from the base of the anterior nasal spine and inserts into the cartilaginous nasal septum. It pulls the tip of the nose inferiorly. Both these muscles are supplied by the buccal branches of the facial nerve.
- The *risorius* muscle arises from the lateral-cheek platysmal thickening or the parotidomasseteric fascia and inserts into the modiolus. It pulls the corner of the

mouth laterally producing an artificial fixed grin (risus sardonicus).
- The *orbicularis oris* is a circular muscle around the mouth, with its fibers interlacing with all surrounding muscles. The buccal and the marginal mandibular branches of the facial nerve supply this muscle. The peripheral part of this muscle gives fibers which insert into the lip vermillion mucosa in the dry part **(Fig. 3)**. This shows externally as the vertical creases we see when we purse or pout our lips. The orbicularis is the only invertor of the lips, and is responsible for various movements of the lips.
    - The orbicularis oris muscle fuses laterally with the SMAS, zygomaticus major, and buccinator muscle. The modiolus forms a tendinous attachment for these muscles and exerts a superior lateral traction to the commissure.[1]
- The *mentalis* muscle arises from the incisive fossa of the mandible and inserts downward into the dermis of the chin. It contracts to elevate and protrude (evert) the lower lip, and also creates dimpling of the skin in the front of the chin (dimply chin).
- The *DAO* arises from the oblique line of the mandible lateral to the DLI. It is a triangular muscle and converges on the modiolus. It depresses the angle of mouth downwards, and also helps evert the outer parts of the lower lip.
- The *DLI* also arises from the oblique line of the mandible in front of the mental foramen, where it is covered by fibers of the DAO. It passes upward and medially as a quadrangular muscle to insert into the skin and mucosa of the lower lip and into fibers of the orbicularis oris. It pulls the outer parts of the lower lip downward in smiling and in showing the teeth. It also helps in everting the outer parts of the lower lip.
- The mentalis, the DAO and the DLI all are innervated by the marginal mandibular branch of the facial nerve.

FAT COMPARTMENTS OF THE MIDFACE

The superficial fat compartments lie superficial to the muscles of facial expression, while the deep fat compartments lie deep to the muscles. The superficial fat compartments were the first to be described in 2007 by Rohrich et al.[15] These consist of the IOF, the lateral orbital fat, nasolabial fat, superficial media cheek fat (SMC), middle cheek fat, and lateral temporal-cheek fat.

The IOF lies immediately cephalad to the SMC. The nasolabial fat, the superficial medial cheek, and the IOF are often collectively referred to as the malar fat and considered the superficial fat of the midface **(Figs. 16A and B)**.

The middle cheek fat compartment lies anterior and superficial to the parotid gland, where the three compartments meet, and forms a dense zone where the zygomatic ligament is described.[17]

The zone where the medial cheek fat abuts the middle cheek fat corresponds to the location of the parotidomasseteric ligaments. The lateral temporal cheek compartment is the most lateral compartment of cheek fat. This fat lies immediately superficial to the parotid gland.[15]

The lateral orbital fat lies subcutaneously below the inferior temporal septum and above the superior cheek septum. The zygomaticus major muscle is adherent to this fat.

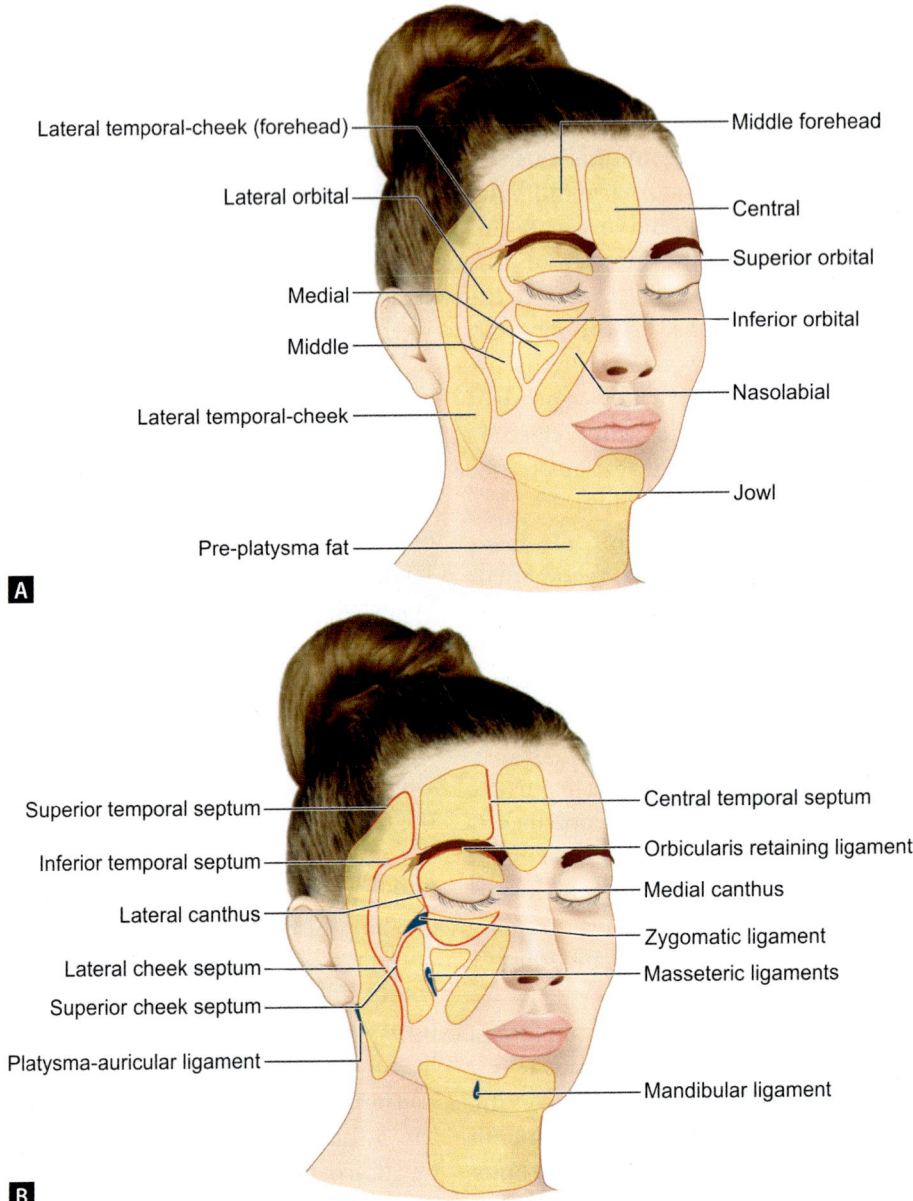

Figs. 16A and B: (A) Superficial fat compartments of the forehead and face, mainly upper face and midface. (B) Ligaments and septa in relation to fat compartments of the forehead and face.
(*Source*: Prendergast PM. Anatomy of the face and neck. Cosmetic Surgery. Schiffman and Guiseppe (Eds). Springer Verlag 2012)

In the upper part of the SOOF represents the deep cheek fat. SOOF has two parts—(1) medial and (2) lateral. The medial part extends from the medial canthus along the inferior orbital rim to the lateral canthus, and the lateral part from the lateral canthus to the temporal fat pad. Deep to the SOOF is a gliding space, the prezygomatic space (described

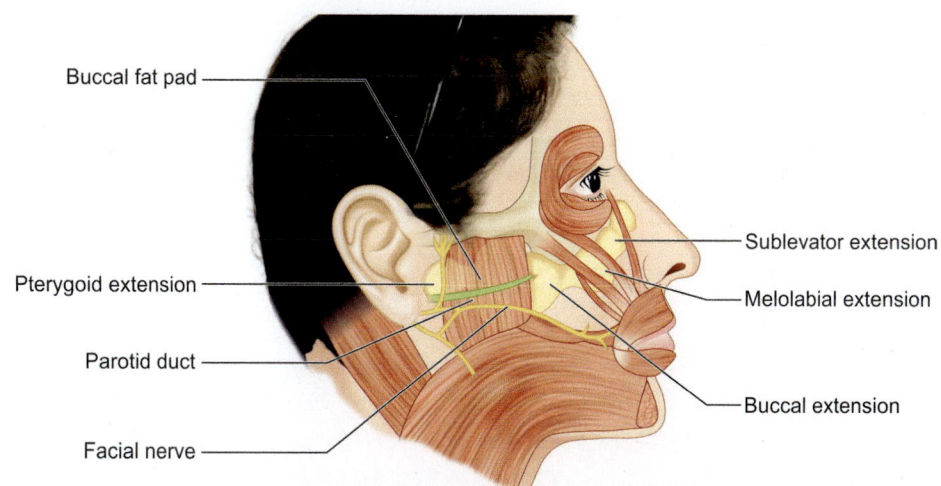

Fig. 17: The buccal pad and its extensions (diagrammatic)–sublevator, melolabial and buccal extensions. Showing relationship with the parotid duct.

earlier). The deep fat compartments consist of the SOOF, the medial cheek fat and the buccal fat with its zygomatic, temporal, and buccal extensions.

The buccal fat pad lies on the posterolateral surface of the maxilla, superficial to the buccinator muscle, and deep to the anterior part of the masseter muscle. The buccal branches of the facial nerve and the parotid duct course over it.

Gassner Rafii et al.[1] gave a completely different concept of the deep fat compartments. They discovered that all deep fat compartments of the midface were actually extensions of the buccal fat pad. So there is the sublevator extension underlying the alaeque nasi, the melolabial extension lying over the maxilla, the LAO, and the buccinator muscle **(Fig. 17)**.

The jowl fat compartment is separate from the nasolabial fat. Jowl fat adheres to the DAO muscle. Medially the boundary is the DLI muscle, and the inferior boundary is a membranous fusion of the platysma muscle. The fusion point between the DAO and the platysma occurs at the site of the mandibular ligament **(Fig. 22)**.

Facial Nerve in the Midface

The facial nerve exits from the stylomastoid foramen and enters the parotid gland. It exits from the parotid gland in the sub-SMAS layer. As the branches course anteriorly they become more superficial. This transition from deep to superficial occurs at locations associated with retaining ligaments, which provide protection to the nerves **(Fig. 18)**.

The *temporal branch (branches)* of the facial nerve can be marked on the surface along the Pitanguy line, which is a line drawn from 0.5 cm below the tragus, to a point 1.5 cm lateral to the supraorbital rim. Contrary to popular teaching, the nerve is deeper at the zygomatic arch where it crosses midway than thought. They exit from the parotid just below the zygomatic arch above the periosteum, and enter the underside of the temporoparietal fascia about 2 cm above the arch, all along protected by a layer of fat and fascia called the parotid temporal fascia.[18]

The *zygomatic branch* exits the parotid gland deep to the fascia just below the zygoma, and slightly superior to the parotid duct. It travels horizontally on the masseter muscle

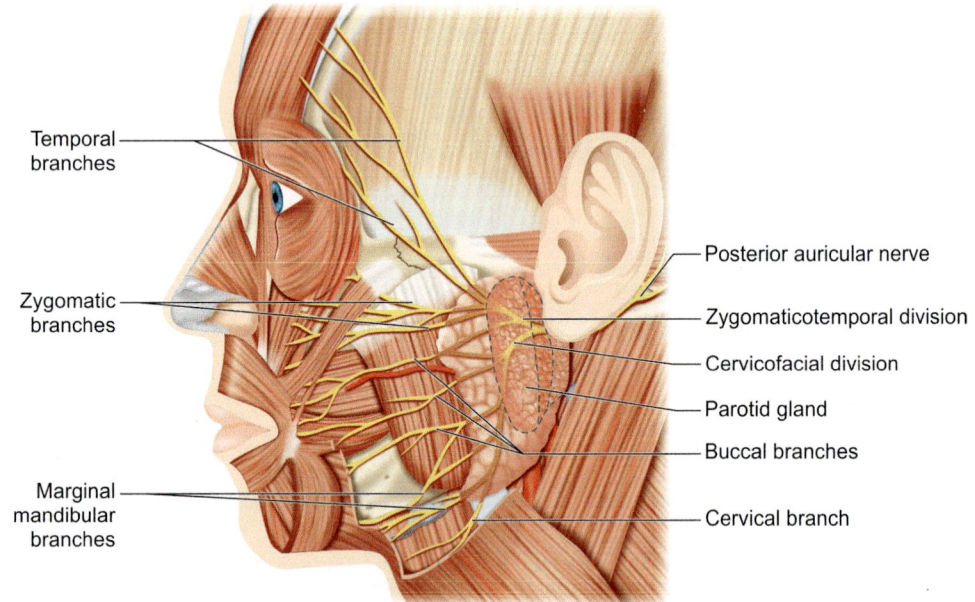

Fig. 18: Facial nerve in the face with its branches.

along with the transverse facial artery. At the lateral border of the origin of the zygomaticus major, it gives off a branch to supply the orbicularis oculi at its inferolateral corner, continues medially, and innervates the zygomaticus major and minor on their deep surface.

The *upper buccal branch* exits the parotid parallel and superficial to the parotid duct still lying deep to the fascia.

The *lower buccal branch* exits the parotid at the level of the earlobe, and travels in the same subfascial plane. At the anterior border of masseter, it comes to lie on the undersurface of the SMAS. At this level, the zygomatic, buccal, and mandibular branches send connecting fibers to each other and then innervate their designated muscles.

The *mandibular branch* exits the parotid, travels on the surface of the masseter, then deep to the platysma just above the lower border of the mandible, crosses over the facial artery at the anterior inferior corner of the masseter, and innervates the DAO, the DLI, and the mentalis.[13]

LIGAMENTS OF THE FACE

The landmark study by Rohrich and Pessa[15] suggests that face subcutaneous fat exists as compartments. These compartments are segregated by thin septae. Fusion points of the septae have been described as ligaments. These areas of fixation or adherence are vascular. Ligaments have been described as true ligaments (which fix the skin to bone) and false ligaments which are condensation of fascia (which fix skin to deep fascia).

True ligaments include the zygomatic ligament, the orbicularis retaining element (ORL), the lateral orbital thickening (LOT), and the mandibular ligament. These are vascular and may have even myocutaneous perforators travelling along them. Even branches of the facial nerve are prone to injury near these ligaments.

- The *zygomatic ligament* connects the inferior border of the zygoma to the skin, and is found just lateral to the origin of the zygomaticus major muscle. The inferior orbital, the lateral orbital and the middle cheek compartments meet at the site. The entry to the prezygomatic space lies above the zygomatic ligament **(Figs. 15 and 16B)**.
- The *ORL* is a circumferential structure is that exists along the upper, lateral, and inferior margins of the orbit. It blends into the medial and lateral canthi, and stabilizes the orbicularis oculi onto the periosteum of the orbital rim. Inferiorly, the ORL separates the preseptal space from the prezygomatic space. Injections into the SOOF cannot travel into the eyelid. In its lateral part just below the frontozygomatic suture, it is thickened to form the LOT **(Fig. 5)**. The LOT fixates the orbicularis and the overlying soft tissues to the periosteum. In the inferior part as the ORL travels medially, it is split into two lamelli and divides the SOOF into a superficial SOOF and the deep SOOF. The medial most part of the ORL is tightly adherent to the periosteum, and has been called the *tear trough ligament* **(Fig. 9)**.
- The *mandibular ligament* lies where the submental increase (point of insertion of the platysma to the skin) fuses with the origin of the DAO at the lower border of the mandible. In an aging face, it appears as the prejowl sulcus, and gives rise to the labiomandibular fold just anterior to the jowl. The marginal mandibular nerve is in close proximity and is prone to injury.

The false ligaments are the parotid-omasseteric ligaments, platysma auricular ligament, and platysmal cutaneous ligaments **(Fig. 19)**.

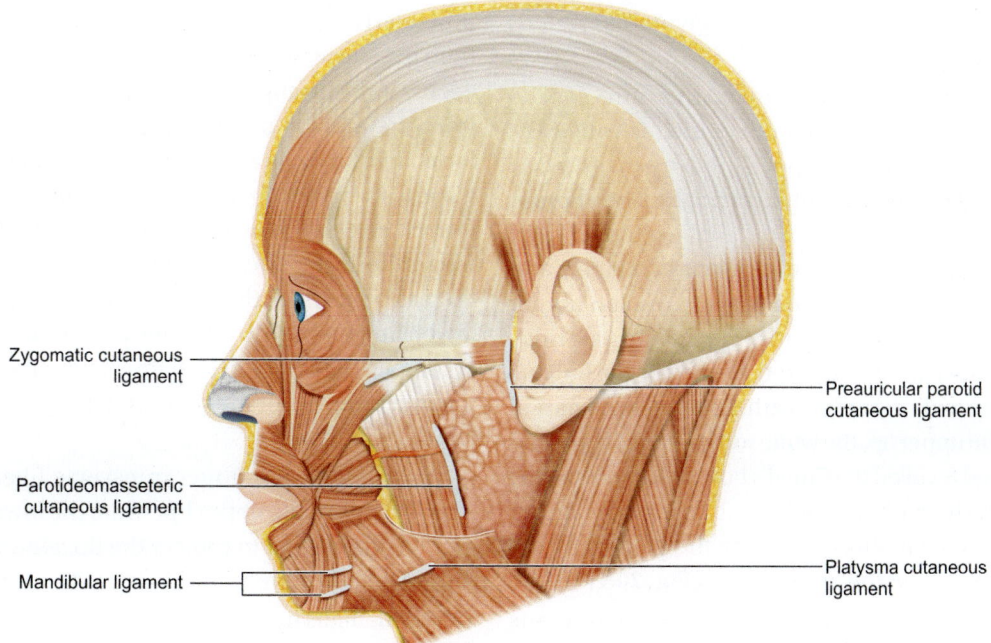

Fig. 19: Ligaments of the face.

- The *parotidomasseteric ligament* arises from the anterior border of the masseter muscle and inserts into the overlying SMAS and dermis. This corresponds to the confluence of the medial and middle cheek fat compartments, as these attenuate, and the SMAS becomes lax, jowls appear.
- The *platysmal auricular ligament* is a vertical line of condensation of fascia under the ear lobule, where the lateral temporal cheek and posterior auricular fat compartments are confluent.

LOWER FACE—LIPS, CHIN, AND JAWLINE

The upper lip extends from the inferior border of the nose above, the nasolabial folds on the sides, the free lip margin below, and up to the upper gingivolabial sulcus posteriorly. Similarly, the lower lip extends from the labiomental groove below, the free vermillion border above, the marionette lines on the sides, and the lower gingivolabial sulcus posteriorly.

The upper and lower lips intersect at the angle of the mouth, which is called the commissure. The upper lip has a pair of vertical ridges called the philtral ridges. They border a central depression called the philtrum, and are consisting of the normal collagen and elastin tissue. Outlining the vermilion border in both the upper and lower lips is a pale ridge known as the white roll, formed by the bulging orbicularis underneath. In the central part of the upper lip, the white roll becomes V-shaped and is called the Cupid's bow, which also forms the lower border of the philtrum. The upper and lower lips connect to the gingiva by the upper and lower frenulum **(Fig. 20A)**.[19]

The vermillion is a modified mucous membrane composed of hairless, highly vascularized, nonkeratinized stratified squamous epithelium. It is 3–5 cell layers thick. It also lacks the skin appendages seen in the skin part of the lip. However, the peripheral part of the orbicularis oris sends fibers to the dry vermillion mucosa and is responsible for the fine folds in the dry part. The red line denotes the division between the dry vermillion and the mucous membrane of the oral cavity, and the transition is marked by the presence of submucous salivary glands and absence of skin lines.

The chin extends from the labiomental groove above, the melomental groove on either side, and the lower border of the mandible inferiorly.

Muscles of the Lower Face

The muscles of the lower face have been discussed earlier. However, the *orbicularis oris* deserves mention again, to learn about the specialized arrangement of muscle fibers around the mouth. The deeper fibers of the orbicularis receive a significant contribution from the buccinator muscle. The medial fibers decussate at the angle of mouth with the fibers from the maxilla passing downward to the lower lip, and those arising from the mandible going to the upper lip. The superficial fibers are formed on either side by the levator and DAO. Fibers from the DAO passing to the upper lip, and fibers from the levator passing to the lower lip **(Fig. 20B)**. The peripheral fibers belonging to the lips are oblique and pass to the mucous membrane to be attached at the wet dry junction.[20]

The *mentalis* has upper transverse fibers which stabilize the upper lip, while the lower oblique fibers help to project the lip, elevate the chin, and produce dimpling in the chin.

The mentalis fibers decussate as they travel downward. A high decussation produces a deep labiomental crease and a bulging upper

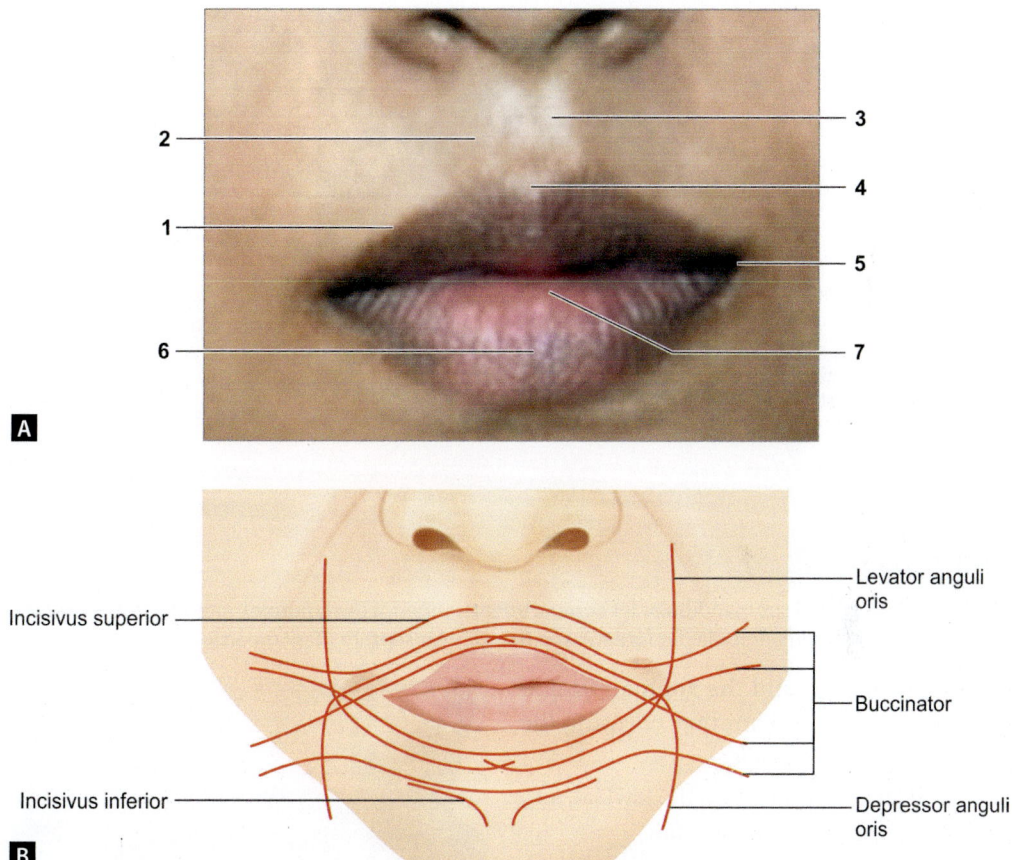

Figs. 20A and B: (A) 1. Vermillion border (white roll), 2. Philtral ridge, 3. Philtrum, 4. Cupid's bow, 5. Oral commissure, 6. Dry vermillion, 7. Wet vermillion; (B) Arrangement of fibers in the orbicularis oris muscle.

part of the chin pad. Failure to decussate in the lower part gives rise to a cleft chin (a muscle free zone).[21]

The *masseter* muscle has a square shape and is located in the inferolateral part of the face. It has distinct superficial and deep heads. The superficial fibers arise from the inferior border of the temporal process of the zygoma, and anterior two-thirds of the inferior border of the zygomatic arch, and insert into the angle and the inferior portion of the ramus of the mandible. The deep head is much bigger and arises from the posterior third of the lower border of the zygomatic arch, and inserts in the upper part of the ramus of mandible. Posterior part of the masseter is covered by the parotid gland, and the anterior margin overlaps the buccinator. The parotid duct and the buccal branches of the facial nerve pass over the masseter from behind to front. It receives its motor supply from the anterior division of the mandibular nerve.

FAT COMPARTMENTS IN THE LOWER FACE

Reece, Pessa, and Rohrich described four fat compartments in the lower face. Two of them over the lower mandibular border, viz. the superior and inferior mandibular

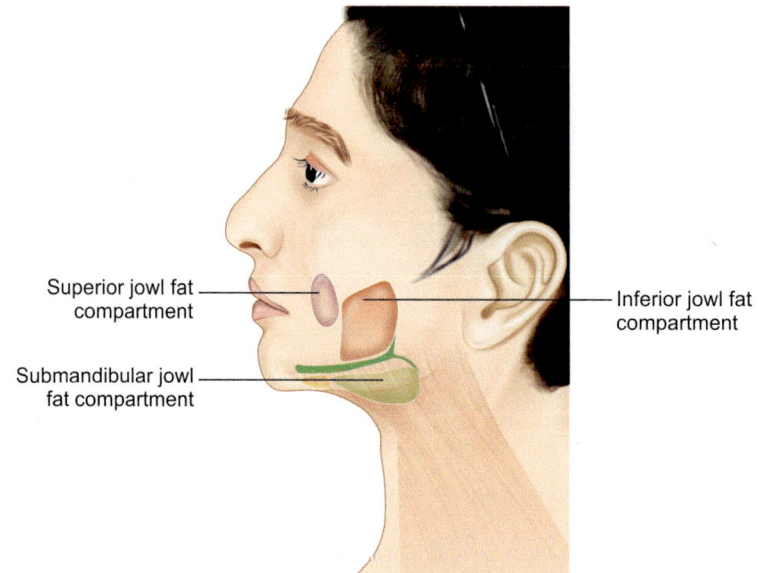

Fig. 21(A): Jowl and submandibular fat compartments, superior jowl (purple), inferior jowl (red) and submandibular fat (green), and mandibular septum (dark green line).

fat compartments, and the submandibular fat compartment and another covering the parotidomasseteric fascia.

Buccal fat is separate from the jowl fat, and jowl fat is separate from neck fat.

The superior mandibular (jowl) fat compartment lies between the nasolabial fat above and the oral commissure anteriorly. The inferior jowl compartment lies inferior and posterior to the superior compartment, and inferiorly reaching the mandibular border.[22]

The mandibular septum is a membranous septum which is located over the mandibular edge and separates the mandibular from the submental fat compartments. It forms a sling for the jowl fat, and is adherent to the lower mandibular border and platysma. The platysma sends some fibers to insert in the middle part of the mandibular lower border. The anterior end of the septum is the mandibular ligament. Posteriorly, the septum ends abruptly at the septum of the fat compartment overlying the parotidomasseteric fascia.

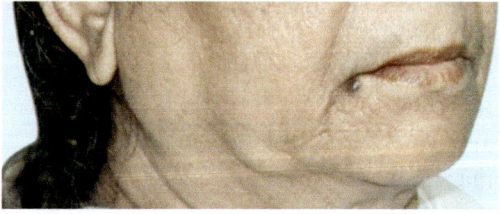

Fig. 21(B): Aging curves of the lower face, viz. chin curve, jowl curve and posterior mandibular curve.

The mandibular septum separates the jowl fat from the submandibular fat **(Fig. 21A)**.

Applied Anatomy

As the mandibular septum attenuates and the jowl fat increases in bulk, the jowl fat ptoses. Three curves can be seen in an aging face-anterior curve is of the contour of the chin ending posteriorly at the mandibular ligament, middle curve representing the jowl fat starting at mandibular ligament and ending at the vertical septum, and the posterior curve from the septum to the angle of mandible **(Fig. 21B)**.

Correction of jowling (middle curve) can be achieved by a vertical vector, and this should be taken into consideration when treating jowls.

CHIN FAT COMPARTMENTS

Pilsl and Anderhuber described fat compartments in the chin in 2010.[23] The superficial fat compartment of the chin lies superficial to the mentalis, DLI, DAO, and the peripheral fibers of the orbicularis oris **(Fig. 22)**. It extends from the labiomental groove to the submental ligaments inferiorly, and from one melomental (labiomandibular) fold to the other.

The deep fat compartment lies deep to the mentalis muscles, but is a small confined space. Deep fat also underlies the labiomental crease, hence the potential for improvement by addressing volume in the groove.[24]

Applied Anatomy

Resorption of lower central alveolar bone and consequent loss of vertical height of the mandible causes the origin of the mentalis muscles to slide inferiorly, causing chin ptosis. Volume replacement in the deep chin compartment corrects chin ptosis partly, but enhancement requires both the superficial and the deep fat compartments to be volumized.

ARTERIES OF THE FACE

The main arterial supply to the soft tissues of the face is the external carotid artery. The branches of the external carotid artery are the facial, internal maxillary, and the superficial temporal arteries. However, a small area in the central forehead, the eyelids and upper part of the nose supplied by the ophthalmic artery, which is a branch of the internal carotid artery.

The superficial arteries of the face arise from the facial artery, and the superficial temporal artery. The deep arteries arise from the internal maxillary artery and the ophthalmic artery.

Facial Artery

The *facial artery* is a direct branch of the external carotid artery. It enters the face after looping around the submandibular gland, about 3 cm anterior to the angle of mandible. It can be palpated on the lower one of the mandible at the anteroinferior angle of the massacre of muscle. Here, as it lies on the mandible, it is deep to the platysma and is accompanied by the marginal mandibular branch of the facial nerve which lies superficial to it **(Fig. 23)**. The facial artery from here courses up words and medially in a zigzag manner toward the media canthus. Initially, it lies deep to the DAO **(Fig. 24)**, zygomaticus, risorius, and then the levator anguli oris muscles. It gives away the inferior labial artery and the superior labial artery and continues as the angular artery.

The *inferior labial artery* arises deep to the LAO muscle and follows a tortuous course

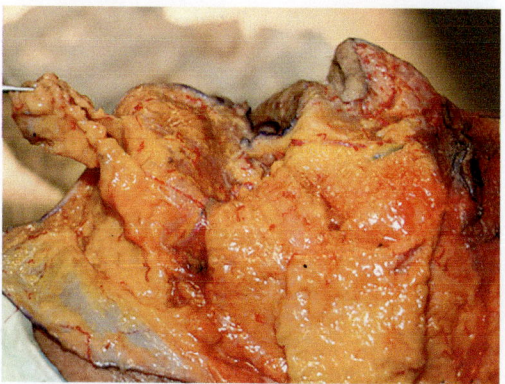

Fig. 22: Chin superficial fat compartments lifted off to show muscles underneath, viz. DAO, DLI, and Orb. oris.

(DLI: depressor labii inferioris; DAO: depressor anguli oris)

along the edge of the lower lip between the muscle and mucosa. It anastomoses with its sister artery from the opposite side, with the mental branch of the inferior alveolar artery and with the sub mental artery.

The *superior labial artery* arises (inferior to the commissure 70%, superior to the commissure 25%, and at the level of the commissure 5%). It is larger and more tortuous than the inferior labial artery. It also travels between the orbicularis oris muscle and the mucosa at the level of the white roll, and anastomoses with the artery from the opposite side. It supplies the upper lip and gives off branches that ascend to the nose, a septal branch, and an alar branch which supplies the end of the nose **(Fig. 25)**.

The *columellar artery* (single 48.9% and double 38.7%) arises from the superficial ascending branches of the superior labial artery which travel between the skin and the muscle **(Fig. 25)**.

The *lateral nasal artery* arises from the facial artery at the level of the nasolabial groove. It runs 2-3 mm above the alar groove, and gives off the superior and inferior alar arteries to the lower nose **(Fig. 26)**. The lateral nasal artery anastomoses with the fellow from

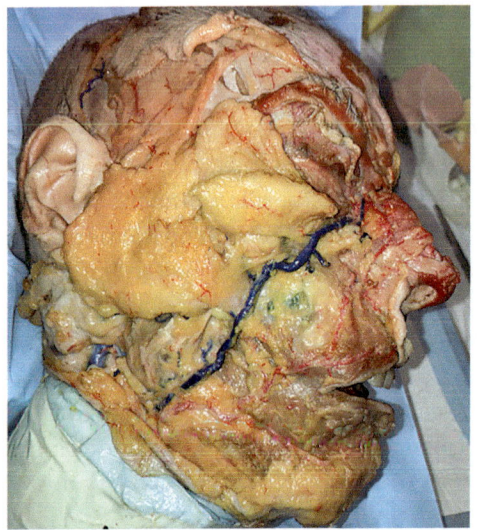

Fig. 23: Course of the facial artery in the face. Marginal mandibular nerve at the lower border, deep to DAO, zygomaticus, LAO, giving off inferior labial, superior labial, alar, lateral nasal, and continuing as the angular artery (in this case).

(DLI: depressor labii inferioris; DAO: depressor anguli oris)

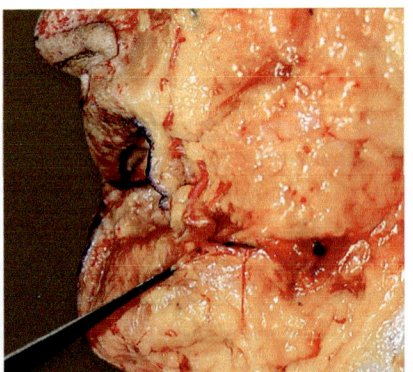

Fig. 24: The depressor anguli oris has been divided to show the facial artery giving off the Inferior Labial and then the superior labial branches (deep to the zygomaticus major muscle, and then continuing as the angular artery.

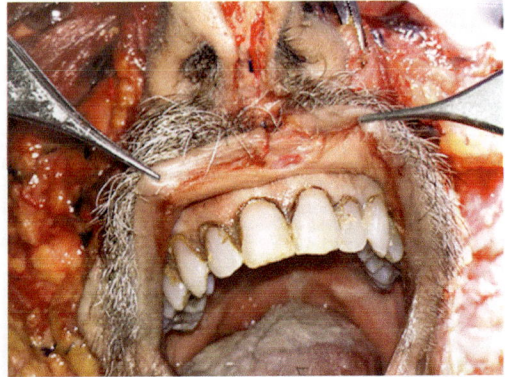

Fig. 25: The superior labial artery seen in the submucosal plane horizontally about a cm above the free margin of the upper lip. Also, can see the columellar artery, a branch of the superior labial.

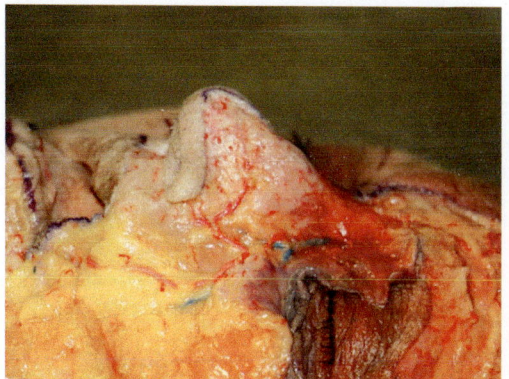

Fig. 26: The facial artery in the midface giving off the lateral nasal artey and the alar branch, before continuing as the angular artery to anastomose with the infratrochlear artery, a branch of the ophthalmic artery.

the opposite side, with the septal and alar branches, the dorsal nasal artery (branch of ophthalmic artery) and the infra orbital artery (branch of maxillary artery) **(Fig. 26)**.

Applied Anatomy

The lateral nasal artery is a risk for embolization for any fillers injected in the alar groove, especially since the artery is relatively fixed in this area.

The *angular artery* is a terminal part of the facial artery. It ascends in the nasolabial groove to the medial canthal region accompanied by the angular vein. It lies 6–8-mm medial to the medial canthus. In only 22%, the terminal branch is formed by the angular artery **(Fig. 26)**, while in 60% by the lateral nasal artery. It anastomoses with the infraorbital artery, and ends by anastomosis with the dorsal nasal artery (branch of ophthalmic artery).

Its branches are—a communicating branch with the dorsal nasal artery (96%), a communicating branch with the supra trochlear artery (67%), the infratrochlear artery, and the paracentral artery. The paracentral artery arises from the angular artery as the main continuation into the forehead in 71% of the cases, and from the communicating branch with the supratrochlear artery in 30%.

Applied—the angular artery runs under the skin in the nasolabial groove in the superficial fat, and is definitely away from bone. So, safe injection plane is on bone or intradermal/just subdermal.

Submental Artery

The submental artery is usually the largest of the cervical branches of the facial artery. It lies deep to the anterior belly of digastric, passes superficial to the mylohyoid nerve, and anastomoses with the artery of the other side in 92%. It anastomoses with the sublingual artery at the symphysis menti, turns upward over the border of the mandible and gives off superficial and deep branches. The superficial branch passes under the skin and anastomoses with the inferior labial artery, and the deep branch runs between muscle and bone, supplies the lip, and anastomoses with the inferior labial and mental arteries.

Internal Maxillary Artery

The external carotid artery divides into two terminal branches behind the neck of the mandible, namely the internal maxillary artery and the superficial temporal artery. Initially, the maxillary artery lies within the substance of the parotid gland **(Fig. 27)**.

It passes horizontally at first, giving off the middle meningeal artery and the inferior alveolar artery. It passes between the two heads of the lateral pterygoid muscle and gives off the anterior and posterior deep temporal arteries and the buccal artery. In its terminal part, it gives off the infraorbital artery. In

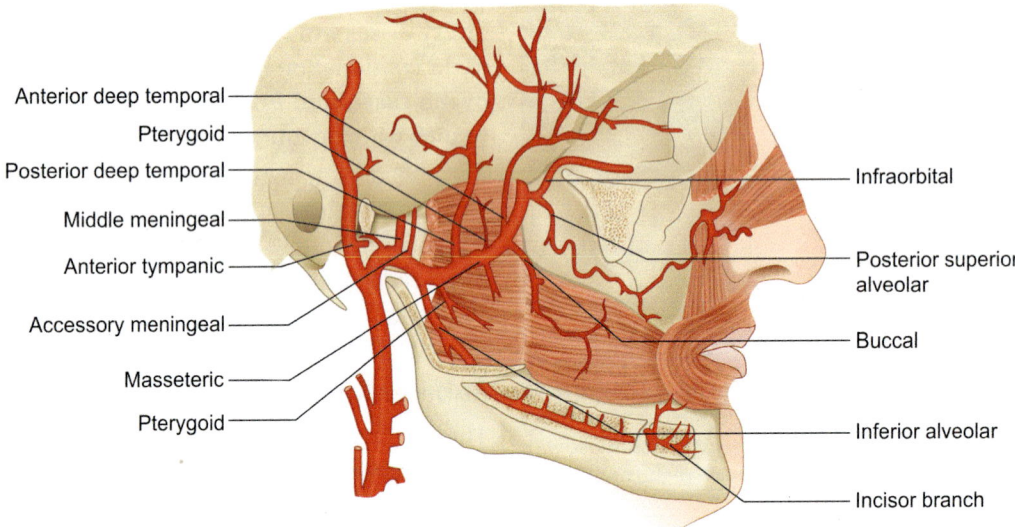

Fig. 27: Arteries of the face showing the internal maxillary artery giving off all its branches, before ending as the infraorbital atery (one of the terminal branches).

addition, in each part there are multiple other branches which will not be discussed here as they are not relevant here.

- The *inferior alveolar artery* enters the mandibular foramen, and on exiting the mental foramen becomes the mental artery. The vertical surface marking of the mental foramen is a straight line dropped from the medial limbus. Another surface marking is a line dropped from between the first and second mandibular premolars, whereas horizontally, it lies between the upper and lower border of the mandible. With age, as the alveolar margin resorbs, the foramen moves closer to the upper border.
- The *deep temporal arteries* (anterior and posterior) ascend between the temporalis muscle and the pericranium and supply the muscle. They anastomose with the middle temporal artery. The anterior temporal artery also anastomoses with branches of the lacrimal artery.
- The *infraorbital artery* is one of the terminal branches of the maxillary artery. It runs in the infraorbital groove along with the infraorbital nerve, and emerges on the face through the infraorbital foramen under the origin of the LLS muscle. Some branches anastomose with the angular artery, others go toward the nose and anastomose with the dorsal nasal artery (branch of the ophthalmic artery). Some branches descend and anastomose with the facial artery, the transverse facial artery, and the buccal artery **(Fig. 27)**.

The arteries on the forehead and the temple region have been discussed in the respective sections.

REFERENCES

1. Gassner HG, Rafii A, Young A, et al. Surgical anatomy of the face. Implications for modern face-lift techniques. Arch Facial Plast Surg. 2008;10(1):9-19.
2. Nemoto M, Uchinuma E, Yamashina S. Three-dimensional analysis of forehead wrinkles. Aesth Plast Surg. 2002;26(1):10-6.
3. Knize DM. An anatomically based study of the mechanism of eyebrow ptosis. Plast Reconstr Surg. 1996;97(7):1321-33.
4. Knize DM. Muscles that act on glabellar skin: a closer look. Plast Reconstr Surg. 2000;105(1):350-61.
5. Hetzler L, Sykes J. The brow and forehead in periocular rejuvenation. Facial Plast Surg Clin North Am. 2010;18(3):375-84.
6. Sykes JM, Cotofana S, Trevidic P, et al. Upper face: clinical anatomy and regional approaches with injectable fillers. Plast Reconstr Surg. 2015;136(5S):204S-18S.
7. Mishra A, Shrestha S, Singh M. Varying positions and anthropometric measurement of supraorbital and supratrochlear canal/foramen in adult human skulls. Nepal Med Coll J. 2013;15(2):133-6.
8. Afifi AM, Sanchez RJ, Djohan RS. Anatomy of the head and Neck. In: Rodriguez ED, Losee JE, Neligan PC (Eds). Plastic Surgery, Volume 3: Craniofacial, Head and Neck Surgery and Pediatric Plastic Surgery, 4th edition. London, UK: Elsevier; 2018.
9. Swift A, DeLorenzi C, Kapoor KM. Injection anatomy: avoiding the disastrous complication. Jones DH & Swift A (Eds). Injection Anatomy-Facial Shaping & Contouring. United States: Wiley Blackwell; 2019. pp. 1-28.
10. Mendelson BC, Muzaffar AR, Adams WP Jr. Surgical anatomy of the midcheek and malar mounds. Plast Reconstr Surg. 2002;10(3):885-96.
11. Michaud T, Gassia V, Belhaouari L. Facial dynamics and emotional expressions in facial ageing treatments. J Cosmetic Dermatol. 2015;14(1):9-21.
12. Prendergast PM. Cosmetic Surgery. In: Shiffman MA, Di Giuseppe A (Eds). Anatomy of the Face and Neck, Heidelberg, Germany: Springer-Verlag Berlin Heidelberg; 2012.
13. Mendelson B, Wong CH. Aesthetic Surgery of the face. Anatomy of the Ageing face. Chapter from. Philadelphia: Elsevier; 2012.
14. Rohrich RJ, Pessa JE, Ristow B. The youthful cheek and the deep medial fat compartment. Plast Reconstr Surg. 2008;121(6):2107-12.
15. Rohrich RJ, Pessa JE. The fat compartments of the face: anatomy and clinical implications for cosmetic surgery. Plast Reconstr Surgery. 2007;19(7):2219-27.
16. Kahn DM, Shaw RB Jr. Aging of the bony orbit: a three-dimensional computed tomographic study. Aesthet Surg J. 2008;28(3):258-64.
17. Furnas DW. The retaining ligaments of the cheek. Plast Reconstr Surg. 1989;83(1):116.
18. Stuzin JM, Baker TJ, Gordon HL. The relationship of the superficial and deep facial fascias: relevance to rhytidectomy and aging. Plast Reconstr Surg. 1992;89(3):441-9.
19. Piccinin MA, Zito PM. Anatomy head and neck, lips. Star Pearls Publishing (Bookshelf ID:507900); 2019.
20. Braz A, Humphrey S, Weinkle S, et al. Lower face: clinical anatomy and regional approaches with injectable fillers. Plast Reconstr Surg. 2015;136(Suppl 5):235S-57S.
21. Garfein ES, Zide BM. Chin ptosis: Classification, anatomy, and correction. Craniomaxillofac Trauma Reconstruction. India: Thieme Medical Publishers; 2008. pp. 1-14.
22. The Mandibular Septum: Anatomical observations of the jowls in ageing—implications for facial rejuvenation. Plast Reconstr Surg. 2008;121(4):1414-20.
23. Pilsl U, Anderhuber F. The chin and adjacent fat compartments. Dermatol Surg. 2010;36(2):214-8.
24. Gierloff M, Stöhring C, Buder T, et al. Aging changes of the midfacial fat compartments: a computed tomographic study. Plast Reconstr Surg. 2012;129(1):263-73.

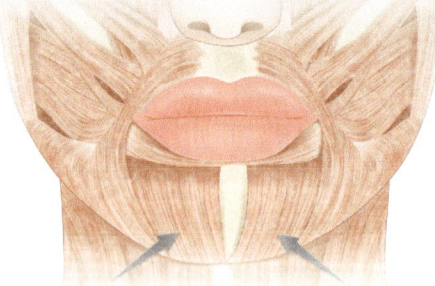

CHAPTER 5

Facial Assessment

Malavika Kohli, Banani Choudhury

INTRODUCTION

Facial assessment is a method to quantify facial aging and evaluates the results of esthetic intervention.

It is important to conduct a full facial assessment for esthetic treatments before proceeding to actual treatment. The aging process involves changes in the facial anatomy. This process mostly affects the bones of the orbits, the cheekbones and chin, as well as changes to the soft tissue, consisting of descent of the fat pads and weakening of the facial ligaments. A sound knowledge of facial anatomy, taking into account facial proportions, is required when assessing a patient for facial treatment.

HIGHLIGHTS OF FACIAL ASSESSMENT

It is worthwhile to consider esthetic ideals when analyzing the face for rejuvenation, as facial proportions, angles, and contours vary with age, sex, and race.

Facial proportions that are deemed ideal are outlined below to facilitate the novice physician with facial analysis **(Fig. 1)**.

Upper One-third of Face

Forehead and Eyebrow

The forehead occupies the upper face, from the hairline to the eyebrows. Its contour, usually convex, is determined by the shape

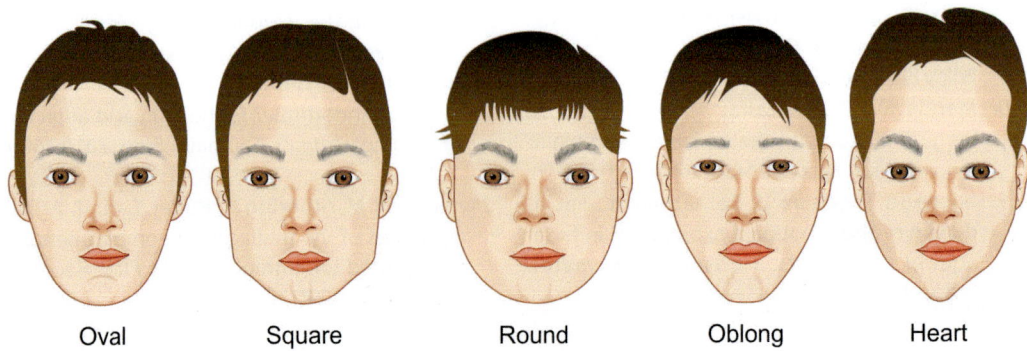

Fig. 1: Facial shapes.

of the underlying frontal bone and distribution of subcutaneous and submuscular fat pads.

The eyebrows are positioned horizontally in males, overlying the supraorbital ridges.

In females, the brows arch slightly from medial to lateral, with the highest part ideally in line vertically with the lateral limbus, or between the lateral limbus and lateral canthus.

Middle Third of Face

Cheeks

The soft tissue of upper lateral cheeks projects anteriorly over zygomatic arch and represents an important feature beauty in all races. Anteriorly, the convexity of cheeks and smooth lip cheek junction is attributable to good deep cheek fact pads supports in young person. Further down, the buccal fat pads give cheeks rounder looks.

Nose

The external nose pyramidal shape attributes attractiveness to face. It projects anteriorly and inferiorly from nasion the dorsum connects the nasion to the apex and nasal tip. The widest part of nose consists of the alae or nostrils, which leads to nasal vestibule. Centrally the columella connects the apex of the nose to philtrum of the cutaneous upper lip.

Lips

One of the highlight of facial analysis is lips. The junction of red part of the lips with the skin is the vermilion border. Immediately adjacent to vermilion border is the white roll, a tube-like structure that runs the length of the lips. In the midline, the top line projects anteriorly as the tubercle. Below the lower lip, the labiomental groove passes between the lip and chin. Between the alae of the nose and lateral border of the lips, the nasolabial grove or fold separates upper lip from cheeks.

Chin and Jawline

Inferior margin of the face runs from the menton in midline at chin, laterally along the inferior and lateral borders of the mandible, to the auricle. Jowl fat and laxity of platysma lead to ptosis and jawline definition is lost.

CONCEPT OF THE GOLDEN RATIO (FIG. 2)

Beauty and facial attractiveness are easy to identify but difficult to quantify. The measurement of esthetically pleasing features, has reproduced a single number or ratio called golden ratio.[1]

The golden ratio, denoted by the symbol (phi), is an number of the order of 1.618033988. The ratio is obtained when a line a + b is sectioned such that

$$a + b/a = a/b$$

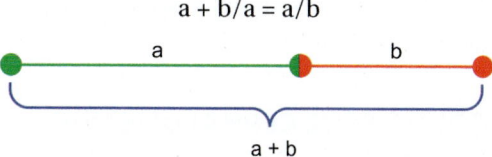

Although Indian mathematicians studied the golden ratio over 2,000 years ago, it first

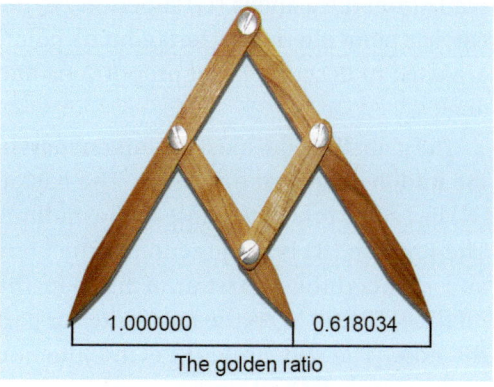

Fig. 2: Concept of golden ratio.

appeared in written documentation in Euclid's elements around 300 B.C.[2] The golden ratio, also called divine proportion, is the basic of most studies on facial esthetics. Ricketts showed the proportion in a face generally perceived as beautiful are related phi ration.[3-6] The width of mouth is phi times the width of nose and distance between lateral canthus is phi time the width of mouth. The height of face from pupil to chin is phi times to the height from hairline to the pupils. Marquardt devised a mathematical model using phi as central measurement to map facial proportion.[7] The result is phi mask that can be used as a tool to analyze facial beauty ad determines its closeness to ideal golden proportion.

However, Holland et al. concluded that our studies have not found relation to the phi concept with facial attractiveness.[8] These observations tell us the though golden ration is prominent and important tool in facial beauty measurement, it may not be applicable in all case scenario and other contributory factors are playing role.

SOFT-TISSUE CEPHALOMETRIC POINTS (FIG. 3)

In the midline, several soft-tissue cephalometric points are defined along the midsagittal plane from the glabella (G) superiorly to the cervical point inferiorly. The landmark points are used to describe facial proportions and angles.[9]

The glabella is the most prominent part in the midline between the brows. The nasion (N) lies at the root of the nose in the midline. The Rhinion (R) is the junction of the bony and cartilaginous dorsum of nose in the midline. The tip (T) is the most anterior part the nose. The subnasale (S) is the junction of the columella and upper cutaneous lips.

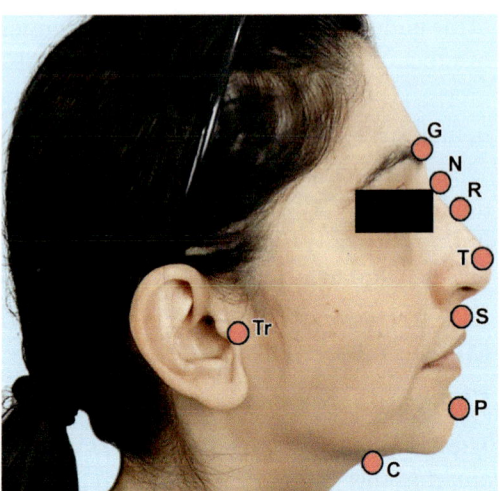

Fig. 3: Soft-tissue cephalometric points.
(G: glabella, N: nasion, R: rhinion, T: tip, S: subnasale, P: pogonion, C: cervical point, Tr: tragus).

The superior labrum (SL) is the junction of the red and cutaneous parts of the lip at the vermillion border in the midline. The stomion (St) is the point where the lips meet at midline. The inferior labrum (IL) is point in the midline of the lower lip at vermilion border. The supramentale (Sm) is the midpoint of the labiomental crease between the lower lip and chin. The pogonion (P) is the anterior point of the chin. The menton (M) is the most inferior point of the chin. The cervical point (C) is the point in the midline where the neck meets the submental areas. The tragion (Tr) is the most superion point on the tragus.

Horizontal Facial Thirds

The upper third extends from hairline to glabella; the middle third from glabella to subnasale and lower third from subnasale to menton **(Fig. 4)**.

The lower third is further divided into thirds: the upper third from subnasale to stomion, middle third from stomion to the

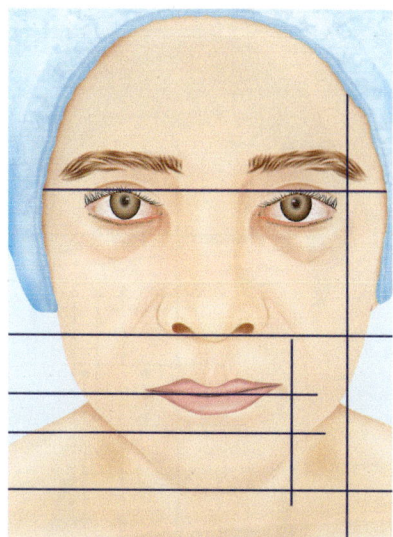

Fig. 4: Horizontal facial thirds.

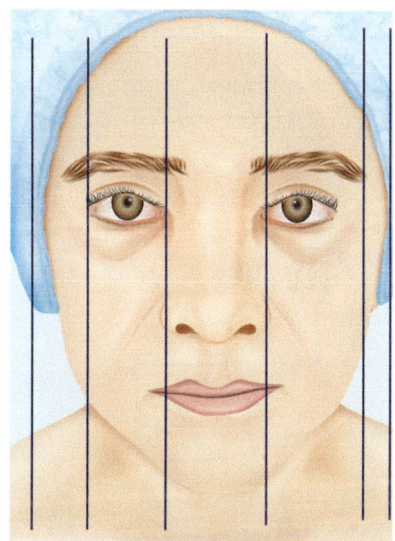

Fig. 5: Vertical fifths.

labiomental crease, and lower third from labiomental crease to menton. Facial thirds are rarely equal. In Caucasians, the middle third is often less than the upper third and middle and upper thirds are less than lower third.[10] The East Asians, the middle third of the face is often greater than upper third and equal to lower third and upper third is less than the lower third.[11]

Vertical Fifths (Fig. 5)

The eye usually measures one-fifth the width of the face. This is discussed more in detail later in the chapter.

Anic-Milosevic et al.[12] compared the proportions of the lower facial third segments in males and females.

The chin represents the largest segment and lower lip height is smallest segment in both sexes. The upper and lower lip heights were larger in males. The heights of upper lip vermilion relative to upper lip were higher in females.

The width of lips should be 40% of width of lower face and usually equal to distance between medial limbi. The width to height ratio of face is typically 3:4 and with oval-shaped face is considered esthetically ideal. The neoclassical canon[13] of facial proportion divides face into vertical fifth, with the width of each eye, intercanthal distance and nasal width all measuring one-fifth.

However, studies using direct anthropometry and photogrammetric analyses in white and Asian subjects found variations in these proportions, with the width of the eyes and nasal widths often being either less than or greater than the intercanthal distance.[12-14]

In a study from India, 100 patients (50 males and 50 females) aged 25–45 years were selected for and facial photographs were analyzed based on the method of Ricketts assessing the divine proportions in vertical and transverse facial planes.[15] Six horizontal and seven vertical ratios were determined, which were then compared with the phi ratio.

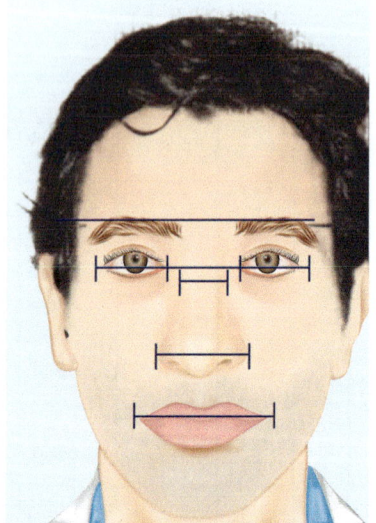

Fig. 6: Seven vertical measurements.

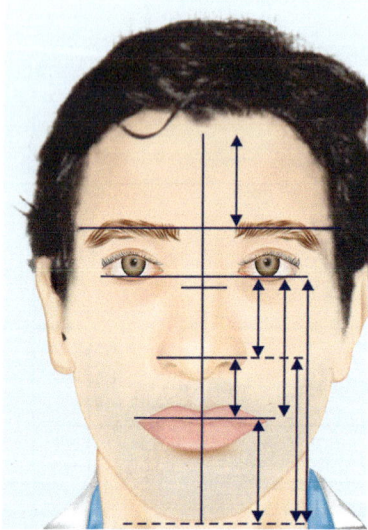

Fig. 7: Six horizontal measurements.

Seven vertical measurements were made along the facial bisecting vertical line (Fig. 6):
1. *Forehead height:* Trichion to the line bisecting the intertemporal plane
2. Intereye point to soft menton
   Menton is the most inferior point on the mandibular symphysis.
3. Intereye point to stomion
   Stomion is a cephalometric landmark defining the contact point of upper and lower lips in mid sagittal line when the mouth is closed.
4. Intereye point to the ala point
5. Ala point to stomion
6. Ala point to soft menton
7. Stomion to soft menton.

Six horizontal measurements were made (Fig. 7):
1. *Intercanthal:* The horizontal measurement from the left lateral canthus of the left eye to the right lateral canthus of the right eye. The midpoint of the measurement was the intereye point.
2. *Interdacryon:* The horizontal measurement between the eyes from the left dacryon to the right dacryon.
   Dacryon is the point of junction of the maxillary bone, lacrimal bone, and frontal bone.
3. *Interalae:* The horizontal measurement between the left lateral rims of the ala of the nose to the right lateral rim of the ala of the nose. The ala point was the midpoint of the line.
4. *Interchilion:* The horizontal measurement from the left chilion to the right chilion of the mouth. The stomion was the midpoint of the line.
   Chilion is the anthropometric term for angle of mouth.
5. *Intertemporal:* The horizontal measurement from the soft tissue lateral border of the left temple to the soft tissue lateral border of the right temple measured along a line that passed through the estimated location of the supraorbital foramen of the of the head.

6. *Nose width:* The horizontal measurement of the bridge of the nose.

In their finding, authors observed that horizontal ratios were similar in males and females. The horizontal mean ratios for both males and females were significantly different from phi ratio indicating that although, the golden proportion is a prominent and recurring theme in esthetics, it should not be embraced as the only method by which human beauty is measured to the exclusion of others factors.[15]

The vertical ratios in male and females were different particularly forehead height/stomion—soft menton ratio and their mean rations were different from phi ration also indicating that golden ratio may not ideal beauty measurement.

Midface Planes

The midface is the key or the foundation point in facial aging process and impacts upper and lower face aging indirectly.[16]

The pathogenesis of midface aging both volumetric and gravitational works in 3 dimensional way to cause aging and sagginess. The tear trough area becomes prominent with loss of deep middle and medial cheek fat and loss of suborbicularis oculi fat (SOOF) support in inferior orbital rim. Orbital retaining ligament becomes lax too and gives the tired look to eyes area.

With the atrophy and decent of deep cheek fat pad, nasolabial groove becomes prominent and impacts on jawline definition in terms of prominence of jowls.

There are objective tools and measurements that have been described by authors for midface esthetics.[17-24]

The ogee curve is a well-known valuable and powerful tool to qualitatively appraise midfacial contour. When seen in the three-quarter view, the soft tissues of the ideal youthful midface form an architectural ogee, or "S"-shaped curve.[24]

Hinderers' lines: It is a line drawn from lateral commissure to the lateral canthus of ipsilateral eye and ala of the nose to tragus **(Fig. 8)**.

Swift and Remington[24] described the ideal midface position as an ovoid, angular cheek mound with an eccentric apex that is measured at 1.618 x from the ipsilateral medial canthus, where "x" is the distance from medial canthus to medial canthus. This corresponds to the intersection of a line drawn from the nasal alar groove to the upper tragus, with a line drawn vertically down from the midpoint of the lateral orbital rim. The youthful face as a whole approximates a double ogee curve, described by Ramirez, with the convexity of the upper ogee at the lateral brow and of the lower ogee at the upper midface.[23] Recreating this curve is an important aspect of midfacial rejuvenation.

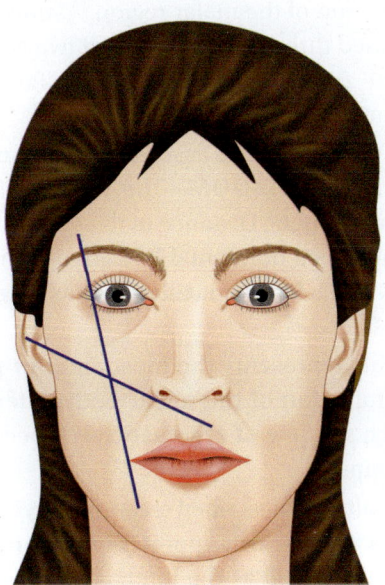

Fig. 8: Hinderers' lines.

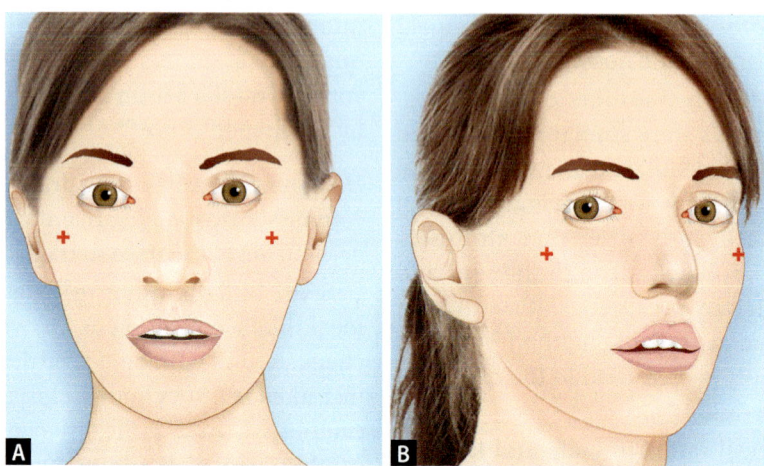

Figs. 9A and B: WIZDOM represents the most anterior point of projection of the malar body, lateral to which the shadow of the zygomatic arch becomes apparent. Red crosses represent the lateral extent of WIZDOM.

Swift and Remington further described the phi relationships and applied them to the midface.[24] The authors of the Juvéderm Voluma trial attempted to divide the cheek into zones[25] as did Binder[26] and Terino.[27] More recently, Marianetti et al. described the "beauty arch," for the assessment of sagittal projection of the malar region.[16] Surek et al. outlined three target zones and two adverse event zones in the midface to facilitate volumizing procedures.[17]

A new midface assessment parameter is called WIZDOM—the Width of the Interzygomatic Distance of the Midface. It is defined as a horizontal line connecting the right and left zygomaxillary points **(Figs. 9A and B)**.[28]

This represents the most anterior point of projection of the malar body, lateral to which shadow of zygomatic arch becomes prominent.

Swift et al. described creating of a youthful cheek apex at Swift's point **(Figs. 10 and 11)**. This is defined as the intersection of a line drawn from the nasal alar groove to the upper tragus and the line drawn vertically down from the midpoint of the lateral orbital rim.

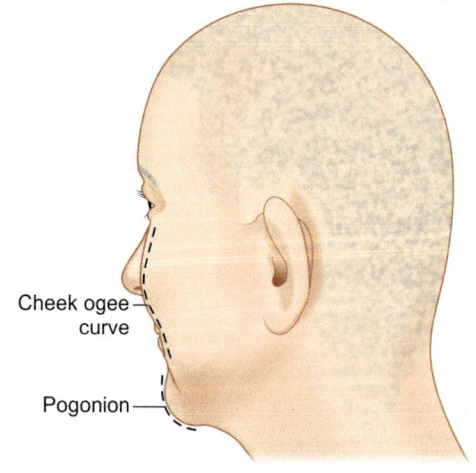

Fig. 10: Cheek apex at Swift's point.
(*Courtesy*: Allergan, Inc (Irvine, CA))

Nose

We have recently experienced lots of queries and request to correct nose tip elevation and projection. So a better understanding of nose anatomy and relation of nose to forehead and

Chapter 5: Facial Assessment

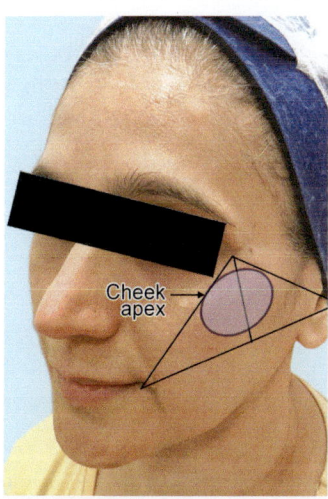

Fig. 11: The triangle is formed by a line from lateral canthus to lateral angle of mouth and from angle of mouth to tragus and from tragus to lateral canthus.

Table 1: Nasal tip projection.	
Baums ratio	2:1
Simons	2.8:1
Nasofrontal angle	115–130°
Nasolabial angle	90–120°

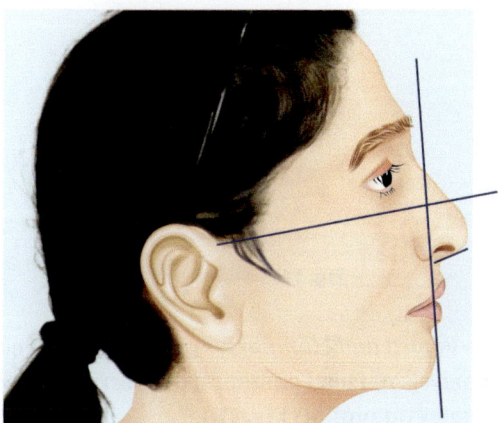

Fig. 13: Nasolabial angle.

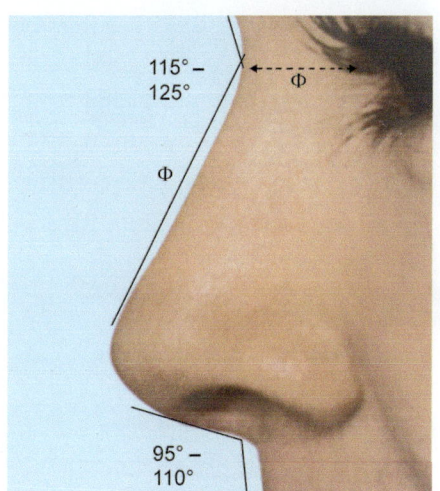

Fig. 12: Nasal tip projection.

nose to lips and chin. Nasal tip projection can be measured using other Parameters **(Fig. 12)**. As listed in the following **Table 1**.[9]

According to Powell and Humphreys the ideal Baum and Simons ratios for whites are 2.8:1 and 2:1, respectively.[29]

Nasolabial Angle

The Frankfurt horizontal plane (FHP) is found by drawing a line from the superior aspect of the external auditory canal to the most inferior point of the orbital rim. The nasolabial angle is formed between a line along the anterior part of the columella and a line perpendicular to the FHP and nasal tip **(Fig. 13)**.

The Simons ratio used to calculate nasal tip projection. A line from the subnasale along the anterior aspect of the columella to the nasal tip (a) divided by a line from the subnasale to the superior labium (b) gives the Simons ratio **(Figs. 14 to 17)**.

FACIAL PROPORTIONS AND ANGLES

These angles facilitate preoperative assessment and planning in facial rejuvenation.

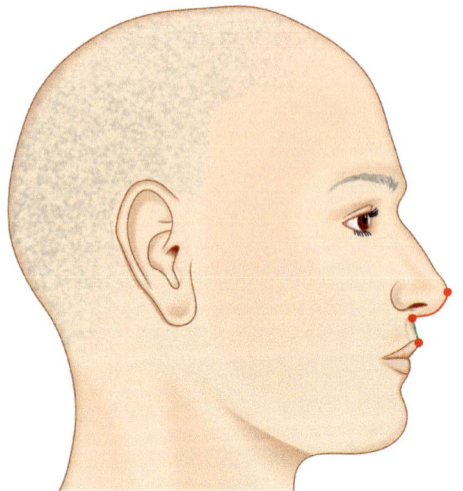

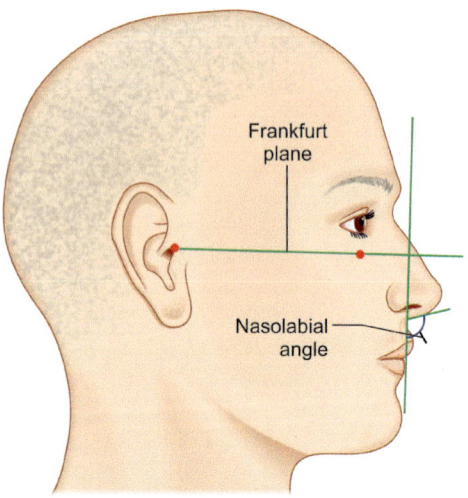

Fig. 14: Simons ratio.

Fig. 15: The Frankfurt plane

Powell and Humphreys provide a detailed analysis of facial contours, proportions, and angles on profile **(Fig. 18)**.[31]

Racial variations exist, Chinese descent has wider nasofrontal angle. The upper and lower lips are posterior to nasofrontal angle in Caucasians, but on or anterior to this line in Africans and Asian descent **(Fig. 19)**.[31]

Peck and Peck describe another orientation plane formed by a line from tragion that bisects a line from nasion to pogonion.[32]

Chin

Chin is an area defined by labiomental crease superiorly and oral commissures laterally and submental cervical crease inferiorly. Position of chin, shape and length, contour and projection, and relation with nose and lip are very important for a n] balanced and propionate face. Consideration of dentition, maxillomandibular skeletal morphology, and soft tissue envelope is essential.[33]

Labiomental fold: The indentation between the lower lip and lower portion of mandible

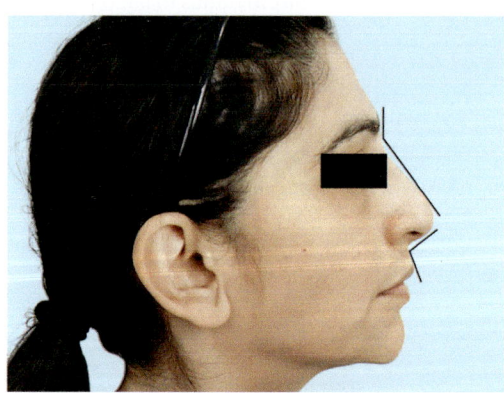

Fig. 16: Nasofrontal angle.

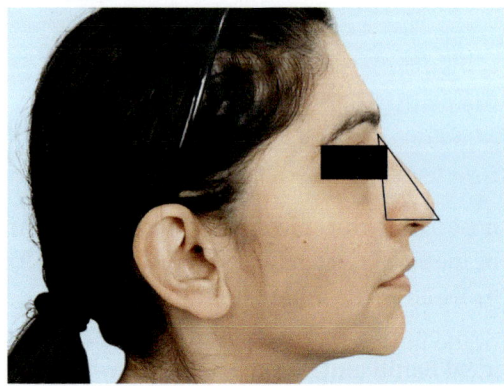

Fig. 17: Nose ratio.

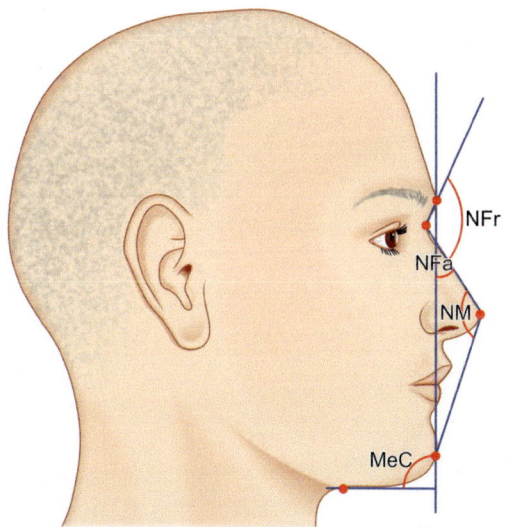
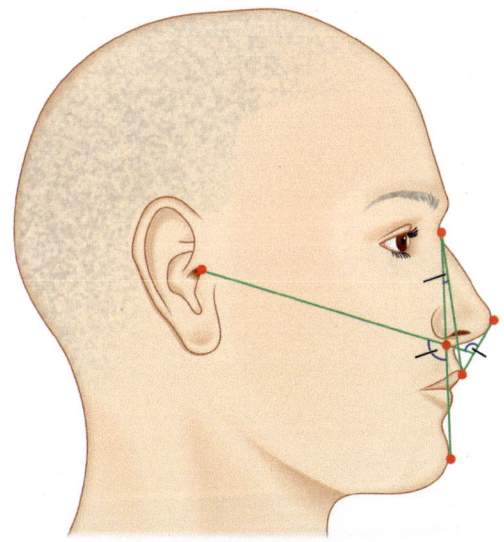

Fig. 18: Powell and Humphreys' esthetic angles.
A line from glabella to pogonion creates the anterior facial plane.
- The angle formed by lines from nasion to glabella and from nansion to nasal tip is nasofrontal angle (NFr): 115–130°
- Nasomental (NM) angle lies between the line along the dorsum to nasion and a line drawn from nasal tip to pogonion: 120–130°
- Nasofacial angle (NFa) is formed between anterior facial plane and the line tangent to dorsum of nose: 30–40°
- A line drawn from cervical point to mention intersecting the anterior facial plane creates mentocervical angle (MeC): 80–95°

Fig. 19: The facial, maxillofacial, and nasomaxillary angles developed from these lines relate upper lip to chin and nasal tip and nasion to chin. Holdaway's H angle describes the degree of soft tissue protrusion of maxilla relative to mandible and is ideally 10°.[32]

pogonion should never project beyond this line **(Fig. 20)**.
- Cervicomental angle—the angle between the chin and the neck should be 105–120°
- Nose-chin evaluation—the esthetics of the nose and the chin should be harmonious. Ideally, chin projection should lie ~3 mm posterior to a line drawn in the nose-lip-chin plane **(Fig. 21)**.

HOW TO LEARN FACIAL ASSESSMENT

As everyone knows, it is very difficult to learn a new practical skill, or to improve upon one that you already have, by simply studying a textbook. To be completely competent in medical esthetic treatments, practitioners must ensure they receive sufficient practical training for each and every procedure. This

is important characteristic in chin esthetics. Ideally the fold should fall at the junction of upper and middle third when the length between stomion and menton is divided into thirds.[33]

Lip-chin relationship—on a balanced face, a line connecting the most prominent portion of the upper and lower lip should touch the pogonion (riedel line). The lower lip should be 2-3 mm posterior to the upper lip and the

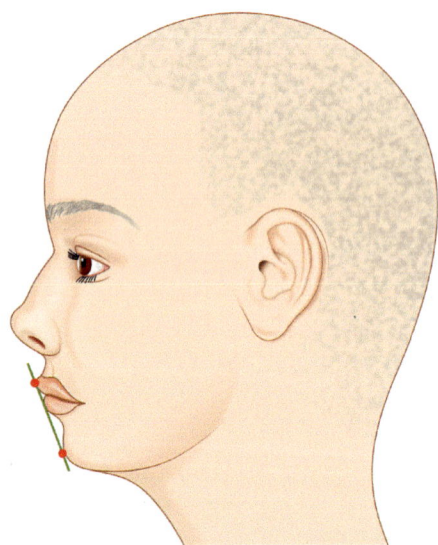

Fig. 20: *Riedel line*: A line drawn vertically down the facial plane connecting the most prominent portion of the upper and lower lip. This line should touch the most prominent anterior portion of the chin in a balanced face.
Courtesy: Edward I lee.

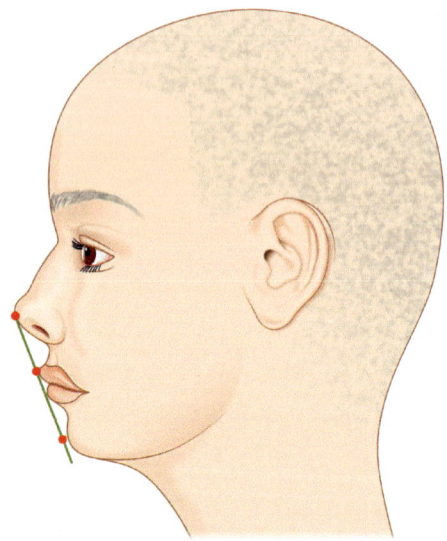

Fig. 21: *Nose-lip-chin line*: A line drawn vertically down the facial plane connecting most projecting point of the nose and most prominent portion of the upper lip. Most prominent anterior portion of the chin should be ~3 mm posterior to this line.
Courtesy: Edward I lee.[33]

training, many practitioners note, is ongoing and essential for safe practice and effective treatments. There are many different ways to learn or stay updated with current practice, but one way is to hear different practitioners with unique experiences speak about their patients to a live audience. It is useful to watch others assess different faces, discuss their most challenging cases, answer audience questions, and perform live demonstrations. A perfect opportunity to get this valuable experience is at congresses.

During pretreatment, a handheld mirror is good way to show patients the changes in their skin and face. Patient can be educated about the changes their face is undergoing and problem areas in each third of face, upper, mid, and lower including the neck area. Any asymmetry in face should be pointed out before the patient undergoes any treatment.

Facial proportions and angles are easily determined in the clinic using photogrammetric analysis. With this information, the physician should educate the patient on the role of facial proportions in esthetics, discuss the most appropriate measures, and tailor a plan to achieve the best results. Once there is an understanding of the importance of proportion in facial esthetics, the proposed plan is usually more acceptable.

Esthetic dermatologist can educate his/her patient how correction of one area of face impacts other areas of face, specially midface impacts lower and upper face proportion and midface acts as foundation point in mature age group patients in facial rejuvenation and augmentation.

Midface volumizing specially in deep middle cheek fat pad improves tear trough area as well as nasolabial fold. Volumizing the lateral fat compartments in cheek area and temporal area has an indirect impact in lower face, making jawline defined and improves sagginess in face. Sharing these knowledge with patient is very important as patient can understand why step-wise correcting face from foundation point to then contouring and refinement is better than correcting one particular area only. Photographic evidence is essential to show patients before and after results and document our data (consent forms) for medicolegal issues.

TIPS AND PEARLS OF FACIAL ASSESSMENT
Assessment: Special Areas
Periocular Rejuvenation (Fig. 22)

A 45-year-old female, thought that he looked tired around the eyes and described herself as "tired in appearance". In our assessment, we noticed that he had deep grooves around the eyes, quite noticeable perioral lines and under-eye bags. We assessed following points: Skin quality, nasojugal groove (tear trough), infraorbital fat pad, malar fat pad, medial cheek fat pad, infraorbital rim and lateral rim, and orbicularis oculi muscle.

Midface Rejuvenation (Figs. 23 to 25)

A 60-year-old patient came to for full-face rejuvenation. Along with upper and lower one-third, we assessed her midface.

We assess the patient with front and side photographic profile and look for the following points:
- Ogee curve, hinderers line, malar prominence or cheek apex, transition of eyes and tear trough into cheeks, submalar area, and nasolabial fold
- Proportion of midface with upper one-third and lower one-third is assessed.

Lower Face (Fig. 26)

A 53-year-old patient's main concern looking old and aged as she had lost weight following bariatric surgery. We assessed her full face.

When we focused on her lower face, the following points need to be looked into.

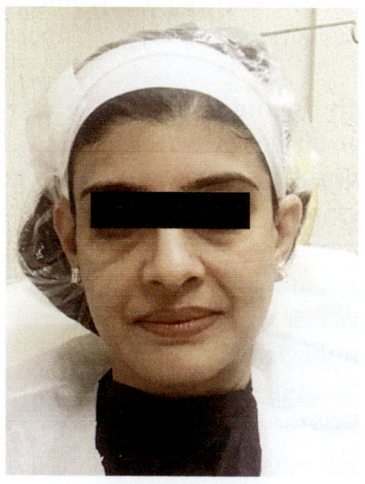

Fig. 22: Periocular rejuvenation.

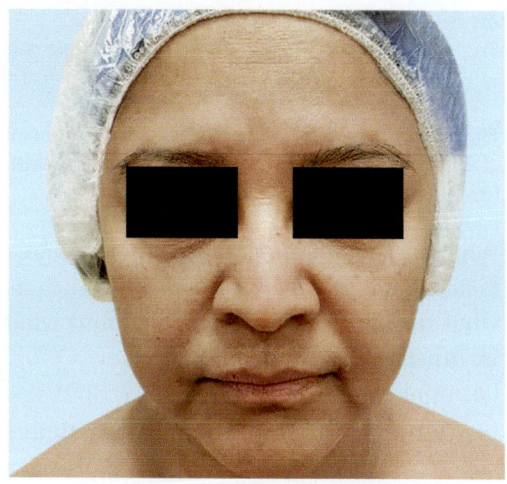

Fig. 23: *Midface assessment*: Front view.

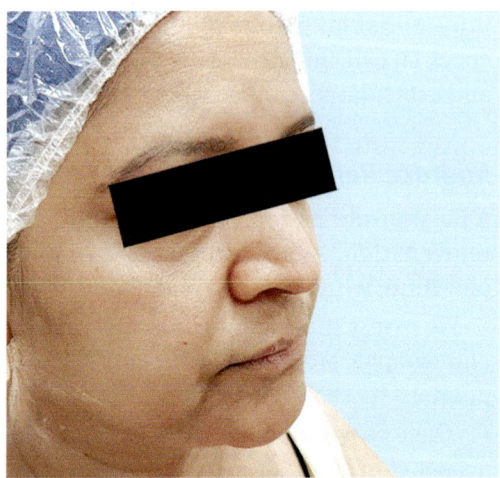

Fig. 24: *Same patient*: 45° profile view: Assessment of ogee curve.

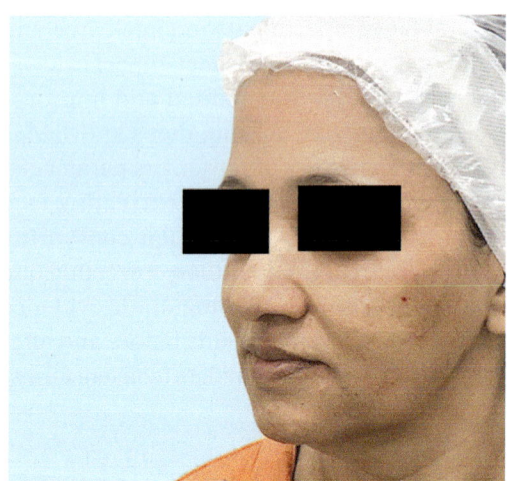

Fig. 26: *Lower face*: Loss of definition of jawline due to jowl formation and chin shortening.

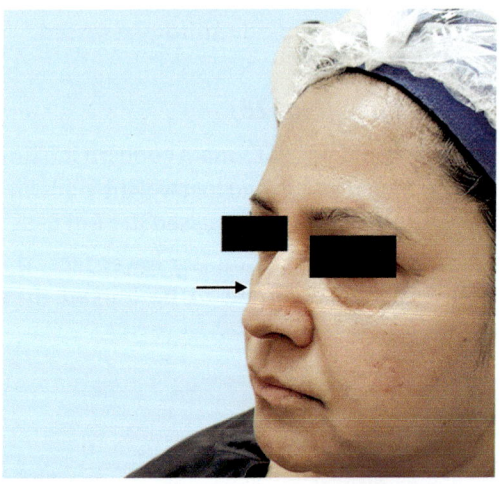

Fig. 25: *Same patient*: Side profile: Assessment of cheek volume and submalar area and relation with lower face.

What you need to look for is how the lower facial shape fits in with the rest of the face, what the structural changes are, and what treatments would be needed to achieve a more harmonious face.

We noticed that although the patient's skin was of good quality, it was a little lax and there was disproportion to the shape of the face. From the frontal view, you can see that, to the side of the chin, she has a jowl and it curves inward quite noticeably. From the side, it is clear her jawline has lost definition and the back of her jaw shape is angulated, rather than 90°. We also noticed that she had a downturned mouth, giving her a slightly sad appearance.

We wanted to focus on changing the lower facial profile and give it more of a V-shape from the front view and define her jawline, anterior projection of jawline and length from the side profile.

In the mandibular region, there are three areas that we usually need to address: the bone, the soft tissue, and the skin. Jawline obliteration can happen due to Bone resorption:

- Ptosis of soft tissue
- Masseter hypertrophy
- Parotid gland hypertrophy.

Lip Augmentation

In every patient assessment, it is important to ask patients what concerns them rather

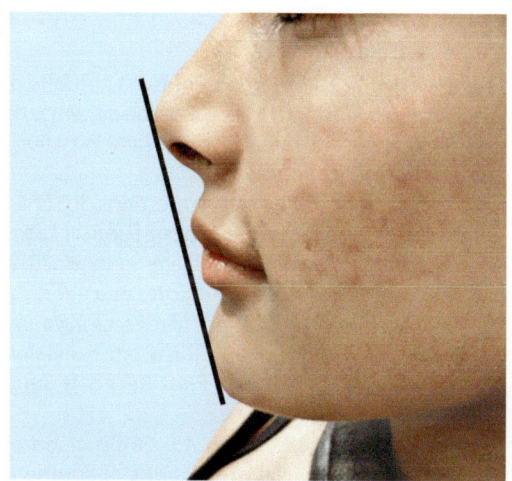

Fig. 27: Correlation of nose, lips, and chin.

total facial dimension and balance with her chin.

Reidel's plane is evaluated.

Correlation of nose, lips, and chin is important for anterior projection of face **(Fig. 27)**.

As we know the understanding of facial aging affects from skin to the bone, so we need to assess all the components. We will need to look into different planes and zones of face. Photographic view of six different views and then focus on the problem zone **(Fig. 28)**. Comparing with the other zones of face is important to keep proportion and symmetry of face.

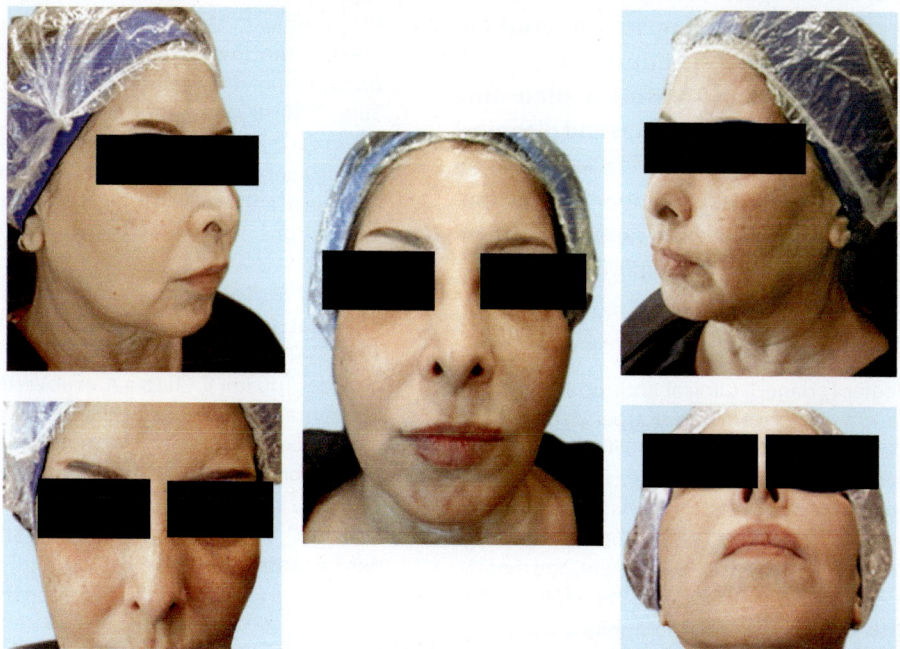

Fig. 28: Photographic view of different zones of face.

than to assume this yourself. Our patient, a 25-year-old informed us what bothered her most was her lips. In our assessment, noticed that her lips were small compared to her

An esthetic facial assessment consultation can last anything between 30 minutes and an hour. This is followed by a written report, then a "cooling off" period for patients to decide whether they want to proceed.

CONCLUSION

Patient often comes to a dermatologist requesting to correct a specific area on face like lip augmentation, nose tip elevation, brow lift, and chin augmentation, or some patients come asking for overall facial rejuvenation.

Knowing the facial assessment skills helps the clinician to understand the facial changes in an individual regardless of male or females. Knowing the average facial ideals and ratios and proportions helps clinicians to apply on patient's face and plan a roadmap for him/her.

Clinician should have adequate knowledge of facial aging changes, changes in bone, muscle, fat compartments (superficial and deep) and skin and their impact in a particular person's aging process. Educating patient should be a part of treatment plan and approaching face in a global way and planning and making a treatment plan is a better way of approach for facial rejuvenation. Satisfaction rate of treatment is high and rapport between treating clinician and patient's is rewarding.

REFERENCES

1. Vegter F, Hage J. Clinical anthropometry and canons of the face in historical perspective. Plast Reconstr Surg. 2000;106(5):1090-6.
2. Bashour M. History and current concepts in the analysis of facial attractiveness. Plast Reconstr Surg. 2006;118(3):741-56.
3. Ricketts RM. Esthetics, environment, and the law of lip relation. Am J Orthod. 1968;54(4):272-89.
4. Ricketts RM. The biologic significance of the divine proportion and Fibonacci series. Am J Orthod. 1982;81(5):351-70.
5. Ricketts RM. The golden divider. J Clin Orthod. 1981;9(11):752-9.
6. Ricketts RM. Divine proportion in facial aesthetics. Clin Plast Surg. 1982;9(4):401-22.
7. Marquardt SR. Dr. Stephen R. Marquardt on the Golden Decagon of human facial beauty. Interview by Dr Gottlieb. J Clin Orthod. 2002;36(6):339-47.
8. Holland E. Marquardt's Phi mask: pitfalls of relying on fashion models and the golden ratio to describe a beautiful face. Aesthetic Plast Surg. 2008;32(2):200-8.
9. Prendergast PM. Facial Proportions. In: Erian A, Shiffman M (Eds). Advanced Surgical Facial Rejuvenation. Berlin, Heidelberg: Springer; 2012.
10. Farkas LG, Hreczko TA, Kolar JC, et al. Vertical and horizontal proportions of the face in young adult North American Caucasians: revision of neoclassical canons. Plast Reconstr Surg. 1985;75(3):328-38.
11. Sim RS, Smith JD, Chan AS. Comparison of the aesthetic facial proportions of southern Chinese and white women. Arch Facial Plast Surg. 2000;2(2):113-20.
12. Anic-Milosevic S, Mestrovic S, Prlić A, et al. Proportions in the upper lip-lower lip-chin area of the lower face as determined by photogrammetric method. J Craniomaxillofac Surg. 2010;38(2):90-5.
13. Wang D, Qian G, Zhang M, et al. Differences in horizontal, neoclassical facial canons in Chinese (Han) and North American Caucasian populations. Aesthet Plast Surg. 1997;21(4):265-9.
14. Crumley RL, Lanser M. Quantitative analysis of nasal tip projection. Laryngoscope. 1988;98(2):202-8.
15. Anand S, Tripathi S, Chopra A, et al. Vertical and horizontal proportions of the face and their correlation to phi among Indians in Moradabad population: A survey. J Indian Prosthodont Soc. 2015;15(2):125-30.
16. Surek CC, Beut J, Stephens R, et al. Pertinent anatomy and analysis for midface volumizing procedures. Plast Reconstr Surg. 2015;135(5):818e-29e.
17. Marianetti TM, Cozzolino S, Torroni A, et al. The "beauty arch": a new aesthetic analysis for malar augmentation planning. J Craniofac Surg. 2015;26(3):625-30.
18. Jacono AA, Ransom ER. Anatomic predictors of unsatisfactory outcomes in surgical rejuvenation of the midface. JAMA Facial Plast Surg. 2013;15(2):101-9.

19. Coleman SR, Grover R. The anatomy of the aging face: volume loss and changes in 3-dimensional topography. Aesthet Surg J. 2006;26(1S):S4-9.
20. Richard MJ, Morris C, Deen BF, et al. Analysis of the anatomic changes of the aging facial skeleton using computer-assisted tomography. Ophthalmic Plast Reconstr Surg. 2009;25(5): 382-6.
21. Zadoo VP, Pessa JE. Biological arches and changes to the curvilinear form of the aging maxilla. Plast Reconstr Surg. 2000;106(2):460-6.
22. Buchanan DR, Wulc AE. Contemporary thoughts on lower eyelid/midface aging. Clin Plast Surg. 2015;42(1):1-15.
23. Little JW. Volumetric perceptions in midfacial aging with altered priorities for rejuvenation. Plast Reconstr Surg. 2000;105(1):252-66.
24. Ramirez OM. Three-dimensional endoscopic midface enhancement: a personal quest for the ideal cheek rejuvenation. Plast Reconstr Surg. 2002;109(1):329-40.
25. Swift A, Remington K. BeautiPHIcation™: a global approach to facial beauty. Clin Plast Surg. 2011;38(3):347-77.
26. Philipp-Dormston WG, Eccleston D, De Boulle K, et al. A prospective, observational study of the volumizing effect of open-label aesthetic use of Juvéderm® VOLUMA® with Lidocaine in mid-face area. J Cosmet Laser Ther. 2014;16(4):171-9.
27. Binder WJ, Azizzadeh B. Malar and submalar augmentation. Facial Plast Surg Clin North Am. 2008;16(1):11-32.
28. Terino EO, Edward M. The magic of mid-face three-dimensional contour alterations combining alloplastic and soft tissue suspension technologies. Clin Plast Surg. 2008;35(3): 419-50.
29. Linkov G, Mally P, Czyz CN, et al. Quantification of the Aesthetically Desirable Female Midface Position. Aesth Surg J. 2018;38(3):231-40.
30. Powell N, Humphreys B. Proportions of the aesthetic face. New York: Thieme-Stratton; 1984.
31. Leach J. Aesthetics and the Hispanic rhinoplasty. Laryngoscope. 2002;112(11):1903-16.
32. Peck H, Peck S. A concept of facial esthetics. Angle Orthod. 1970;40(4):284-318.
33. Lee EI. Aesthetic Alteration of the Chin. Semin Plast Surg. 2013;27(3):155-60.

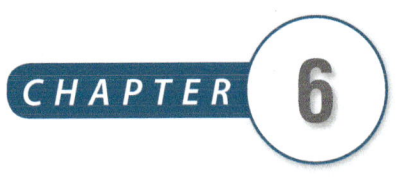
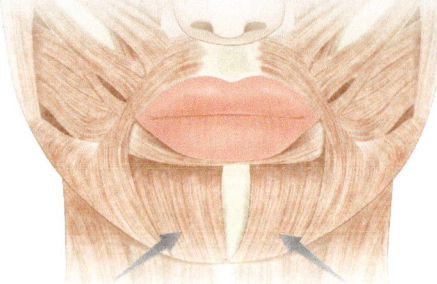

Patient Selection and Esthetic Consult

Latika Arya

INTRODUCTION

Appropriate patient selection and a detailed esthetic consult are absolutely essential for a successful outcome with cosmetic injectables. A perfect treatment may be perceived unsatisfactory by the patient if correct patient selection and pretreatment counseling are not paid enough attention to. The physician should be able to identify ideal patients who will benefit from volume replacement or neuromodulation procedures, and conduct effective individualized counseling for each patient to not only set realistic expectations, but also achieve more successful outcomes, minimize complications, and hence increase patient satisfaction.[1,2] This chapter aims to summarize the factors that should be borne in mind for patient selection for cosmetic injectables, including the contraindications. The chapter also covers pretreatment precautions, patient counseling, and other important considerations during esthetic consultation.

IDEAL PATIENT

The ideal patient for cosmetic injectables is one who has an understanding of the nature of these treatments, realistic expectations about the esthetic outcomes possible, and a willingness to comply with appropriate pretreatment and post-treatment instructions as well as follow-up examinations.[3] The patient should have reasonable skin elasticity and firmness and should preferably be following a skin type appropriate preventive skin care regimen. The ideal candidate should not be having any contraindications to the procedure.[4]

FIRST INTERVIEW

It is important to determine the reasons why the patient wants to undergo cosmetic therapy. Hence, a comprehensive consultation is essential prior to any treatment to not only determine the facial aging changes but also to establish realistic goals for the patient and at the same time making them aware of the limitations and risks of cosmetic injectables treatment to avoid disappointment after the procedure.[2] Mismatched physician and patient expectation can lead to an unhappy patient despite a good result achieved by the injector. It is also helpful to develop a rapport with the patient and be alert to any underlying mental disturbance or dysmorphophobic tendency.[5]

CONTRAINDICATIONS

A complete medical history should be elicited in order to identify patients who have contraindications to the use of dermal fillers or neurotoxins (**Box 1**). It is more important not to treat an inappropriate patient than to treat an ideal patient in order to prevent complications with cosmetic injectables.[5] The medical history should include enquiry into any medical illnesses, allergies, medications used, and prior esthetic procedures.

Treatment should be avoided if there is a history of severe allergy or anaphylaxis to the material or to the lidocaine mixed in the syringe of the filler.[6]

Any patient with an infection in or adjacent to the site of treatment should not be treated, since the infecting organism may populate the site of filler use.[6] These conditions include the following: viral infections such as herpes simplex virus (HSV), perioral human papilloma virus (HPV), and mollusca contagiosa; bacterial infections with streptococci or staphylococci, such as impetigo; presence of excessive amounts of *Propionibacterium acnes*; yeast infections or extensive pityrosporum folliculitis; and parasitic mite infections, such as massive Demodex folliculorum infestation.[2]

Patients with infections such as sinusitis, periodontal or dental infections and ear, nose, or throat infections should also not be treated until the condition has resolved to avoid complications like biofilm reactions.[7]

Caution needs to be exercised in disorders of hemostasis or coagulation, uncontrolled hypertension or when anticoagulants like aspirin, clopidogrel or warfarin are being taken, as the risk of bruising may be higher.[5]

If there is a history of pre-existing neuromuscular disease or intake of aminoglycosides or other agents interfering with neuromuscular transmission (e.g., curare-like compounds), botulinum toxin injections should only be performed with caution as the effect of the toxin may be potentiated.[8]

Cosmetic injectables treatment may not be suitable in patients with a keloid predisposition or inflammatory skin diseases that cause Koebner response such as lichen planus and active psoriasis.[2]

No causal relationship has been established between the use of filler and autoimmune diseases like dermatomyositis/polymyositis, lupus erythematosus, rheumatoid arthritis or scleroderma. Their use is, therefore, not contraindicated in patients suffering from those diseases, whose wound healing is normal.[6] However caution is needed, especially if disease is active. Patients with immunosuppression can undergo treatment with fillers, although poly-L-lactic acid should be avoided.[6]

It is advisable to avoid these treatments during pregnancy/lactation since there are no adequate and well-controlled studies in pregnant or lactating women.[2,8]

PRETREATMENT PRECAUTIONS

Drugs like aspirin and nonsteroidal anti-inflammatory agents and vitamins/herbal

---

Box 1 Contraindications to the use of cosmetic injectables.

Absolute contraindications:
- History of severe allergy or anaphylaxis to the material or to the lidocaine mixed in the syringe of the filler
- Infection in, or adjacent to, the site of treatment

Relative contraindications:
- Bleeding disorders
- History of neuromuscular disease
- History of intake of drugs or supplements which have anticoagulant action or interfere with neuromuscular transmission
- Keloid predisposition
- Inflammatory skin diseases
- Autoimmune diseases
- Pregnancy/lactation
- Unrealistic expectations/dysmorphophobia

supplements with anticoagulant effects should preferably be discontinued 10 days before treatment to minimize the risk of bruising and swelling.

It is preferable to defer treatment in patients with any active skin infection, acne or inflammation until the infection or inflammation has been treated. Further, it is recommended to start prophylactic antiviral therapy (acyclovir, valaciclovir, or famciclovir) in patients who have a history of HSV to prevent virus reactivation.[2]

A history of previous facial surgeries, dental procedures or previous cosmetic injectables as well as the type of filler and their response should be enquired as that may affect the treatment plan.[5]

Further, it is helpful to elicit history about lifestyle e.g., sun exposure, alcohol intake, smoking, and sleeping history. **Box 2** shows the required checklist to be completed in every patient before scheduling the treatment.

Box 2	Checklist for cosmetic injectables procedure.

- Patient motivation
- Patient expectation
- Any dysmorphophobia
- Occupation
- Lifestyle factors
- Medical history
- Drug history
- Contraindications to procedure
- Previous facial surgery/dental treatments
- Previous esthetic treatments
- Previous reactions to treatments
- Discontinuation of anticoagulant medication or herbal supplements unless medically warranted
- Prophylactic antiviral in patients with history of herpes simplex
- Clinical assessment
- Treatment plan—choice and quantity of product, use of anesthesia, cost
- Post procedure care and recovery
- Pretreatment photographs
- Informed consent

ESTHETIC CONSULTATION

Pretreatment Counseling

The most important part of the esthetic consultation is patient counseling. The objectives of this session are to determine the patient's concerns, expectations, and motivations for the cosmetic procedure.

The physician needs to carefully assess the patient's face with an educated eye, including analysis of tissue quality, area and extent of volume loss, any bone loss, extent and pattern of muscular contraction, and surface skin changes. Also, the proportions of the face should be observed taking into account facial height, width and symmetry, by dividing the face into horizontal one-third and vertical one-fifth. Measurements can also be made with calipers. Facial symmetry should be checked and asymmetry, if any, should be pointed out so that the patient does not attribute it to the treatment.[9] At the same time the physician must remember that the definition of an attractive and beautiful face is subjective, depending upon social, cultural, and ethnic factors as well as age and gender.[10]

Photographs

Pretreatment photography is essential not only for the purpose of documentation but also helps in understanding the changes happening in the face, checking proportions and symmetry, assessment of treatment effects and any adverse effects and for medicolegal purposes. Photographs of patients at a younger age may aid in goal-setting, and help to convey the potential benefits and limitations of each treatment.[11]

Treatment Plan

Based on the patient's requirement and the outcome agreed upon, the range of options then need to be discussed in detail. The treatment plan is made regarding the use of neuromodulators and fillers. It is recommended to give the patient a road map of their esthetic improvement journey keeping their long-term rejuvenation goals in mind.

The appropriate soft tissue augmentation product that meets the patient's overall objectives is identified. Its benefits, limitations, and safety profile are discussed. Many physicians as well as patients prefer the hyaluronic acid fillers due to their more favorable safety profile, natural composition, and their possibility of reversal by use of hyaluronidase whereas others may prefer longer lasting products.[1]

The financial cost is also discussed in this session as it is an important factor influencing the treatment plan and product selection.[1]

Discuss the pain tolerance of the patient and plan if topical anesthesia is desired. Moreover, it is also important to discuss with the patient the postprocedure precautions and possible events in the recovery period such as pain, swelling, bruising etc. in order to prepare them for "social down-time".[12]

Consent

Before the treatment procedures are carried out an informed consent is signed and witnessed. This consent should be as complete as possible, including all the necessary information about the treatment and should also mention potential problems or complications, and should be explained to the patient.[5]

CONCLUSION

Proper patient selection and detailed esthetic counseling are essential to identify patient desires and goals, review potential risks, and establish realistic expectations. It is the foundation to a successful outcome with cosmetic injectables.

REFERENCES

1. Day D. Counseling patients on facial volume replacement and adherence with post-treatment instructions. Patient Prefer Adherence. 2010;4:273-81.
2. De Boulle K, Heydenrych I. Patient factors influencing dermal filler complications: prevention, assessment, and treatment. Clin Cosmet Investig Dermatol. 2015;8:205-14.
3. Gladstone HB, Cohen JL. Adverse effects when injecting facial fillers. Semin Cutan Med Surg. 2007;26(1):34-9.
4. Buck DW 2nd, Alam M, Kim JY. Injectable fillers for facial rejuvenation: A review. J Plast Reconstr Aesthet Surg. 2009;62(1):11-8.
5. Urdiales-Gálvez F, Delgado NE, Figueiredo V, et al. Preventing the Complications Associated with the Use of Dermal Fillers in Facial Aesthetic Procedures: An Expert Group Consensus Report. Aesthetic Plast Surg. 2017;41(3):667-77.
6. Lafaille P, Benedetto A. Fillers: contraindications, side effects and precautions. J Cutan Aesth Surg. 2010;3:16-9.
7. Narins RS, Coleman WP, Glogau RG. Recommendations and treatment options for nodules and other filler complications. Dermatol Surg. 2009;35 Suppl 2:1667-71.
8. Vartanian AJ, Dayan SH. Complications of botulinum toxin A use in facial rejuvenation. Facial Plast Surg. Clin North Am. 2005;13(1):1-10.
9. Milutinovic J, Zelic K, Nedeljkovic N. Evaluation of facial beauty using anthropometric proportions. Sci World J. 2014;2014:428250.
10. McKnight A, Momoh AO, Bullocks JM. Variations of structural components: specific intercultural differences in facial morphology, skin type, and structures. Semin Plast Surg. 2009;23(3):163-7.
11. Vedamurthy M, Vedamurthy A, Nischal KC. Dermal fillers: do's and dont's. J Cutan Aesthet Surg. 2010;3:11-5.
12. Brennan C. The "nuts & bolts" of becoming an aesthetic provider: part 3- maximizing your aesthetic practice and client outcomes. Plast Surg Nurs. 2014;34(2):62-9.

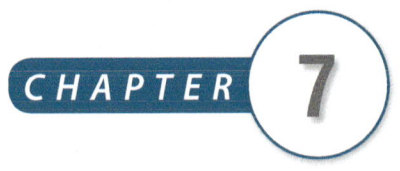
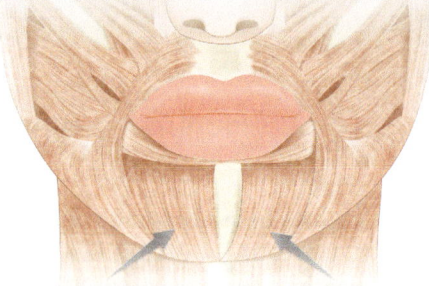

CHAPTER 7

Pre-requisites for Filler Treatment

Rashmi Sarkar, Vivek Nair

INTRODUCTION

Documentation is perhaps the most important part of doing a filler or toxin procedure. This is because good standardized photographs reflect before and after changes much better than a patient's memory, and at the same time serve as a record for future treatment planning. Documentation consists of getting written informed consent from the patient regarding the procedure, a treatment chart which documents the type and technique of filler/toxin used, and most importantly pre- and post-treatment photographs.

METHODS[1]

While designing the consent form, it is essential to list all the commonly observed side effects; this facilitates a discussion of any concerns the patient may have prior to doing the injection procedure. A sample consent form for both fillers and botulinum toxin is attached in the appendix. Many filler/toxin companies also provide a standardized consent form which can serve as a template for clinical use.

Photography

Regarding photographs it is best to take them with a DSLR camera with standardized overhead lighting. This is often not possible and practically the camera in most smart phones available today can do a decent job provided the lighting is okay. The authors find it best to take pictures without flash use since a flash can wipe out contoural details. Five standard angles are taken for each patient—front on, 45° from each side, and 90° from each side. Using an overhead lighting source with an off-face focal point on the lower trunk with equal illumination from both sides at about a 45° angle provides the best results.[2] The author also uses the Canfield Vectra system which provides a 3-dimensional representation of the patients face with various advanced measurement options. This is great for research work but not essential for day to day practice since taking and storing the pictures in systems such as these is a time consuming process. There are smartphone apps available for both the android and iOS system which facilitates taking standardized photographs using aids such as onscreen grids and these can be very useful.

The other thing which is essential with photographs is to have a safe way of storing them and an efficient retrieval system where it does not take more than 30–60 seconds to access old photographs. Cloud hosting and local hosting are the two methods available for storage and each have their advantages and disadvantages.

Cloud hosting provides automatic back up by the online service provider as well as ease of accessibility. However, privacy is becoming an issue with this method as online servers are prone to hacking as well as unethical use of photographs by the software or online service provider. For this reason, the authors prefer *local hosting* of the photographs on portable hard drives. Any photograph management software like iOS Photos, Picasa, etc. can be used to organize the photographs. It is essential to have backups for all the data on a local hosting system to prevent data loss on account of hardware failure. At least two backups are recommended and these should be updated weekly.

Procedural notes are very important and must be maintained for every procedure done in clinic. Again, it helps to have standardized forms for this. The notes can be brief but should be done as soon as possible after the procedure to avoid recording errors. Suggested data for fillers are the points of injection, type of filler used, cannula or needle or both, any areas of layering different fillers, type of anesthesia used, and any obvious or suspected bruising. For botulinum toxin, data is much simpler and basically consists of the points of injection and dose per site. Any pre-existing asymmetry should be recorded in the form. Well maintained treatment records permit fine tuning of toxin dose for subsequent sessions; thereby, producing consistently excellent clinical outcomes. Sample filled forms are included in the appendix. If possible, these forms should also be digitalized and stored securely. In case there are multiple doctors in a clinic, the treating physicians name should be clearly mentioned on both the consent and procedural forms, and he or she should sign the forms.

REFERENCES

1. Mang WL, Neidel F, Becker A, et al. (2010). Informed Consent in Aesthetic and Plastic Surgery. In: Manual of Aesthetic Surgery. Springer, Berlin, Heidelberg. pp. 7-11.
2. Prantl L, Brandl D, Ceballos P. A proposal for updated standards of photographic documentation in aesthetic medicine. Plastic and Reconstr Surg Glob Open. 2017;5(8):e1389.

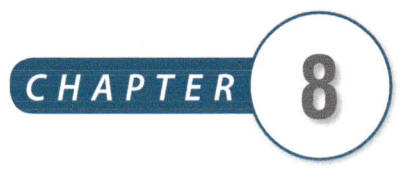
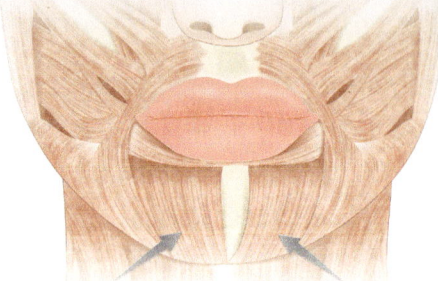

Anesthesia

Tanvi Gupta Arora

INTRODUCTION

Providing sufficient anesthesia is a crucial part of a successful cosmetic injectable practice. Good anesthesia offers the patient a better procedural experience, minimizes discomfort with better precision and improved outcomes.

Type of anesthesia depends on the level of pain expected with the procedure and also the duration and patient tolerance. It can be achieved in the following ways:

- With the use of injectable anesthetics (lignocaine or bupivacaine as regional block or local infiltration)
- Topical anesthesia (EMLA)
- Contact cooling
- Vibration devices as pain reducing devices.

INJECTABLE ANESTHETICS

Lidocaine or bupivacaine reduces pain by blocking neural cell membrane sodium channels and thus inhibiting propagation of nerve impulses. Pain and temperature sensation go faster than pressure.[1]

Local infiltration can lead to distortion of the local anatomy and thus minimum amount is to be injected. Injectable anesthesia has the advantage of faster onset of action and lower chances of bruising when used in combination with epinephrine.

Regional nerve blocks are beneficial when full face or multiple areas are to be treated.[2] Another advantage is lesser distortion of local tissue as anesthetic is injected away from the treatment area. Infraorbital and mental nerve blocks are most commonly deployed and the nerves are easily found by palpating the respective foramina.

As seen in **Figure 1**, the infraorbital nerve supplies upper lip, lower eyelid, lateral portion of nose, and inner cheek. We use a short 0.5-inch needle so that we reach the distal ends of the nerve and without entering the foramen. Always palpate the foramen and keep the finger there during injection to prevent accidental needle entry into the foramen which can damage the infraorbital nerve as well the lower intraorbital contents. Philtrum and corners of the mouth may not be anesthetized well and additional local infiltration might be needed. Mental nerve supplies chin and part of lower cheek. The zygomaticofacial and zygomaticotemporal blocks are two other useful blocks for injecting the zygomatic and temporal area respectively **(Fig. 1)**.[2]

For the last few years, dermal filler preparations have lidocaine (0.3%) and only the skin prick is painful which can be adequately anesthetized with topical anesthesia. So regional

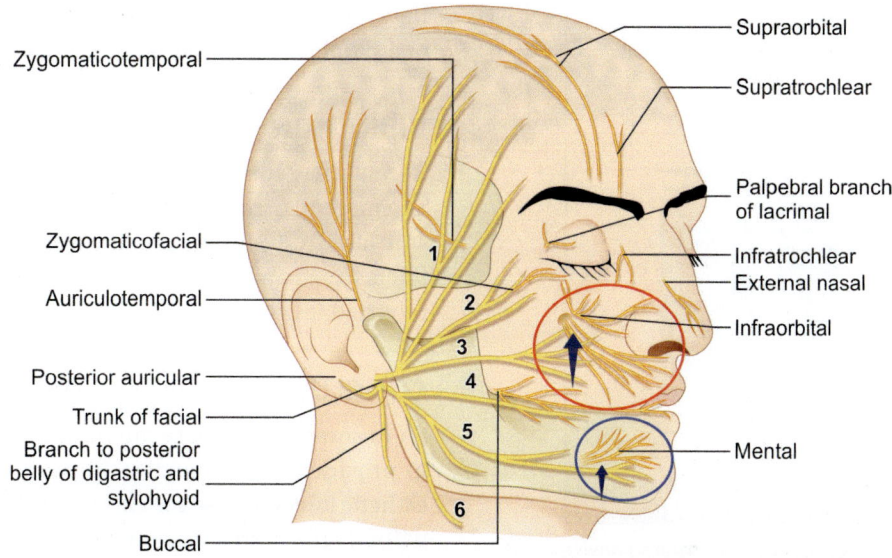

Fig. 1: Shows the area supplied by the infraorbital nerve and mental nerve and points of injection.

nerve blocks are seldom done nowadays. Local infiltration is still commonly used for the entry point of cannulas during dermal filler injection.

TOPICAL ANESTHESIA

Ease of application and a needleless procedure have made topical anesthesia, the anesthesia of choice for fillers and botulinum toxin injection. EMLA (eutectic mixture of 2.5% lidocaine and 2.5% prilocaine) is most commonly used.[3] The skin is degreased with spirit and the product is applied as a thick layer and then occluded with a plastic sheet or micropore **(Fig. 2)**.

Duration of application depends on the procedure and generally 45 minutes–1-hour application is sufficient for most patients. Disadvantages include relatively less pain control as compared to an injectable anesthetic, longer visit time, occasional skin irritation, and also more cost.

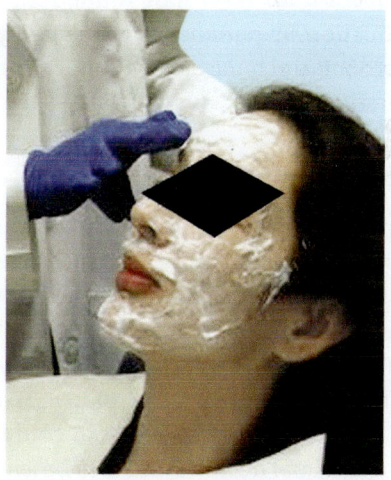

Fig. 2: Face with EMLA applied under occlusion.

Major side effects result from systemic absorption which can be negated by restricting the surface area of application. Systemic toxicity can manifest as dizziness in mild cases and respiratory depression when severe. There has been one case of methemoglobinemia reported recently after extensive EMLA

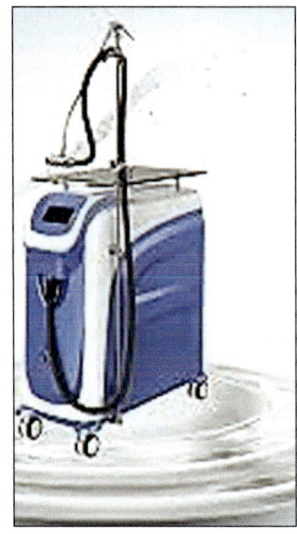

Fig. 3: A contact cooling device.

application for laser hair reduction.[4] Self-application by patients at home can prove hazardous and hence clinic application is to be preferred.

CONTACT COOLING

Ice packs or cooling gels can be used alone or in conjunction pre- or postprocedure to alleviate pain sensation. Anesthesia is achieved by cooling the area for 1–3 minutes till numbness is felt or erythema appears. The desired temperature is 5°C. Prolonged contact and excess cooling can result in cold burns and epidermal necrosis and is to be avoided. Generally, 15–30 seconds of contact followed by a 10–15 seconds break is well tolerated. Repeat this cycle for 2–3 minutes before injecting. A specialized contact cooling device or a simple icepack may be employed **(Fig. 3)**.

VIBRATION

Recently few authors have described vibration as a method of reducing pain sensation.[5] In a split face study design, the side where dermal fillers were combined with vibration patients reported less pain.

CONCLUSION

So to summarize, there are numerous ways to provide effective analgesia during facial esthetic injectable treatments and these once painful procedures are now very comfortable for the patient.

REFERENCES

1. Joshi GP, Schuq SA, Kehlet H. Procedure-specific pain management and outcome strategies. Best Pract Res Clin Anaesthesiol. 2014;28(2):191-201.
2. Bosenberg AT. Blocks of the face and neck. Tech Reg Anesth Pain Manag. 1999;3:196-203.
3. Shahid S, Florez ID, Mbuagbaw L. Efficacy and safety of EMLA cream for pain control due to venipuncture in infants: a meta-analysis. Pediatrics. 2019;143(1):e20181173.
4. Lerner RP, Lee E. EMLA-induced methemoglobinemia after laser-assisted hair removal procedure. Am J Emerg Med. 2019;37(11):2119.e1-2119.e2.
5. Bourdier S, Khelif N, Velasquez M, et al. Cold vibration (buzzy) versus anesthetic patch (EMLA) for pain prevention during cannulation in children: a randomized trial. Pediatr Emerg Care. 2019. [Epub ahead of print].

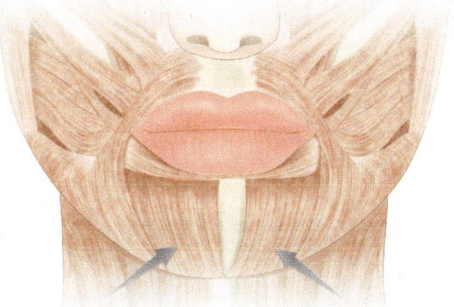

CHAPTER 9

Filler Injection Techniques

Richa Ojha Sharma

INTRODUCTION

Dermal filler injections are becoming increasingly popular for esthetic enhancement. The results of filler injections are highly dependent upon two factors—(1) choice of filler type for the indication and (2) injection technique. In this chapter, we will discuss how adopting the right injection technique results in superior esthetic outcome, with lesser product volume. Also of importance is the fact that correct injection technique can minimize or avoid side effects such as nodules, tyndallization, ecchymoses, and the much dreaded vascular injections.[1]

BASIC INJECTION TECHNIQUES

The main techniques are:

- *Serial puncture*: Material is deposited in multiple injections serially along the length of the wrinkle **(Fig. 1A)**
- *Linear threading:* First the entire needle length is inserted into the wrinkle, then material is deposited in a line while needle is being pulled out **(Fig. 1B)**
- *Fanning:* Material is deposited by linear threading fashion along multiple lines in a fan like arrangement after entering the plane through a single point of entry and changing direction of needle **(Fig. 1C)**
- *Crosshatching*: First the material is injected in a linear thread at one edge of the area, subsequently along many lines 5–10 mm apart. The process is repeated perpendicularly to make a grid **(Fig. 1D)**
- *Depot:* Material is deposited in a bolus and then massaged gently to fill the gap **(Fig. 1E)**
- *Tower technique:* Material is deposited in multiple columns perpendicular to the tissue plane, gradually reducing the amount of product as the needle is withdrawn **(Fig. 1F)**.[2]

Most often, a combination of the above techniques is used depending upon the anatomy of the location and the expected outcome. With experience, every injector devises his/her favorite technique, while sticking to these basics.

Needle versus Cannula

Filler packs are accompanied with needles for injection. The bore and length depend upon the type of the filler, such that the product is extruded with minimal effort, yet keeping the bore size the least possible. Most often a 27–30 G, 0.5 inch needle is supplied. In order to minimize bruising and risk of intravascular spread, blunt-tipped metal cannulas with a side bore may be preferred **(Fig. 2)**. The cannula length and bore is chosen by the injector as per the injection technique and site. 25, 27, and 30 G cannulas of length 19 mm,

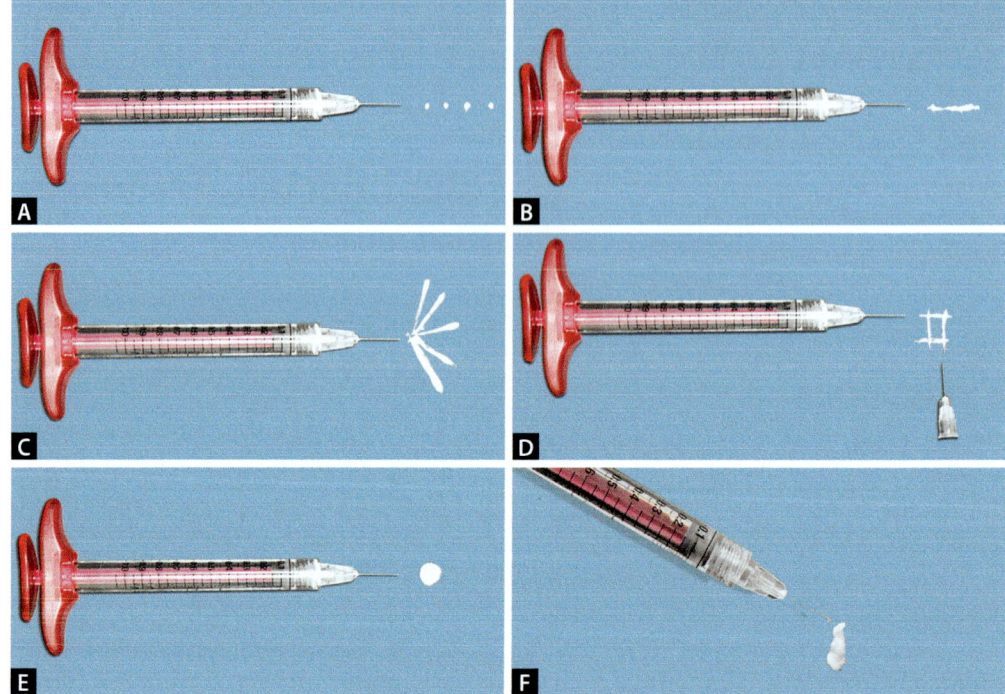

Figs. 1A to F: Basic filler injection techniques: (A) Serial puncture; (B) Linear threading; (C) Fanning; (D) Crosshatching; (E) Depot; (F) Tower technique.

25 mm, and 38 mm are chosen from. First a puncture with a larger bore needle is made and then the cannula is inserted through that puncture. This port of entry serves to inject a large area simply by moving the cannula in different directions and planes.[1]

There is lesser risk of intravascular product migration when cannula is used. There is also evidence that after placement of product with a needle, the material can migrate backward along the trajectory of the needle[3] and thus can get deposited superficially in multiple planes.[4]

It is important to point out that incidents of vascular compromise have been reported with use of cannula too. A recent consensus report therefore advises using cannulas of wider bore, i.e. 25 G or more to prevent such events.[5]

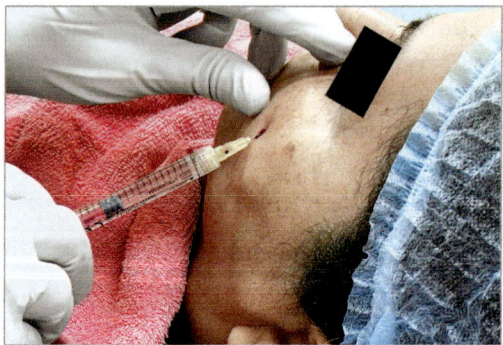

Fig. 2: Blunt tipped metal cannula being used for midface injection.

INJECTION TECHNIQUES FOR DIFFERENT SITES

Tear Trough

Bolus of 0.1–0.2 mL of material is placed supraperiosteally at 2–3 locations in tear trough. The product is then gently massaged medially. Linear threading may be done with caution to avoid the angular artery near the medial canthus.

Lip

Linear threading is done to accentuate the borders and lip roll, if it appears effaced. The tubercle should receive a bolus, but the area just lateral to it must be little less full. Vermillion enhancement is done by small boluses in the submucosal or intramuscular plane. The volume of the product being injected should be gradually tapered going laterally to give a natural appearance.

Nasolabial Fold

When just the nasolabial (NL) fold needs to be filled, such as in individuals in whom the inferomedial cheek is not overhanging, a fanning technique in deep dermis is used to correct the lower two-third of the fold. Subsequently, in the very apex of the fold, at the base of the nose, subcutaneous crosshatching or supraperiosteal bolus deposit may be done. In the presence of inferomedial cheek overhang, crosshatching for creating a scaffold is recommended. In most cases, cheek augmentation is done simultaneously.

Marionette Line

Linear threading in the crease (in mid-dermis for superficial and subcutaneous for deeper lines) and crosshatching across the area gives the best support and fill. Subcutaneous fanning lateral to the labiomental crease and support of the corner of the mouth with fanning and or bolus deposit is also recommended.

Prejowl Sulcus

The tower technique works well in the prejowl sulcus. Linear threading in subcutaneous plane along the inferior border of the mandible to fill the sulcus, crosshatching, fanning, and bolus are all performed with some success depending on the depth of the sulcus.

Nose

Linear threading with tiny amounts of product is recommended. On the tip, the plane of injection should be deep dermal, while on the dorsum, it can be deeper. The gel can then be molded gently to deposit it into position.

Cheek

Bolus injections at supraperiosteal location at the highest points of the malar eminence, and along the zygomatic arch serve to lift the cheek area. For submalar hollowing, fanning, or crosshatching the product subcutaneously works well.

Jawline

To accentuate the angle of the jaw, crosshatching with vertical alignment along the ramus, and horizontal alignment along the body is preferred. Tower technique or pillars of filler to reconstruct severe hollowness in this area is often preferred too.

Temples

Bolus deposits in deep supraperiosteal position, followed by massaging to evenly distribute the product are recommended.

Brow Lift

Linear threading in subcutaneous plane in the lateral brow improves volume loss here, lifting the brow.

Hands

Multiple small, subcutaneous blebs, carefully avoiding tendon sheaths, and vessels followed by massaging the product evenly are recommended.[6]

Glabella

This is an area prone to the danger of intravascular injection into supraorbital and supratrochlear vessels. Very superficial, intradermal linear threading is advised in the glabellar lines.

Forehead

Tiny boluses at the level of the bone followed by massage, ensuring that no bumpiness or bead remains the technique that works best for hollow areas of the forehead.

Acne Scars

Subcision and intradermal placement of filler successfully improve appearance of some types of acne scars.

USEFUL TIPS

- The correct injection technique determines the volume of product required and the degree of correction achieved.
- Intravascular injections and subsequent vaso-occlusive episodes can be minimized by correct injection techniques such as slow injection, minimal pressure, and correct plane of injection.
- Postinjection edema can be minimized by appropriate filler selection and controlled injection volume.
- Nodules can be prevented by avoiding intradermal injections of thicker fillers and using modest volumes.
- Although traditional teaching has been to aspirate before injecting, there may not always be a flashback of blood upon hitting a vessel, owing to high viscosity of the gel and small bore of the needle, implying that one cannot safely eliminate the possibility of intravascular placement of the needle even when no blood is seen in the hub upon aspiration.[7] Nevertheless, a cautious approach of aspiration and holding till a count of 10 to see for a flashback of blood is still recommended.
- Cannulas may be preferred for injection over needles as they are less likely to cause intra-arterial injections and minimize the risk of bruising.

REFERENCES

1. Alam M, Tung R. Injection technique in neurotoxins and fillers: Indications, products, and outcomes. J Am Acad Dermatol. 2018;79(3):423-35.
2. Bartus CL, Sattler G, Hanke CW. The tower technique: a novel technique for the injection of hyaluronic acid fillers. J Drugs Dermatol. 2011;10(11):1277-80.
3. van Loghem JAJ, Humzah D, Kerscher M. Cannula versus sharp needle for placement of soft tissue fillers: an observational cadaver study. Aesthet Surg. 2017;13;38(1):73-88.
4. Frank T, Erlbacher K, Erlbacher K, et al. Precision in Dermal Filling: a comparison between needle and cannula when using soft tissue fillers. J Drugs Dermatol. 2017;116(9):866-72.
5. Humzah MD, Ataullah S, Chiang C, et al. The treatment of hyaluronic acid aesthetic interventional induced visual loss (AIIVL): a consensus on practical guidance. J Cosmet Dermatol. 2019;18(1):71-6.
6. Bass LS. Injectable filler techniques for facial rejuvenation, volumization, and augmentation. Facial Plast Surg Clin North Am. 2015;23(4):479-88.
7. Carey W, Weinkle S. Retraction of the plunger on a syringe of hyaluronic acid before injection: are we safe? Dermatol Surg. 2015;41(Suppl 1):S340-6.

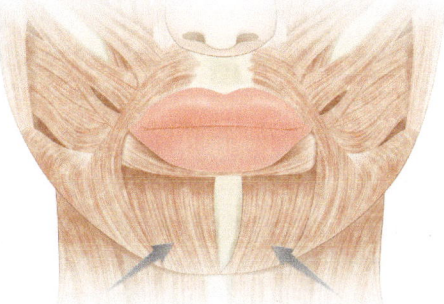

CHAPTER 10

Fillers for Upper Face—Forehead and Temporal Region

Vanravi Vachatimanont, Rungsima Wanitphakdeedecha

FOREHEAD AND TEMPORAL
Indications

Signs of aging on the upper face include wrinkles (horizontal forehead lines and glabellar lines), irregular surface, flattening of the forehead, and prominent eyebrows and/or brow ptosis. These are consequences of photodamage and also a natural aging process, reflecting as skin atrophy and elastosis, as well as loss of volume. Unlike dynamic wrinkles, static wrinkles cannot be diminished by using botulinum injection. The dynamic lines are emphasized and become more prominent due to the loss of volume as we age, thereby making filler the complementary choice of treatment to compensate these defects as shown on **Figure 1**. A smooth and convex forehead is highly desirable in many Asian women.

Anatomic Considerations
Forehead

The forehead is composed of five layers, skin (layer 1), superficial fat compartments (layer 2), superficial fascia of the frontalis and the frontalis muscle (layer 3), deep fat compartments (layer 4), galea aponeurosis, and periosteum (layer 5).[1] The skin and subcutaneous fat of the forehead are very thin layers.

The supratrochlear artery and supraorbital artery are the main blood supply of the forehead; together with their related veins and nerves they emerge through the supratrochlear foramen and supraorbital foramen, respectively. Furthermore, a cadaveric study has shown that the supratrochlear artery and supraorbital artery comprise of two main types of anatomical variation. Type I has superficial

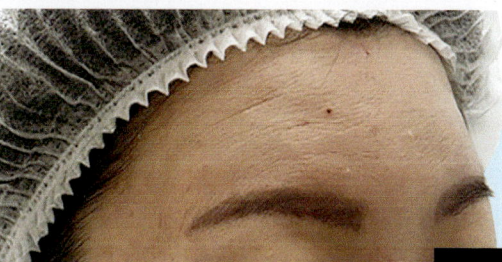

Fig. 1: A smooth and contoured forehead. An ideal youthful forehead for many Asian women is the smooth surface and convex forehead. Filler injection replaces the lost volume, and improves superficial rhytides, giving an optimal esthetic result when used in conjunction with botulinum toxin injection.

and deep branches for both the supratrochlear and supraorbital arteries. There is an absence of the deep branch of supratrochlear artery in type II. Furthermore, type I is subcategorized further to two subtypes. Type Ib consists of an additional arterial branch, either central artery (deriving from dorsal nasal artery) or the paracentral artery (deriving from angular artery)[2-4], whereas they are absent in type Ia.[1] Additional contributing blood supply is the frontal branch of the superficial temporal artery, which forms an anastomosis with the superficial branch of the supratrochlear artery and the deep branch of the supraorbital artery that penetrates the frontalis and emerges as the superficial branch.[1] In respect to the aforementioned, the deep branch of the supraorbital artery has been shown to emerge superficially to the subcuticular level approximately 20 mm above the orbital rim. This landmark is important as the injection sites on the forehead should be above this level on the supraperiosteal plane and lateral to the supraorbital foramen line.

The superficial temporal artery runs along the superficial temporal fascia and passes medially in front of tragus and bifurcates approximately 9.5 mm anterior to the posterior margin of the mandibular condyle, and 21.7 mm above the superior margin of the zygomatic arch, and approximately 53.2 mm posterior to the pterion.[5] Most importantly, the frontal branch runs across the temporal crest approximately 2 cm above the supraorbital margin.[6] As mentioned above, the frontal branch of superficial temporal artery eventually anastomoses with the supratrochlear and supraorbital arteries, which originate from the ophthalmic artery. Therefore, injection into this artery may also lead to blindness.

Temporal Area

The temporal area can be separated into two parts, upper and lower part. The upper temporal part consists of eight layers **(Table 1)**, starting from the most superficial layer, the skin, subcutaneous temporal fat, temporoparietal fascia or superficial temporal fascia. This layer encloses a very important structure, the superficial temporal artery, which crosses this plane and supplies the forehead. However,

Table 1: Fascial anatomy and related structures of the upper temporal region.	
Layers of temporal area	**Related important structures**
Skin	
Subcutaneous fat	
Superficial temporal fascia	Superficial temporal artery runs within this fascia
Loose areolar tissue layer	This is the desirable plane for filler placement
Deep temporal fascia (superficial and deep layer)	• Superficial layer fascia is the continuation of the galea aponeurosis from the forehead that further extends as a superficial musculoaponeurotic system. • There is a fatty tissue between the superficial and deep layer, where middle temporal vein runs horizontally approximately 2 cm in parallel above the zygomatic arch
Temporalis fascia (superficial part)	
Temporalis muscle (deep part)	
Temporal bone	Supraperiosteum is the desirable plane for filler placement

there is no important anatomic structure in between the superficial temporal fascia and the superficial layer of the deep temporal fascia, as it is only a loose areolar tissue layer. Thus, making this space a safe plane to place filler.

Furthermore, the deep temporal fascia composes of two layers, superficial and deep. It is important to note that the superficial layer of the deep temporal fascia is the continuation of the galea aponeurosis from the forehead that is further extending across as a superficial muscular aponeurotic system (SMAS). There is a fatty tissue between these layers, where middle temporal vein runs horizontally approximately 2 cm above in parallel to the zygomatic arch.

Subsequently, the temporalis muscle is enveloped tightly by the temporalis fascia, which is located beside the temporal bone. Temporalis muscle consists of two parts, the superficial and deep part. In addition, another plane that filler can be safely deposited is the supraperiosteum, just below the temporalis muscle.

Injection Techniques

Forehead

As the forehead is a highly vascularized area, the use of a cannula sized 22 G to 25 G is highly advised to avoid intravascular injection. Make an entry from the superior temporal septum, approximately 1 cm above the supraorbital margin and enter slightly medial to the septum. Subsequently, advance the cannula medially along the periosteum and inject minimally (0.1–0.2 cc on each side) in a fanning manner to avoid undulation.[7] A recommended choice of filler is the medium viscosity filler with high G. Try to avoid passing too medially beyond the supraorbital foramen to prevent penetration of the deep branch of supratrochlear artery.

Temporal Area

As aforementioned, the temporal area can be separated into two parts, upper and lower part. The upper part is shallower in depth, in comparison to the lower part of the temporal. As a result, the upper temporal part is the only safe area to use sharp needle technique with the needle length of 3 mm. Firstly, palpate along the superior temporal septum, 1 cm. above the orbital rim. Then place filler within 1 cm posterior to the orbital rim. Inject in perpendicular to the temporal bone and deep in contact with the periosteum. Minimally deposit approximately 0.3–0.5 mL per side.[8] It is recommended to use 27 G needle with high G' and hard viscosity filler.[7] Moreover, placing too large of a volume of filler at this layer may cause the filler to migrate inferiorly to the buccal region as the buccal fat pad is an extension of the deep temporal fat pad **(Table 2)**.

Alternatively, cannula technique can also be used for temporal augmentation. As mentioned earlier, the galea aponeurosis of the forehead runs continuously with the superficial layer of the deep temporal fascia, thereby inserting the cannula from the same entry as for forehead augmentation should allow the cannula to approach to the desired plane, in between the superficial temporal fascia and deep temporal fascia. Make an entry at 1 cm above the supraorbital margin, along the superior temporal septum, and enter slightly medial to the septum. Insert the cannula deep and glide along the periosteum, diverting the cannula laterally towards the temporal area. It may require a minimal force to go through the superior temporal fascia. Once the cannula is passed through, the cannula should be easy to maneuver along this plane. However, if there is a strong resistance

Table 2: Fascial anatomy and related structures of the lower temporal region.

Layers of temporal area	Related important structures
Skin	
Subcutaneous fat	
Superficial temporal fascia	
Superficial temporal fat pad	
Superficial layer of deep temporal fascia	
Deep temporal fat pad	
Deep layer of the deep temporal fascia	
Temporalis muscle	
Buccal fat pad	• Buccal fat pad is an extension from the deep temporal fat pad • Inappropriate placement or too large quantity of filler injected into this layer may result in the migration of filler down to the buccal area
Superficial layer of masseter	
Deep layer of masseter	
Periosteum	

while gliding through the plane, that means the cannula may be located on the wrong plane. It is recommended to use cannula sized 22 G to 25 G with medium viscosity filler,[7] and inject minimally (0.3–0.5 mL) in advancing and fanning manner to avoid undulation.

Postinjection Instructions

Forehead

Mold the filler as appropriate on the forehead to prevent an uneven surface. However, some palpable masses may occur during the first couple of days and usually, gradually smoothen out with time. Reassurance is all that is required.

Temporal

Mold the filler as appropriate on the temple to prevent an uneven surface. Some patients may have a slight headache or tension-headache after the injection. The patient may take some pain reliever such as paracetamol, though avoid using nonsteroidal anti-inflammatory drugs (NSAIDs). In the authors' experience, some may feel sensation of heaviness around the injected area.

Precautions

The forehead is a highly vascularized area, hence is a risky zone for filler injection. Good knowledge of the vascular anatomy is a must prior to injection to prevent vascular complications. It is advised to use blunt cannulas rather than sharp needles to decrease the chance of intravascular injection. Moreover, it is important to place the filler in the correct plane, down deep just above the periosteum as most of the blood vessels runs superficially or intramuscularly. Slow injection with minimal volume of injection is recommended. Aspiration prior to initiating the injection is a useful habit, though it does not guarantee nonvascular placement.[9]

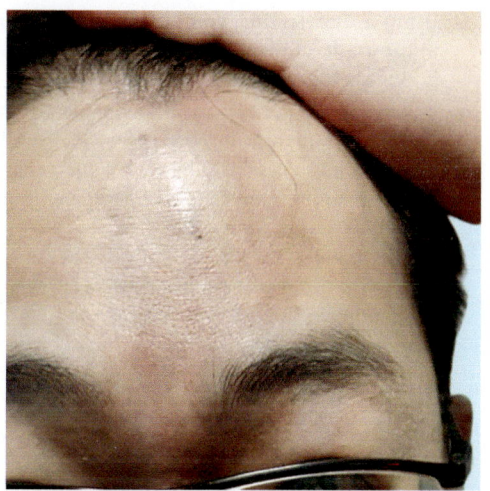

Fig. 2: Intravascular complication. Accidental filler injection into supratrochlear and supraorbital arteries, causing ischemia around the injected site and vision loss.

Accidental intravascular injection into supratrochlear and/or supraorbital arteries may lead to ischemia or infarction of the surrounding tissues as shown in **Figure 2**. Also, a retrograde flow of filler could embolize to the central retinal artery via the ophthalmic artery, leading to blindness of the effected eye. This event may occur in a matter of seconds.[9] Visual loss due to occlusion of the ophthalmic artery often presents with severe ocular pain. However, occlusion of the central retinal artery or the related branches may cause visual loss without any ocular pain.[10] Therefore, be cautious for any sign of blanching at the injection site and stop the injection immediately if the patient complains of any unusual pain.

The frontal branch of superficial temporal artery also anastomoses with the supratrochlear and supraorbital arteries thereby connecting to the ophthalmic artery system. Therefore, injection into this artery may also lead to blindness. To minimize any uneventful accident, it is recommended to inject slowly with low pressure, and place multiple small amounts of filler rather than a large bolus.[9,10] Aspiration prior to every injection is always useful. Furthermore, perpendicular injection is recommended if using a sharp needle to reduce risk of intravascular injection. However, a retrograde backflow of filler through the needle track was observed in a cadaveric study, despite careful perpendicular injection deep on to the supraperiosteum.[8] Thus, there is no absolutely safe technique and always be mindful for signs of intravascular complication.

USEFUL TIPS

- Forehead is a very risky area as it is highly vascularized. The importance of good knowledge of vascular anatomy cannot be overstated. Therefore, only cannulas should be used in this area.
- For temporal augmentation, avoid placing filler more than 0.5 mL per side as it may cause tension-headache.
- Either sharp needle or cannula technique can be used for temporal augmentation. Nevertheless, always be cautious for any signs of intravascular complication.
- The following techniques have been recommended to reduce the risk of intravascular accident.[9,10]
    - Choice of a cannula is preferred rather than using a sharp needle.
    - It is always helpful to aspirate every time before injection.
    - Injecting slowly with low pressure is essential.
    - Avoid injecting a large bolus in one area as it increases more risks of injection into the blood vessels. Instead, place multiple deposits of very small amount of filler.

- Beware of any signs of intravascular complications such as severe pain, blurred vision, or blanching on the skin.

REFERENCES

1. Cong LY, Phothong W, Lee SH, et al. Topographic analysis of the supratrochlear artery and the supraorbital artery: implication for improving the safety of forehead augmentation. Plast Reconstr Surg. 2017;139(3):620e-627e.
2. Faris C, van der Eerden P, Vuyk H. The midline central artery forehead flap: a valid alternative to supratrochlear-based forehead flaps. JAMA Facial Plast Surg. 2015;17(1):16-22.
3. Skaria AM. The median forehead flap reviewed: a histologic study on vascular anatomy. Eur Arch Otorhinolaryngol. 2015;272(5):1231-7.
4. Kleintjes WG. Forehead anatomy: arterial variations and venous link of the midline forehead flap. J Plast Reconstr Aesthet Surg. 2007;60(6):593-606.
5. Kim BS, Jun YJ, Chang CH, et al. The anatomy of the superficial temporal artery in adult koreans using 3-dimensional computed tomographic angiogram: clinical research. J Cerebrovasc Endovasc Neurosurg. 2013;15(3):145-51.
6. Kim HJ, Seo KK, Lee HK, et al. General anatomy of the face and neck. In: Kim HJ, Seo KK, Lee HK, Kim J (Eds). Clinical Anatomy of the Face for Filler and Botulinum Toxin injection. Seoul: Springer Nature; 2015. pp. 45-8.
7. Sundaram H, Liew S, Signorini M, et al. Global aesthetics consensus: hyaluronic acid fillers and botulinum toxin type A–recommendations for combined treatment and optimizing outcomes in diverse patient populations. Plast Reconstr Surg. 2016;137(5):1410-23.
8. van Loghem JAJ, Humzah D, Kerscher M. Cannula versus sharp needle for placement of soft tissue fillers: an observational cadaver study. Aesthet Surg J. 2017;38(1):73-88.
9. Loh KT, Chua JJ, Lee HM, et al. Prevention and management of vision loss relating to facial filler injections. Singapore Med J. 2016;57(8):438-43.
10. Park SW, Woo SJ, Park KH, et al. Iatrogenic retinal artery occlusion caused by cosmetic facial filler injections. Am J Ophthalmol. 2012;154(4):653-62.

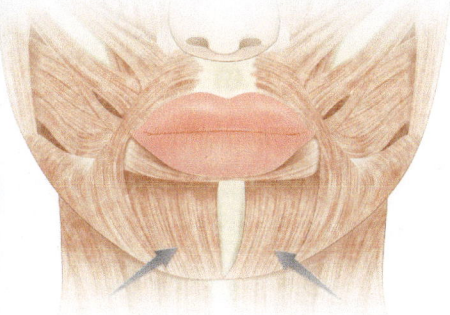

CHAPTER 11

Fillers for Upper Face—Temples

Gulhima Arora, Sandeep Arora

INTRODUCTION

Esthetic rejuvenation and reflation with fillers have enjoyed immense popularity owing to the advances in product development and techniques of administration with fewer complications. However, unlike other areas of face, the temple area has no set ideal esthetic standards.[1] This in part, provides flexibility to the injector to suit each face with its own unique shape. There are, of course, a few guidelines that an injector follows to restore the volume of the aged temple. Unlike the other areas of the face, the patient is usually unaware of the effect of temple rejuvenation on the overall improvement of the aging face.

ANATOMIC CONSIDERATIONS

According to the Consensus Meeting held at Korea,[2] one of the scales of beauty is a regular, oval-shaped face, which encompasses a full and smooth-contoured temple.

Temporal region in the young presents with upper face convexity and is responsible for the transition of the upper into the midface. It lies in the temporal fossa, which is one of the largest anatomical regions of the skull. This fossa is bordered by the superior temporal line superiorly and posteriorly, the zygomatic arch inferiorly and the frontal process of the zygomatic and the zygomatic process of the frontal bone anteriorly.

Temporal region surface anatomy on the other hand is well-delineated anteriorly (lateral orbital rim), anterosuperiorly by the superior temporal line palpated as the temporal crest and inferiorly (zygomatic arch), while the posterosuperior and posterior aspects are obscure as they are covered by the hair line. Floor is formed by the pterion—an area formed by the frontal, parietal, temporal, and the greater wing of the sphenoid.

Anatomical layers in this region an injector must keep in mind from outside to within are the skin, subcutaneous fat, temporoparietal fascia, loose areolar tissue, deep temporoparietal fascia, temporalis muscle, pericranium, and the bone. The superficial temporal fascia is the cephalic extension of the superficial musculoaponeurotic system (SMAS). The deep temporal fascia splits into two layers to enclose the superficial temporal fat pad. The deep temporal fascia is highly adherent to the muscle at younger age. The large fan-shaped temporal muscle is a muscle of mastication intertwined with the masseter below, deeply adherent to the temporal bone.

The vasculature of the temple is present in three planes **(Fig. 1)**. All are branches of the external carotid artery. The superficial temporal artery and vein are located in the superficial temporal fascia. The temporal branch of the facial nerve accompanies them. The middle temporal vessels are located

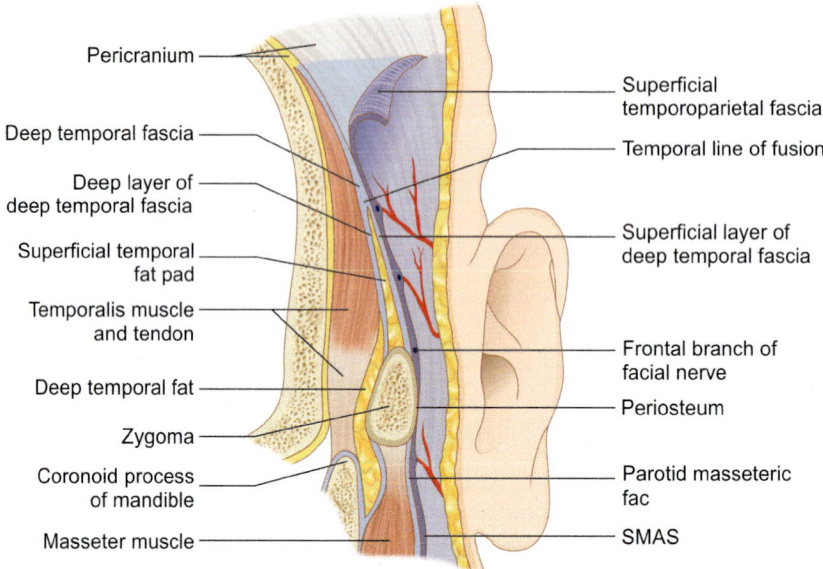

Fig. 1: Coronal section with anatomical relationship of layers with vessels in temporal region.
(SMAS: superficial musculoaponeurotic system)

along the deep temporal fascia, and the deep temporal vessels are located deep to the deep temporal fascia.

The middle temporal vein is a large vessel which drains into the jugular and has a potential for emboli if injected directly into it.[3] A number of perforators traverse this region with the highest density reported at the junction of zygomatic arch with the lateral orbital rim and 18–32 mm superior to the anterior half of the zygomatic arch **(Fig. 2)**.[4] The injectors must also be alert to the variations in course of temporal artery and its branches in this region.[5]

Retaining ligaments of this region are the superior temporal septum, inferior temporal septum, orbicularis retaining ligament, and zygomatic cutaneous ligament. The inferior temporal septum divides the subcutaneous fat layer into the lateral temporal fat compartment and the lateral orbit fat compartment, and the areolar tissue into the upper and lower temporal compartments.[4,6]

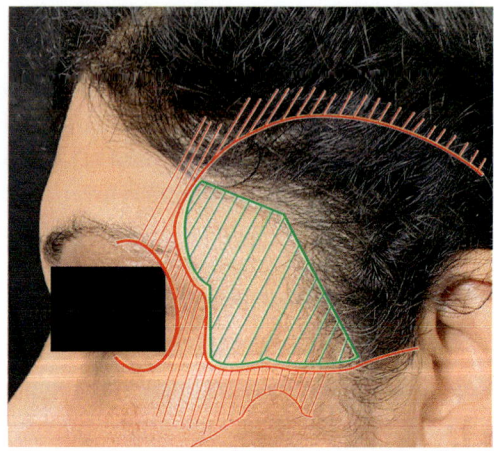

Fig. 2: The upper and lower temporal compartment and the dangerous area of perforators.

Temporal muscle atrophy with aging along with bone resorption, atrophy and thinning of the subcutaneous fat results in temple hollowing and at the same time opens up a potential space for "filler" augmentation.[7]

Due to these changes, the temples look hollow, the eyebrow tail drops down, and

Table 1: Stages of temporal aging.[9]	
Stage	Features
Stage 1	Temporal fossa shows no volume changes and is linear or convex
Stage 2	First aging signs can be perceived, with a slight depression
Stage 3	Temporal fossa concavity is evidenced, with some vessels becoming visible and the eyebrows drooping
Stage 4	Major "skeletonizing" and concavity of the temporal fossa are observed, making bones, veins and arteries clearly visible

the fullness goes away. The tail is no longer visible from the front view. Veins become more prominent due to dermal thinning. The orbital ridge and the temporal crest also become more visible. The hairline recedes or may even become sparse with age.[1,8]

Raspaldo[9] rated the temporal aging in four stages **(Table 1)**.

INJECTION TECHNIQUES

Injections to the temple can be made in three, relatively avascular planes. A superficial subcutaneous plane, one slightly deeper in the loose areolar tissue, and a deep, submuscular supraperiosteal plane.[10,11]

The superficial potential space formed by the loose areolar tissue and the deeper periosteal region has their own cautionary points. The deeper injection plane has the deep temporal arteries while the superficial space has the frontal branch of the superficial temporal artery and vein along the temporal branch of the facial nerve. These superficial vessels may become prominent initially till the filler settles and integrates with the surrounding tissue.[7] More superficial injections can cause contour irregularities, which need to be massaged over days to iron out.[12]

A filler with high cohesivity and high G' should be used when giving a supraperiosteal

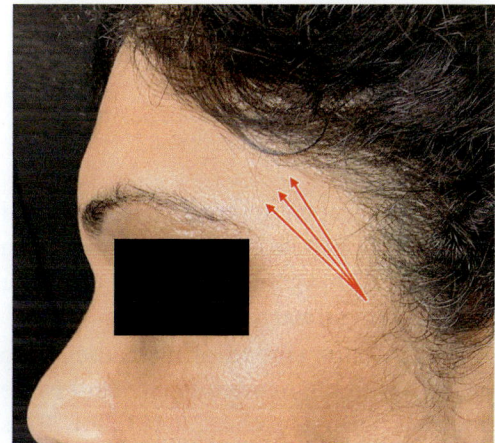

Fig. 3: Cannula approach for filling the temple region.

bolus injection. Lower viscosity, lower G' fillers should be used if injecting subcutaneously.

Both bolus or fan techniques can be used to fill the temples. Use of cannula or needle is the injectors' choice. The authors' recommendation is to use a needle while giving supraperiosteal bolus injections, and to use a cannula when injecting in a more superficial plane, using the fan technique **(Fig. 3)**. By far, the safest injection point in this high-risk area, is the "swift point".[13] This is a point 1 cm above and 1 cm lateral to the tail of the eyebrow **(Fig. 4)**. It is considered to be a very safe point, high up in the temporal fossa, as it is relatively avascular and with the muscle fibers being very thin here.[12] The second

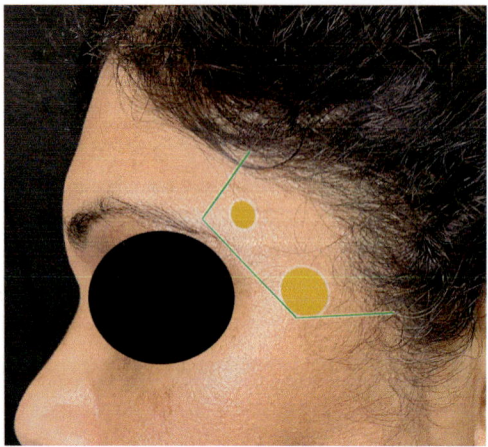

Fig. 4: Supraperiosteal bolus points for temple filler injection.

supraperiosteal bolus point is determined at the center of a circle 2 cm in diameter drawn superior to the zygomatic arch and posterior to the lateral orbital rim **(Fig. 4)**.

Blocking the spread of filler above the hairline with the nondominant hand while injecting is a good technique to follow. This makes the injection more economical.

Visualizing or palpating the superficial temporal vessels and even marking them before injecting, is a good practice to follow. The Valsalva maneuver can be used to make them more prominent.

Aspiration before injecting is a must for injections to the temple. The patient is asked to open the mouth to loosen the temporalis muscle just before injecting the bolus, to make the injection more comfortable. Slow injections are recommended.[1] Typically, depending on the grade of hollowness, 0.5–1 mL, sometimes even more, of filler may be required for each side.

Piercing the layers containing vessels, ensure the filler is placed deep to the vessels. Inadvertent piercing the vessels does not create delayed bruising if pressure is maintained for a minute or two after injection.[12] Massaging the area after injecting gives a smooth contour. A more superficial injection in the loose areolar tissue between the superficial and deep temporal fascia is made using a cannula of 25 or 27 G calibre.[12] An entry point can be made either above or below the area to be filled. Filling should be slow, perpendicular to the vessels. Pressure after the injection is recommended. With caution, a cannula may also be used to deposit filler deeper to the subcutaneous plane over the muscle.

PRECAUTIONS

Iatrogenic blindness is the most serious possible complication owing to the rich vascularity of this region. It is proposed the retrograde flow into the central retinal artery leads to its occlusion and subsequent blindness. However, it is also proposed that with enough force, microdroplet spread may infiltrate the smaller vessels and subsequently have the same devastating effect.[14]

Palatal necrosis is a possibility[12] if injections are given in the lower or posterior fossa of the temple near the zygomatic arch, and there is a compromise of the internal maxillary artery.

Supraperiosteal technique using a perpendicular injection approach using either a cannula or needle may also result in intracranial penetration of the filler material, if excessive force is used, as the cranial bone is thinnest in the temple region.[15]

POSTINJECTION INSTRUCTIONS

Moderate pain and edema, especially on jaw movements are expected sequelae and settle within 48–72 hours. In the cases, requiring post-treatment analgesia acetaminophen is the drug of choice. Ask the patient to avoid steam, sauna, and facial massage for the first 7 days after treatment. Heavy exercise should be avoided for at least 3 days.

USEFUL TIPS

- The temple area is an often neglected region for filler injection. Injected skillfully, it can make a remarkable difference to an aging face.
- The safest plane of injection is on the bone, and this is easiest done with a needle.
- Just a few points of injection can fill the entire temporal hollow as the zygomatic ligament prevents further downward migration of the filler.
- The "swift point" is the easiest landmark to remember for novice injectors—it is a 1 cm above and lateral to the tail of the eyebrow.
- The superficial temporal vessels may look more prominent after temple filler injections—this settles with time.

REFERENCES

1. Rihani J. Aesthetics and rejuvenation of the temple. Facial Plast Surg. 2018;34(2):159-63.
2. Sundaram H, Liew S, Signorini M, et al. Global aesthetics consensus: hyaluronic acid fillers and botulinum toxin type A—Recommendations for combined treatment and optimizing outcomes in diverse patient populations. Plast Reconstr Surg. 2016;137:1410-23.
3. Sieber DA, Scheuer JF, Villanueva NL, et al. Review of 3-dimensional Facial Anatomy: Injecting Fillers and Neuromodulators. Plast Reconstr Surg. 2016;4:e1166.
4. Huang RL, Xie Y, Wang W, et al. Anatomical Study of temporal fat compartments and its clinical application for temporal fat grafting. Aesthet Surg J. 2017;37:855-62.
5. Imran FH, Yong CK, Das S, et al. Anatomical variants of the superficial temporal artery in patients with microtia: a pilot descriptive study. Anat Cell Biol. 2016;49:273-80.
6. Fitzgerald R, Carqueville J, Yang PT. An approach to structural facial rejuvenation with fillers in women. Int J Womens Dermatol. 2019;5:52-67.
7. Hotta TA. Understanding the anatomy of the upper face when providing aesthetic injection treatments. Plast Surg Nurs. 2016;36:104-9.
8. Ross JJ, Malhotra R. Orbitofacial rejuvenation of temple hollowing with perlane injectable filler. Aesthet Surg J. 2010;30:428-33.
9. Raspaldo H. Temporal rejuvenation with fillers: Global faceculture approach. Dermatol Surg. 2012;38:261-5.
10. Suwanchinda A, Webb KL, Rudolph C, et al. The posterior temporal supra SMAS minimally invasive lifting technique using soft-tissue fillers. J Cosmet Dermatol. 2018;17:617-24.
11. Almeida AR, Sampaio GÂ de A, Queiroz NPL (2017). Hyaluronic acid in the rejuvenation of the upper third of the face: review and update. Part 2: temporal and supraorbital regions. Surg Cosmet Dermatol. [online] Available from: http://www.gnresearch.org/doi/10.5935/scd1984-8773.20179201 [Last accessed on December, 2019].
12. de Maio M, Swift A, Signorini M, et al. Facial Assessment and injection guide for botulinum toxin and injectable hyaluronic acid fillers: Focus on the upper face. Plast Reconstr Surg. 2017;140:265e-76e.
13. Carruthers J, Humphrey S, Beleznay K, et al. Suggested Injection Zone for Soft Tissue Fillers in the Temple? Dermatol Surg. 2017;43:756-7.
14. Li X, Du L, Lu J. A Novel Hypothesis of Visual Loss Secondary to Cosmetic Facial Filler Injection: Ann Plast Surg. 2015;75:258-60.
15. Philipp-Dormston WG, Bieler L, Hessenberger M, et al. Intracranial penetration during temporal soft tissue filler injection—Is it possible?. Dermatol Surg. 2017;84-91.

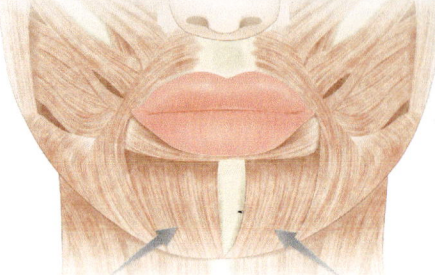

CHAPTER 12

Fillers for Upper Face—Eyebrow

MK Shetty

INDICATIONS

Fillers in the region of the brow have the ability to enhance or restore lost volume and curvature creating a more youthful and rejuvenated look. However, it is best left in the hands of advanced injectors, blurred as that line might be. It is pertinent to reiterate the importance of sound anatomical knowledge, understanding the plane of injection, the choice of product, and its delivery. Given the virtues and robustness of hyaluronic acid (HA), the author recommends its almost exclusive use in a facial filler practice and in the current context for the brows.

RELEVANT ANATOMY[1]

The characteristics of the ideal brow differ between the sexes. The female brow is located above the supraorbital margin arching gracefully, with its peak in line with the lateral limbus of the iris. The tail of the brow is positioned slightly higher than its medial end. The male brow in contrast is positioned more horizontally at the supraorbital margin with minimal arching and less anterior projection.

Structurally from superficial to deep, brow tissue comprises of the epidermis, dermis, subcutaneous fat, superficial fascia and muscle, loose areolar tissue and submuscular fat, periosteum, and bone. The vascular network is driven by the supratrochlear and supraorbital arteries, which are terminal branches of the ophthalmic artery arising from the internal carotid artery.

And while the hair appendage in the brow is sacrosanct and perhaps its crowning glory, aging changes lead to a loss in skin elasticity, bone resorption, and fat depletion. There is a resultant supraorbital hollowing, reduction in brow volume, deflation, and descent.

INJECTION TECHNIQUES[3,4]

When planning enhancement or correction, brow structure should be assessed in three dimensions. Appropriate projection of the brow with some elevation would be the desired end points. The role of neuromodulators in brow shaping is beyond the scope of this chapter. In a large majority, it is the tail of the brow that needs correction.[2] While a lateral brow injection may be facilitated through a needle, medial brow filler placement is best delivered via a cannula. Before injection, the orbital rim must be identified to prevent inadvertent placement of product in the orbital cavity. The technique here involves placing HA gel supraperiosteally in the retro-orbicularis oculi fat (ROOF) **(Fig. 1)** using small aliquots although subcutaneous fat may be the site of injection with a low viscous product. Mid and

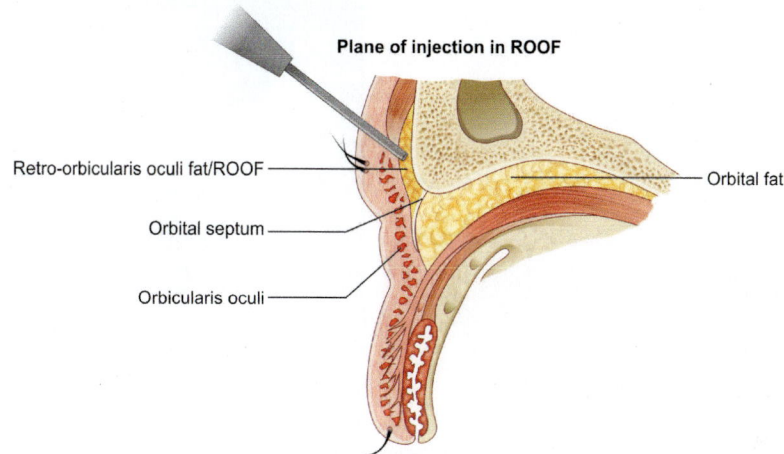

Fig. 1: Diagram demonstrating the anatomical plane of injection—the hyaluronic acid gel filler is injected into the ROOF plane in order to augment the contour of the eyebrow fat pad.
(*Source*: Mustak H, Fiaschetti D, Gupta A, et al. Eyebrow Contouring with Hyaluronic Acid Gel Filler Injections. The Journal of Clinical and Aesthetic Dermatology.2018, 11(2):38-40)

medial brow injections through a cannula are placed similarly.

A stiff 22 G cannula is the preferred choice as 25 G and above could behave as needles allowing for accidental intravascular placement. The injection technique should be measured, slow, and precise. A lateral bolus with a needle should always be preceded by aspiration to observe for a flashback **(Figs. 2 and 3)**. Multiple punctures run the risk of bruising. An anterograde placement may be adopted. Less is more in this region and lateral injections in the tail, the site of the most common brow correction, consumes no more than 0.1–0.2 mL of filler. The amount rarely exceeds 0.3–0.4 mL for the whole length of the brow on each side. Excessive placement could lead to an over prominent brow with potential lid swelling.

PRECAUTIONS[3,4]

Palpate for the orbital rim to avoid inadvertent placement of filler in the orbital cavity. One can use a needle or cannula for the tail of the brow but always use a cannula for the mid and medial brow. Inject smoothly and slowly, and always aspirate before doing so. Watch for pain or blanching. The plane of injection should be supraperiosteal in the retro orbicularis oculi fat. If a less viscous gel is used, it may be placed subcutaneously. Limit the amount of product injected to prevent an unesthetic outcome. There has been eyelid edema reported with repeated injection of the brow region.

USEFUL TIPS[3,4]

- The area around the eye represents a vascular danger zone and the injector must be very well versed with the anatomy of the area before injecting.
- Always keep in mind the differences between male and female brow shape while injecting.
- Before injection, the orbital rim must be identified to prevent inadvertent placement of product in the orbital cavity.
- Cannulas are preferred as much as possible.

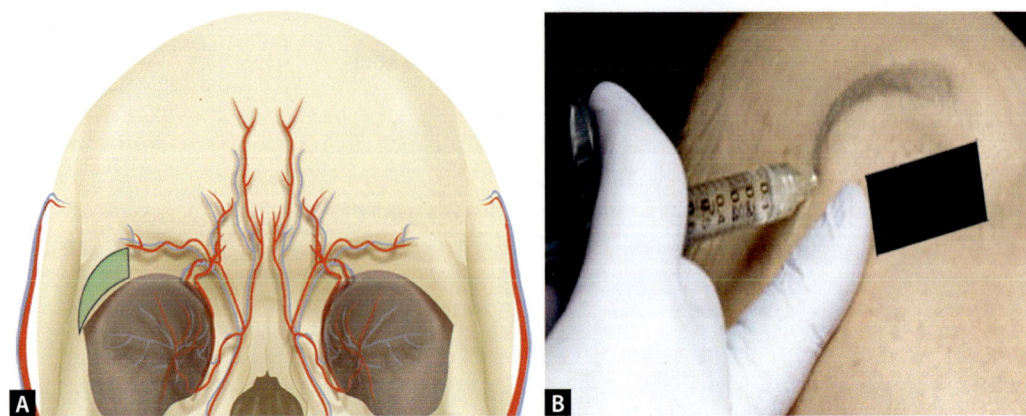

Figs. 2A and B: Eyebrow shaping using a hyaluronic acid filler (e.g. Juvéderm Ultra plus or Volift). Each filler is delivered by means of injections at two sites (A). Aspiration is mandatory before each injection, and a finger should be placed to avoid migration of the filler into the upper eyelid (B).

(*Source*: de Maio M, Swift A, Signorini M, Fagien S. Facial assessment and injection guide for botulinum toxin and injectable hyaluronic acid fillers: focus on the upper face. Plast Reconstr Surg. 2017;140(2):265e-76e)

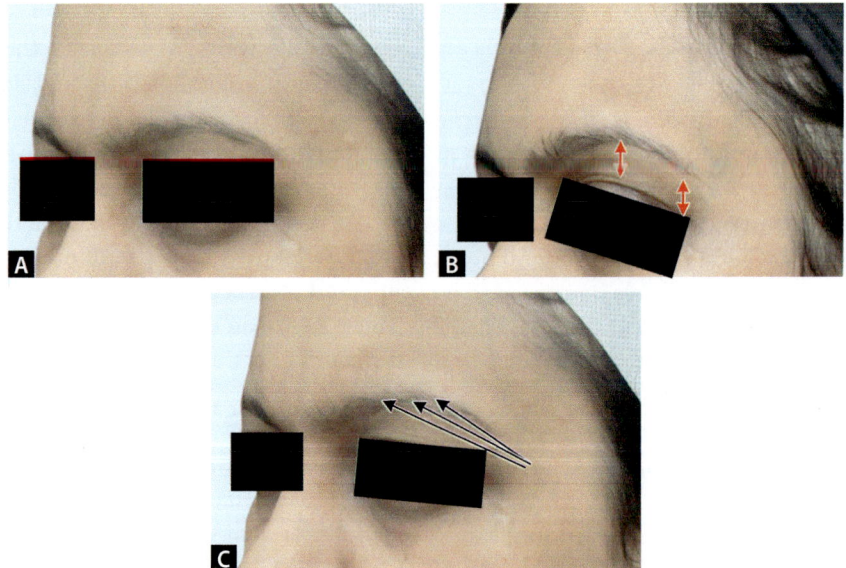

Figs. 3A to C: 0.1 mL hyaluronic acid filler injected via a cannula using a linear retrograde technique.

(*Courtesy*: Dr Chytra V Anand)

- The plane of injection is supraperiosteal in the ROOF.
- The eyebrows which play the role of a lighthouse keeper in the upper third often skip the attention of the mid-level injector but enthuse an experienced one, whose hands could make a subtle, yet telling difference to the esthetics of the face.

REFERENCES

1. Woodward J. Review of periorbital and upper face: pertinent anatomy, aging, injection techniques, prevention, and management of complications of facial fillers. J Drugs Dermatol. 2016;15(12):1524-31.
2. Van Loghem JAJ. Use of calcium hydroxylapatite in the upper third of the face: Retrospective analysis of techniques, dilutions and adverse events. J Cosmetic Dermatol. 2018;17(6):1025-30.
3. Mustak H, Fiaschetti D, Gupta A, et al. Eyebrow Contouring with Hyaluronic Acid Gel Filler Injections. The Journal of Clinical and Aesthetic Dermatology. 2018;11(2):38-40.
4. Sundaram H, Kiripolsky M. Nonsurgical rejuvenation of the upper eyelid and brow. Clin Plast Surg. 2013;40(1):55-76.

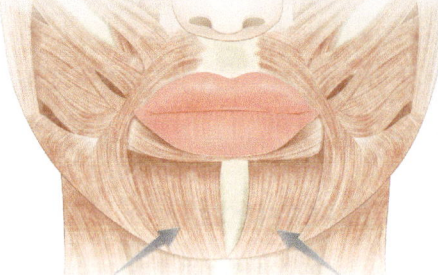

CHAPTER 13

Fillers for Upper Face—Upper Eyelid

Indu Ballani

INTRODUCTION

The eyes are the first part of the face to show visible signs of aging. Shifting of fat pad from the tear trough leads to a hollow or puffy look which can be corrected with fillers. The upper eyelid is also an integral part of the eye unit and without treating this part a fully rejuvenated look cannot be achieved. Usually, the eyebrow can be lifted with botulinum toxin; thus, rejuvenating it at a younger age but with age, there is loss of volume in the upper eyelid fat (mainly the retroseptal fat) which leads to laxity and wrinkles or skinfolds. In the past, upper eyelid rejuvenation was a surgical process but now fillers are being increasingly used to treat the upper eyelid, even after surgery if a hollow look is created due to removal of fat pads and extra skin.

ANATOMY

Classification

Assessment of eyebrow unit (independent of eyebrow hair) must be done. Three-dimensional shape is to be observed and identification of volume loss is important to get good results by filling. Hollow look mainly on medial side or lateral flattening of the eyebrow with age maybe observed. Romeo et al. has given a classification based on pretarsal skin show. An ideal pretarsal skin m should be

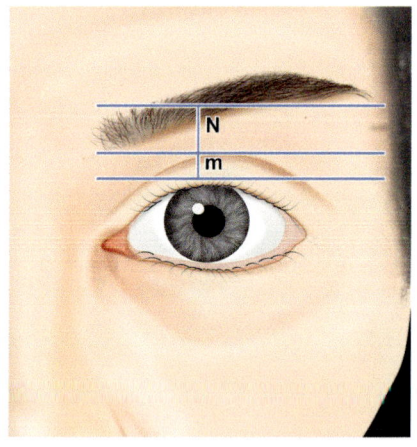

Fig. 1: Ratio of pretarsal to preseptal skin.

2 mm < m < 7 mm (**Fig. 1**) and it is half of the orbital portion of lid n (preseptal skin) both m and n are defined along the mid pupillary line. Ratio between m and n should be 1:2 with an optimal value of m being 3–4 mm. With age, this ratio changes and may reverse. Any rejuvenation procedure on the eye should aim at restoring the correct ratio between m and n. Hollow eye with skin fold or dermatochalasis is not an indication for eyebrow filling.

The bony orbit holds the orbital globe surrounded by intraocular muscles, surrounding this is the orbital fat held by orbital septum. The orbital fat is divided into two compartments central and nasal. The retro orbicularis oculi fat (ROOF) pad is centrally located in the supraorbital area and this

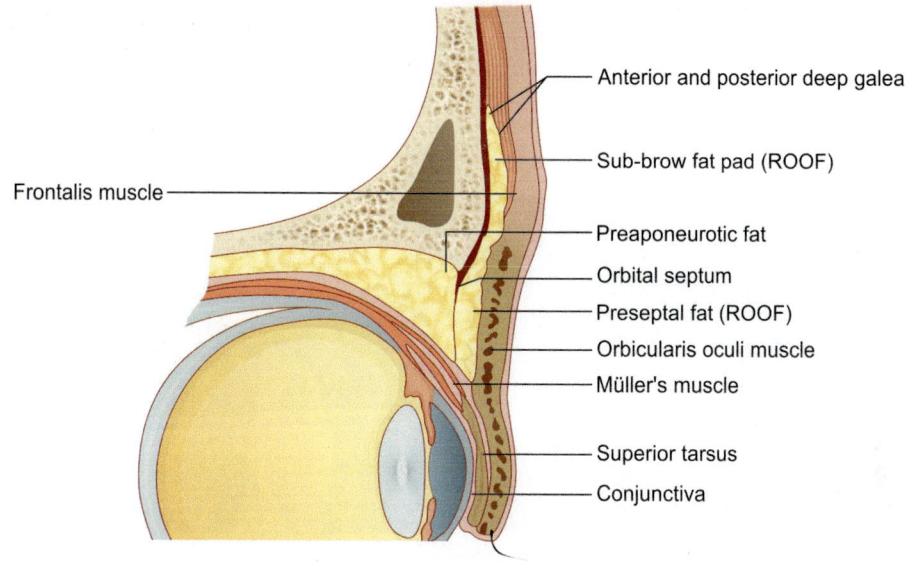

Fig. 2: Anatomy.[1]
(ROOF: retro orbicularis oculi fat)

is the fat pad which requires the filling **(Fig. 2)**. If we look at tissue planes under the brow from superficial to deep are the epidermis, dermis, superficial fascia, subcutaneous fat and muscle, subgaleal loose areolar tissue and periosteum and bone. The eyelid has a thickened sheet of connective tissue which extends to bony orbit and is known as arcus marginalis where it inserts into orbital rim. Fat at the roof of the orbit lies below the arcus.[2]

INJECTION TECHNIQUES

Injecting the temples automatically lifts the lateral side of our eyebrow; hence, in most cases it is combined with injection of eyebrows.

Fillers preferred for injection of eyebrow are the low viscosity fillers like Juvéderm ultra or restylane.

MD Codes for Injection

Recently, MD codes have been created by Dr Mauricio de Maio for injections on different regions of face. These specify location of

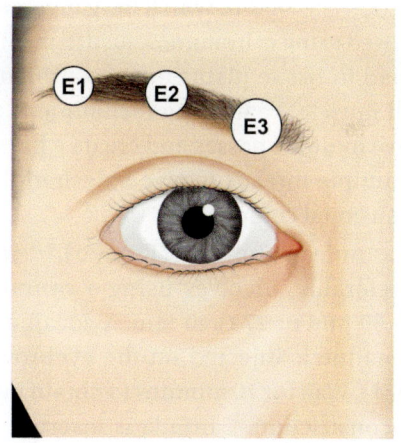

Fig. 3: MD codes for injecting eyebrow.

point to be injected for specific filling. For the eyebrows, these points are labeled as E1, E2 and E3 **(Fig. 3 and Table 1)**.

Injections E1, E2, and E3 are given deep into the fat pad, though not reaching the periosteum because of presence of supraorbital and supratrochlear vessels at E2 and E3; preferred quantity is 0.1 mL at each point.

Section 1: Dermal Fillers

Table 1: MD codes for injection of eyebrows.

E1	Eyebrow tail	Can be injected with needle or cannula
E2	Eyebrow center	Preferably done with cannula
E3	Eyebrow head	Preferably done with cannula

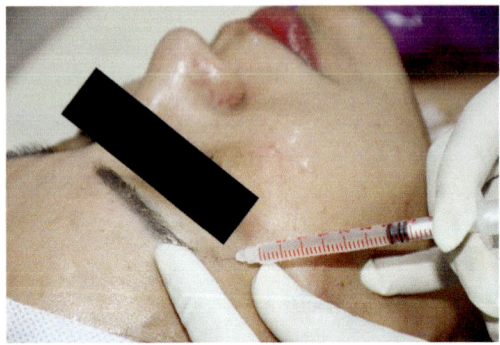

Fig. 4: Injection of xylocaine at the tail.

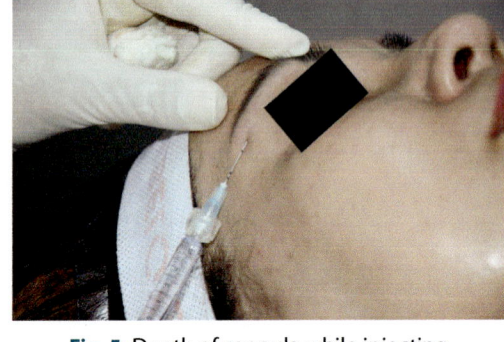

Fig. 5: Depth of cannula while injecting.

Hamzah Mustak et al.[3] have described an injection method in which 30-gauge needle was used to inject hyaluronic acid in the ROOF fat pad in tissue plains deep to orbicularis oculi muscle. Feathering technique is used to give multiple passes and create a haystack of multiple threads to give a desired three-dimensional contour.

Cannula technique (Romeo),[4,5] which is preferable, involves using a cannula of 25 G 50 mm or 27 G 40 mm. Xylocaine with adrenaline is injected on the eyebrow tail **(Fig. 4)**. Wait for 10 minutes to obtain proper vasoconstriction. Cannula is inserted after making a needle puncture at the tail. It is maneuvered through the muscle tissue and fascia to enter the correct plane (ROOF) till it reaches the lateral compartment of nasal fat pad. Cannula is deep and it is not normally visible but becomes visible only on tilting it **(Fig. 5)**. Boluses are deposited on all three points (E1, E2, E3) or else a linear thread is deposited all along in the deep plane. Over correction should be avoided and about 0.35–0.5 mL is the maximum amount of HA filler deposited on each side.[6]

PRECAUTIONS

Bruising may occur, especially if procedure has been performed with a needle. Icing before and after the procedure reduces this risk. Injection site inflammation including erythema, swelling, pain, and tenderness can occur. These resolve in 3–4 days. Lumpiness at the injection site can also be felt at times. This again resolves in 3–4 days.

Intravascular injection is most dreaded complication in this area. This is possibly more commonly with needle especially on medial side, due to the location of supratrochlear and supraorbital vessels on the bone, where they emerge from their respective foramen **(Fig. 6)**. Injecting very small boluses and aspiration may avoid this complication. Vision threatening complications due to emboli reaching the central retinal artery have been reported but are rare.

Chapter 13: Fillers for Upper Face—Upper Eyelid

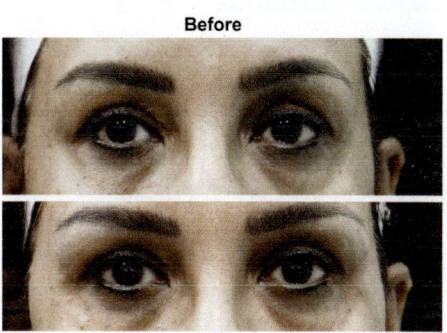

Fig. 7: Results.

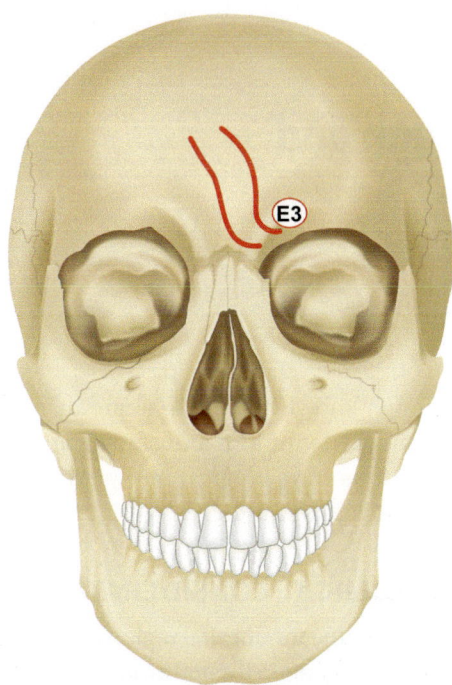

Fig. 6: Location of supratrochlear and supraorbital vessels.

- A wrong choice of filler viscosity can make the eyebrow appear too projected or thick.[7]
- Cannula injection is better than needle in this area.
- The retro orbital fat has to be filled for giving optimal results.
- Never overfill the eyebrow as too much projection would not give an esthetically pleasing result.[7]

POSTINJECTION INSTRUCTIONS

Patient should be counseled about swelling which subsides in 3–4 days. Lumps can be massaged. Icing the area is advised in case of swelling or bruising. Exercises should be avoided for 48 hours. Steam, sauna, and facials are avoided for 7 days. Painkillers and anti-inflammatory may be given in some cases. Patient should be instructed to report immediately for any bleeding, visual blurring or headache.

Results usually last for more than a year in this area **(Fig. 7)**.

USEFUL TIPS

- Proper assessment is the key—if there is dermatochalasis, injecting the eyelid can make it appear heavier than before.

REFERENCES

1. Finn JC, Cox S. Fillers in the periorbital complex. Facial Plast Surg Clin North Am. 2007;15(1): 123-32.
2. Buckingham ED, Bader B, Smith SP. Autologous fat and fillers in periocular rejuvenation. Facial Plast Surg Clin North Am. 2010;18(3): 385-98.
3. Mustak H, Fiaschetti D, Gupta A, et al. Eyebrow contouring with hyaluronic acid gel filler injections. J Clin Aesthetic Dermat. 2018;11(2): 38-40.
4. Sundaram H, Kiripolsky M. Nonsurgical rejuvenation of the upper eyelid and brow. Clin Plast Surgery. 2013;40(1):55-76.
5. Romeo F. Upper eyelid filling with or without surgical treatment. Aesth Plast Surg. 2016.
6. Romeo F. Upper Eyelid Filling Approach [U.E.F.A.] Technique: State of the Art after 500 Consecutive Patients. Aesth Plast Surg. 2019.
7. Lambros V. Volumizing the brow with hyaluronic acid fillers. Aesthet Surg J. 2009;29(3):174-9.

CHAPTER 14

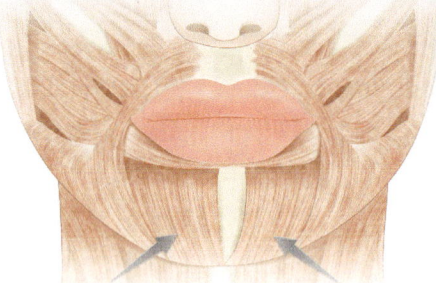

Fillers for Midface—Tear Trough and Infraorbital Areas

Rajat Kandhari, Deepak Jhakar

INDICATIONS

The esthetic of the periorbital region plays an important role in the perception of general facial attractiveness and there appears to be certain common trends or anthropometric differences between average and attractive eyes according to racial background.[1] The periorbital region is one of the first to demonstrate the effects of aging, possibly due to significant recession in the periorbital skeleton reducing soft tissue support around the eyes. Further, loss of volume, skin laxity, attenuated ligaments, and loss of muscle tone in this area result in the formation of "grooves" and/or "hollows" imparting a "sad", "tired", or "fatigued" look in the individual. The infraorbital region of the face including the tear trough is a distinct area of the face owing to its typical anatomical considerations. Correction of tear trough deformity (TTD) is a commonly asked for indication in daily clinical practice although it is also an indication which has a steep learning curve and requires experience for the injecting physician. Soft tissue fillers appear to be the most commonly used modality for the correction of grooves and hollows in this region. The type of filler, amount to be injected, injection method, and depth of injection should be appropriately selected in order to achieve optimal results. This goal can be easily achieved by having a thorough knowledge of the anatomy of this region; and definitions and classifications of the various physiological and pathological alterations in this area.

ANATOMICAL CONSIDERATIONS

A groove in the infraorbital region (GIR) refers to a fine indentation located around the orbital rim at the lid-cheek junction, and has several names, including nasojugal groove (or fold), TTD, and/or the palpebromalar groove.[2] On the other hand, hollowness in the infraorbital region (HIR) refers to a relatively broad depression in the infraorbital area, including the medial and central cheek region, and an area of the orbital rim. It can occur with or without GIR **(Fig. 1)**.[2]

The TTD is defined as the indentation of the medial third of the orbital rim from the medial canthal area to the mid-pupillary line.[3] The groove at the lateral lid-cheek junction based on the mid-pupillary line is called as the palpebromalar groove.[3] The tear trough ligament (TTL) is a true osteocutaneous ligament arising from the maxilla and inserting into the skin, along the location of tear trough **(Fig. 2)**.[4]

The TTL exists in the medial suborbital region between the palpebral parts and the orbital parts of the orbicularis oculi muscle

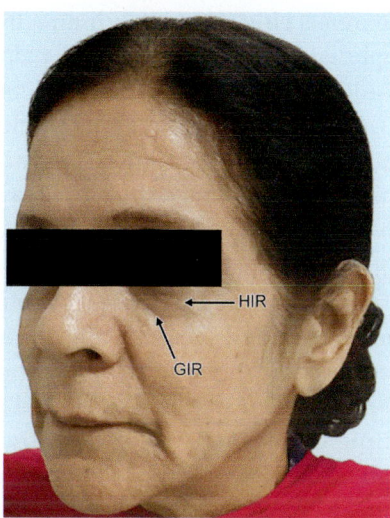

Fig. 1: The arrows demonstrate a groove in the infraorbital region (GIR) and hollowness in the infraorbital region (HIR).

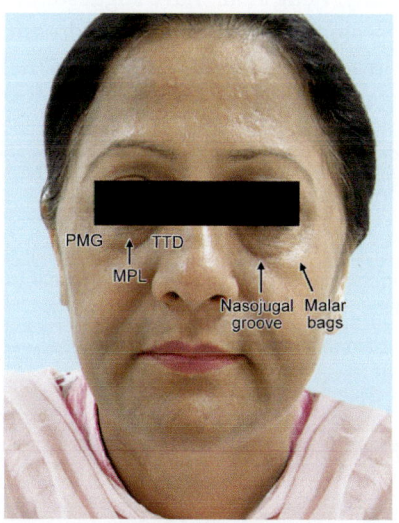

Fig. 2: Demonstration of the nasojugal groove, malar bags. The tear trough deformity continues laterally as the palpeabromalar groove.

(TTD: tear trough deformity; PMG: palpeabromalar groove; MPL: mid-pupillary line)

(OOM), originating from the level of the insertion of the medial canthal tendon to the mid-pupillary line. The TTL becomes continuous as the bilayered orbicularis retaining ligament (ORL) laterally. The ORL of the lateral orbital rim plays a significant role in the formation of the groove in the lateral portion of the lid-cheek junction. The ORL arises from the lateral orbital thickening and ends lateral to the mid-pupillary line at the junction between the palpebral and orbital part of the OOM.[3] The ligamentous attachment formed medially by the TTL continuing laterally as the ORL manifests as a cutaneous groove on the skin essentially due to the tethering effect of the ligamentous system and is referred to as the "prominent lid-cheek junction".

The nasojugal groove in its medial aspect includes the tear trough and typically refers to a drooping of the area extending from the medial canthus to the anterior zygomatic region. The OOM separates the malar fat pad in the anterior zygomatic region into superficial malar fat pad and a deeper fat compartment below the orbicularis oculi referred to as the suborbicularis oculi fat (SOOF), which undergoes drooping and resorption with aging.[5]

Many anatomical theories[2-6] have tried to explain the causes of GIR and HIR—(1) herniation of the intraorbital fat, (2) attachment of the orbital septum to the inferior orbital rim, (3) the prominence of the orbital rim, (4) atrophy of the skin and subcutaneous fat, including the bone in the suborbital area, (5) the presence of the ORL and TTL, (6) the gap between the OOM and levator labii superioris alaeque nasi (LLSAN) muscles, and (7) surface puckering caused by contraction of the OOM. The periorbital fat pads and SOOF are important structural considerations in this region as they can result in herniation and out-pouching leading to groove and hollow formation.

In addition to the muscle, ligament, fat pads, and bone in this area, it is of utmost importance for the injecting physician to have a thorough knowledge of the vascular supply of this region. Important vessels in this region include the angular artery; angular vein; zygomaticofacial artery; infraorbital artery; infraorbital trunk of facial artery; facial vein; and facial artery. One must be acutely aware of the anastomosis between the angular artery (a branch of the facial artery) and the dorsal nasal artery (a branch of the ophthalmic artery), which connect the internal and external carotid systems. The angular artery demonstrates variable patterns and injectors must practice caution while injecting the periorbital/medial cheek region in order to avoid intravascular injections into the angular artery which may lead to serious sequelae such as blindness owing to the aforementioned anastomosis. The zygomaticofacial and infraorbital arteries also connect either directly or indirectly with the ophthalmic artery. The inferior palpebral vein and the angular vein also traverse the tear trough region adding to its prominent vascular network. The venous supply in this region in addition to the thin skin may lead to the appearance of "dark circles".[5]

Hirmand in 2010 classified tear troughs into three clinical categories **(Table 1)**.[2] Whereas Hirmand's classification is useful in determining the severity and extend of tear trough, its usefulness is limited when multiple deformities other than the tear trough are encountered in the infraorbital region. The Allergan infraorbital hollow scale is the most widely used scale and has been validated by various studies.[7] The scale grades the severity from grade 0 to grade 4 **(Table 2)**. Recently, Peng et al.[8] have suggested a novel ABL scale for classifying and addressing the tear trough area. The ABL scale includes

Table 1: Hirmand's classification of tear trough abnormaility.[1]

Class	Characteristics
I	Volume loss only in the medial infraorbital region
II	Volume loss in the lateral infraorbital and the medial orbit regions, with the tear trough connected to the palpebromalar grooves
III	Characteristics of both Class I and Class II, along with volume deficiency in the anteromedial cheek

Table 2: Allergan infraorbital hollows scale descriptors.[4]

Grade	Term	Descriptor
0	None	No visible hollowing or volume loss medially or laterally
1	Minimal	Presence of hollowing with some volume loss medial to the midpupillary line; smooth lateral lid–cheek transition
2	Moderate	Defined hollowing extending laterally beyond the midpupillary line with moderate volume loss; smooth lateral lid–cheek transition with mild volume loss
3	Severe	Defined hollowing extending laterally beyond the midpupillary line with moderate volume loss creating a defined groove along the lid–cheek junction
4	Extreme	Defined hollowing extends from medial to lateral canthus; severe volume loss creates a marked step along the lid–cheek junction

Table 3: ABL categorization of various deformities that occur alongside tear trough.[5]

Category	Description
A (Atrophy)	• *A0*: Neither tear troughs nor volume loss of the anteromedial cheek • *A1*: Medial tear troughs only • *A2*: Both medial tear troughs and visible palpebromalar grooves (PMGs) • *A3*: Medial tear troughs, visible PMGs, and anteromedial cheek volume deficiency
B (Bulging)	• *B0*: Neither lower eyelid bags nor malar festoons • *B1*: Only lower eyelid bags • *B2*: Only malar festoons • *B3*: Both lower eyelid bags and malar festoons
L (Laxity)	• *L0*: Neither lower eyelid laxity nor cheek laxity • *L1*: Only cheek laxity • *L2*: Only lower eyelid laxity • *L3*: Both lower eyelid and cheek laxities

three categories—(1) category A (atrophy), (2) category B (bulging), and (3) category L (laxity) **(Table 3)**.

A careful evaluation of the patient including any medical or treatment history along with an informed consent is essential prior to injection. Simple tests like tilt test, snap test, smile test, squint test, pull test, and push test may help plan out the treatment sessions.[8] Preinjection counseling is crucial while addressing this area as a moderate TTD may do well with the sole use of hyaluronic acid fillers (HAFs), whereas a more severe deformity may require a combination approach or surgical intervention. Further, patients must be forewarned regarding the frequent occurrence of bruising and/or transient swelling postinjection. Pre- and post-treatment photographic documentation is essential.

INJECTION PROTOCOLS

The injection protocol employed typically takes into consideration the type of filler used, site of injection, depth/level of injection, amount to be used, and the use of needle or cannula for injection. HAFs with a low water retention capacity and low viscoelasticity are preferred while injecting the periorbital area. While HAFs with high water retention capacity may lead to a nagging swelling and "unnatural" appearance postinjection, those with a high viscoelasticity or a high g prime may lead to lumpiness postinjection and are better avoided. The depth or the layer of injection while injecting the periorbital region involves essentially two layers, namely the SOOF layer of the prezygomatic space, which requires restoration particularly in cases with severe atrophy, and the subcutaneous tissue located on the upper aspect of the OOM.[5]

The use of blunt cannula for injecting is highly recommended in this region owing to its high vascularity. While our preference while injecting this region is a 25 G cannula, one may consider a cannula of any size between 23 G and 30 G. A 30 G cannula may be preferred for more superficial filling.[5]

Filling of the TTD involves addressing the following regions:

- *Tear trough and nasojugal groove:* The tear trough or the medial aspect of the nasojugal groove is addressed with a 25 G cannula and the entry point of the cannula should be in a straight line 1 cm away from the end of the tear trough. While injecting the nasojugal groove, the injection depth should be at the level of the prezygomatic space deep to the SOOF layer. Restoration of volume to the SOOF addresses the sunken portion of the groove and subsequently more superficial injections may be carried out in the subcutaneous layer in order to provide natural contours to the area. 23–27 G cannulas are recommended for this region and the usually the point of cannula insertion corresponds to the point where the perpendicular line starting from lateral canthus intersects with the horizontal line passing the inferior border of nasal ala **(Fig. 3)**. The tethering effect of the ligamentous structures can be reduced by undermining and releasing the dense fibrotic tissue with the help of the cannula being used.[1,9-12]

- *Palpebromalar groove:* The palpebromalar groove is injected slowly with a sharp needle in the supraperiosteal location. The authors prefer a 30 G needle and a bolus injection followed by gentle massage in order to layer the filler along the groove.

A cannula may also be used for injecting this region, wherein the insertion point of the cannula is placed 0.5 apart from the lateral canthus **(Figs. 4 and 5)**.

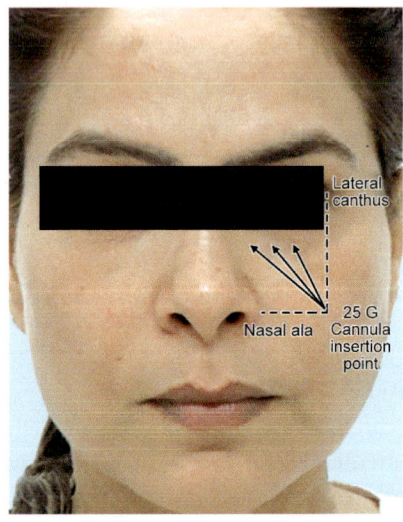

Fig. 3: The cannula entry point for replacing volume in the SOOF (suborbicularis oculi fat) coincides with the point of intersection of a vertical line drawn down from the lateral canthus and a horizontal line drawn from the nasal ala.

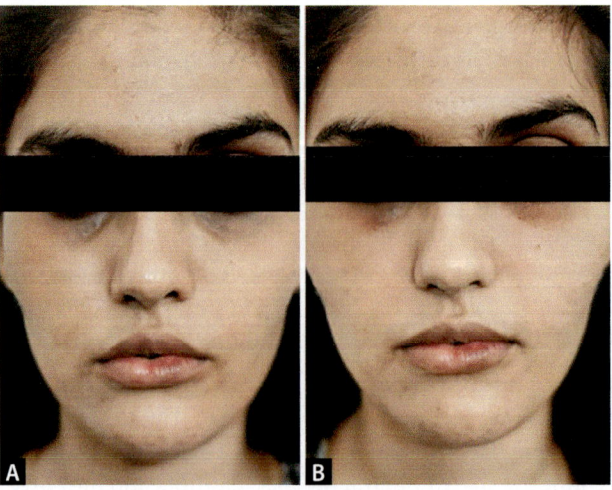

Figs. 4A and B: (A) Groove and hollowness in the infraorbital region preinjection; (B) immediately postinjection with 1 mL of Juvederm Ultra Plus XC.

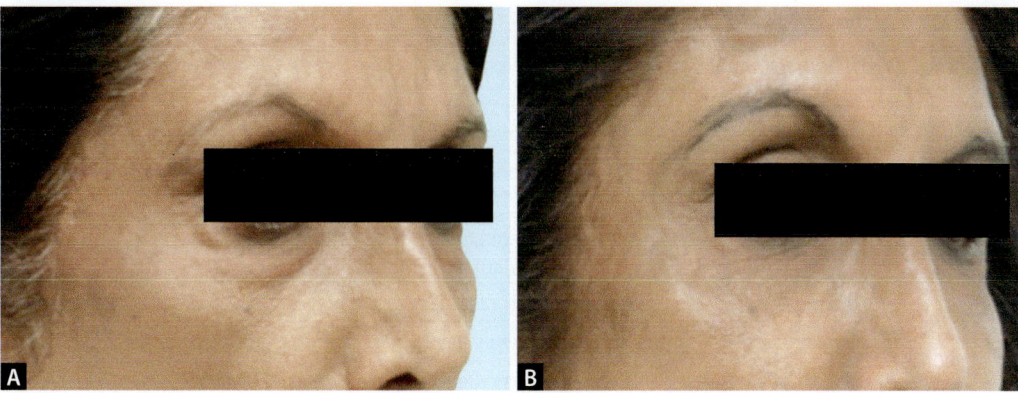

Figs. 5A and B: (A) Tear touch deformity and the palpeabromalar groove along with eye bags preinjection; (B) Post two sessions of hyaluronic acid fillers.

Table 4: Typical tear trough and anterior and lateral cheek injection points face map.		
Code	Injection area	Treating the emotional attributes
Tt1	Central infraorbital	Patient desire
Tt2	Lateral infraorbital	To look less sad
Tt3	Medial infraorbital	MD codes formula T1 + T2 + T3
Ck1	Zygomatic arch	Ck1 + Ck2 + Ck3
Ck2	Zygomatic eminence	May or may not be combined with codes for the eyebrow and neurotoxin
Ck3	Anteromedial cheek	

Courtesy: Allergan and Dr Mauricio de Maio.[6]

While the aforementioned methods are one way of injecting the periorbital region, various points or "codes" (MD Codes™) have also been described for correction of the TTD. The injection area codes defined in **Table 4**.[9] The preferred method used for injection, injection level, and injection amount are shown in **Table 5**.[8]

While the preferred method is one the injector is comfortable with the product selection and depth of injection and is crucial while injecting the periorbital region owing to the thin skin and its distinct anatomy. As mentioned above, HAFs with low water retention capacity and a low g-prime are suitable for the region. The authors preference for HAF injections in this region have been elucidated **(Box 1)**.

POSTINJECTION INSTRUCTIONS

Application of ice packs and gentle massage may be done postprocedure. Patient should be counseled for the potential swelling and bruising; and no further manipulation should be carried out for the next 2 weeks.

PRECAUTIONS

Complications of postfiller administration in the periorbital region typically involve:

- *Wrong product selection*: The use of high water retaining fillers may lead to persistent

Table 5: Injection methods, technique, and amount of filler used.[5]

Injection site	Needle/cannula	Injection level	Injection amount/per side
Tt1	Needle or cannula	Subperiosteal or under orbicularis oculi muscle	0.1–0.3 cc
Tt2	Needle or cannula	Subperiosteal or under orbicularis oculi muscle	0.1–0.2
Tt3	Cannula	Subperiosteal or under orbicularis oculi muscle	0.05–0.1
Ck1	Needle	Subperiosteal	0.1–0.3 cc
Ck2	Needle	Subperiosteal	0.1–0.3 cc
Ck3	Needle or cannula	Subperiosteal or deep medial cheek fat pad	0.3–.05 cc

Box 1 Preferred fillers available in India for filling the periorbital area.

- Juvéderm Ultra (Hylacross), Volbella (Vycross), (Allergan, Inc., Irvine, CA)
- For severe deformities—Juvederm Ultraplus (Hylacross), Volift (Vycross) may also be used (Allergan, Inc., Irvine, CA)
- Restylane (Ipsen Ltd., Berkshire, UK)
- Mild deformity—Belotero Soft (Merz Pharma, Frankfurt)
- Moderte—severe deformity—Belotero Balance (Merz Pharma, Frankfurt)
- Yvoire Classic (LG Chem Life Sciences)
- Princess filler (Croma-Pharma GmbH, Austria)
- Perfectha Complement, Perfectha Derm (Sinclair Pharma, France)
- Mona Lisa Mild Type (Genoss Co., Korea)

swelling postfiller administration, whereas high G-prime or highly viscoelastic fillers may lead to lumpiness in the area **(Fig. 6)**.

- *Amount of filler used*: Excessive amount of product in this region can lead to "overcorrection" or an un-natural appearance. Excessive product placement may also lead to decrease in the aperture of the eye **(Fig. 6)**.
- *Placement of filler in the wrong plane*: Superficial filler placement in this region leads to appearance of a bluish gray discoloration owing to the "Tyndall effect".

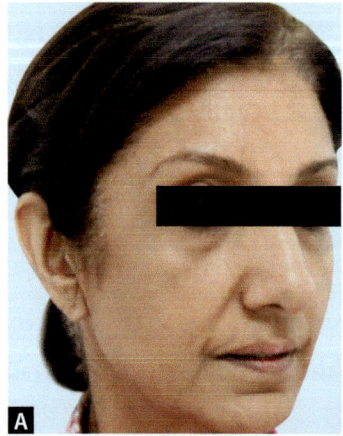 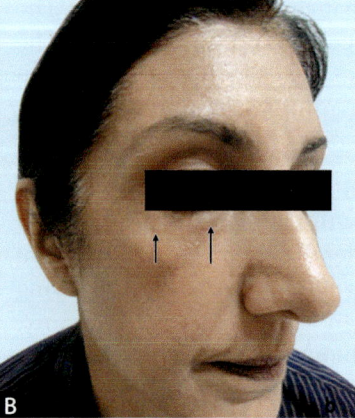

Figs. 6A and B: (A) Nasojugual groove with eye bags in the periorbital region; (B) Wrong product selection leading to lumps and "overcorrection".

Table 6: Potential complications in the periorbital areas and their prevention and management.

Complication	Tips and management
Wrong product selection/excessive filler/placement of filler in the wrong plane (lumps, nodules, and tyndall effect)	• Use the right product (not highly water retaining fillers), be judicious in administration of filler in this area as the margin for error is minimal • Hyaluronidase (1,500 U vial) post-/pretest • No correction post hyaluronidase for at least 2 weeks • Manual removal of filler after nicking the skin with a 30 G needle or surgical scalpel
Bruising	• Use of small gauge needles (27–30 G) • Injecting slowly • Injecting small volumes • Using blunt cannulas (23–30 G as per preference) • Limiting number of transcutaneous puncture sites • Discontinuing blood thinning medications in the week prior to treatment (providing it is safe to do so)[13] • Firm pressure at the first sign of bruising, cold compress and Vitamin K cream.[14,15] • Arnica—200 TDS, Bromelain—400–500 mg BD/TDS • Best started few days prior to procedure and continued for 5–7 days postprocedure • Topical arnica can be allergenic
Vascular complications	• No hyaluronidase pretest needed • Keep epinephrine at bed site • Use of hyaluronidase in a conventional or pulsed manner

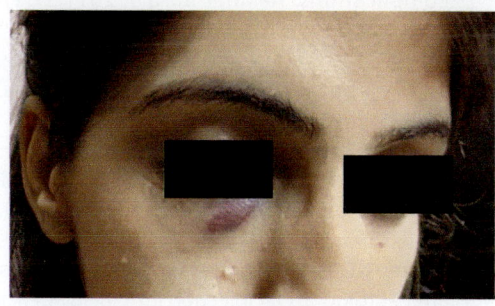

Fig. 7: Bruising in the periobital region postinjection with a 27 G, sharp needle.

- *Vascular complications:* While the occurrence of bruising in this region is common **(Fig. 7)**, the less commonly occurring (although more severe) complications include vascular compromise which maybe a result of excessive injection of filler (compression effect of filler on the vessels), embolization of filler into the artery (can potentially lead to blindness)[16] and direct vascular injury to the vessel due to the needle or cannula. Cutaneous necrosis following fillers has also been reported.

Tips to avoid such complications and management strategies have been enumerated **(Table 6)**.[13-15]

USEFUL TIPS

- Use the right product (not highly water retaining fillers), be judicious in administration of filler in this area as the margin for error is minimal.
- Using blunt cannulas (23–30 G as per preference).
- Discontinue blood thinning medications in the week prior to treatment (providing it is safe to do so).
- If a needle is used for injection limit number of transcutaneous puncture sites. Icing the area can also help prevent bruising.

- Avoid trying to correct the tear trough completely since this can lead to swelling later. A 70% correction at the time of injection is sufficient for most patients.
- If hyaluronidase is used to correct badly placed filler the reinjection of the area should only be done after 2 weeks.

REFERENCES

1. Rhee SC, Woo KS, Kwon B. Biometric study of eyelid shape and dimensions of different races with references to beauty. Aesthetic Plast Surg. 2012;36(5):1236-45.
2. Hirmand H. Anatomy and nonsurgical correction of the tear trough deformity. Plast Reconstr Surg. 2010;125(2):699-708.
3. Yang C, Zhang P, Xing X. Tear trough and palpebromalar groove in young versus elderly adults: a sectional anatomy study. Plast Reconstr Surg. 2013;132(4):796-808.
4. Wong CH, Hsieh MK, Mendelson B. The tear trough ligament: anatomical basis for the tear trough deformity. Plast Reconstr Surg. 2012;129(6):1392-402.
5. Kim HJ, Seo KK, Lee HK, et al. Clinical Anatomy of the Midface for Filler Injection. In: Seo KK, Kim J (Eds). Clinical Anatomy of the Face for Filler and Botulinum Toxin Injection. Singapore: Springer; 2016. pp. 119-51.
6. Haddock NT, Saadeh PB, Boutros S, et al. The tear trough and lid/cheek junction: anatomy and implications for surgical correction. Plast Reconstr Surg. 2009;123(4):1332-40.
7. Donofrio L, Carruthers J, Hardas B, et al. Development and validation of a photonumeric scale for evaluation of infraorbital hollows. Dermatol Surg. 2016;42(Suppl 1):S251-8.
8. Peng PH, Peng JH. Treating the tear trough: A new classification system, a 6-step evaluation procedure, hyaluronic acid injection algorithm, and treatment sequences. J Cosmet Dermatol. 2018;17(3):333-9.
9. de Maio M, DeBoulle K, Braz A, et al. Facial assessment and injection guide for botulinum toxin and injectable hyaluronic acid fillers: focus on the midface. Plast Reconstr Surg. 2017;140(4):540e-50e.
10. Carruthers J, Carruthers A, Humphrey S. Introduction to Fillers. Plast Reconstr Surg. 2015;136(Suppl 5):120S-31S.
11. Cotofana S, Schenck TL, Trevidic P, et al. Midface: clinical anatomy and regional approaches with injectable fillers. Plast Reconstr Surg. 2015;136(Suppl 5):219S-34S.
12. Scheuer JF 3rd, Sieber DA, Pezeshk RA, et al. Anatomy of the facial danger zones: maximizing safety during soft-tissue filler injections. Plast Reconstr Surg. 2017;139(1):50e-8e.
13. Bailey SH, Cohen JL, Kenkel JM. Etiology, prevention, and treatment of dermal filler complications. Aesthet Surg J. 2011;31(1):110-21.
14. Alam M, Dover JS. Management of complications and sequelae with temporary injectable fillers. Plast Reconstr Surg. 2007;120(Suppl):98S-105.
15. Funt D, Pavicic T. Dermal fillers in aesthetics: an overview of adverse events and treatment approaches. Clin Cosmet Invest Dermatol. 2013;6:295-316.
16. Dreizen NG, Fram L. Sudden unilateral visual loss after autologous fat injection into the glabellar area. Am J Ophthalmol. 1989;107:85-7.

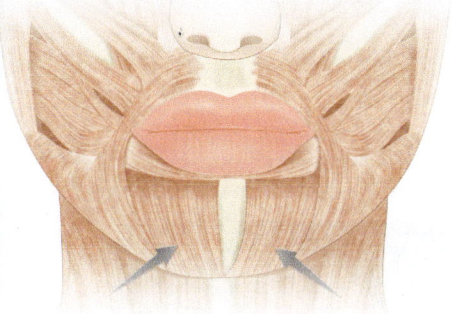

CHAPTER 15

Fillers for Midface—Cheeks

Madhuri Agarwal

INDICATIONS

The youthful face is a symphony of gentle curves, largely due to plentiful volume. As we age, volume loss (combined with other aging changes) produces a deflated and drawn appearance. Complex interaction of gravitational pull, loss of structural elasticity, and volumetric loss of bone, muscle and fat overtime contribute to aging. Midface is considered to be the support system of a youthful face. The rejuvenation of the midface with volumizing fillers has marked a turning point in the treatment of the region. Deep understanding of facial anatomy and changes that occur through aging contributes to achieving optimal patient satisfaction.

ANATOMIC CONSIDERATIONS

Midface comprises of the middle one-third of the face, lying between two parallel lines drawn through the nasion and subnasale (**Fig. 1**). Aging leads to anteromedial decline of skin and fat along with loss of underlying volume. The descent ends at subcutaneous skin attachments leading to skin folds. Studies have verified about the concept of volume loss from both dynamic (midfacial descent) and static (bone and fat) sources. Before notable loss of density in lumbar spine there is decrease in bone density in maxilla and

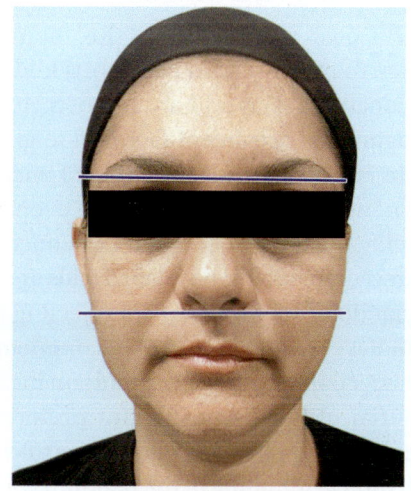

Fig. 1: Midface—nasion to subnasale.

mandible in both sexes.[1] Loss of bony volume increases the depth of the alar crease, and loss of maxillary projection leads to midfacial deflation and descent. These add up to the three-dimensional (3D) deflation of the midface. Loss of orbital volume contributes to the sunken and hollow appearance of eyes. Thus volumetric shifts from the midportion of the face to the lower face is seen as an overall contribution of loss of fat in deep and subcutaneous midface along with ligamentous stretching.[2] Reinflation is done to address the concern and a multilayered, and sometimes multiproduct, approach is often needed to accomplish individual improvements.

Allergan Photometric Midface Volume Deficit Scale is easy and straightforward to use in clinical practice. The scale grades are 5 = severe, 4 = significant, 3 = moderate, 2 = mild, 1 = minimal, and 0 = none. Injectors can use this to evaluate and assess the levels of improvement before and after injection and it can be applied to track the longevity of results.

INJECTION TECHNIQUE

In the past two decades, the focus has shifted to midface from nasolabial folds and marionette lines, as primary area of correction for aging and sagging of face due to gravity. There is a better understanding of anatomy and newer, safer techniques have evolved to simplify the filler injections. The concept of indirect correction of nasolabial folds and tear trough deformity by virtue of injecting filler in midface is propagated and recommended. The injection technique depends on the filler material utilized and injector preference. Needle injections can be made more tolerable with topical numbing of the region. Typically prepackaged injectable fillers come with needles of recommended sizes commonly 27-gauge needle. A 30-gauge needle allows precise contouring for the new Vycross range of fillers.

The concept of cheek filler should be to deliver optimum cheek contour restoration and reshape. It must not just volumize or fill it. The conventional technique of injecting midface was with the help of Hinderer's lines. Hinderer's lines comprise of two intersecting lines, one from the ala to the tragus and the other one from the lateral canthus to the commissure of the ipsilateral lip, as seen in **Figure 2**. The intersection of these two lines denotes the apex of the malar

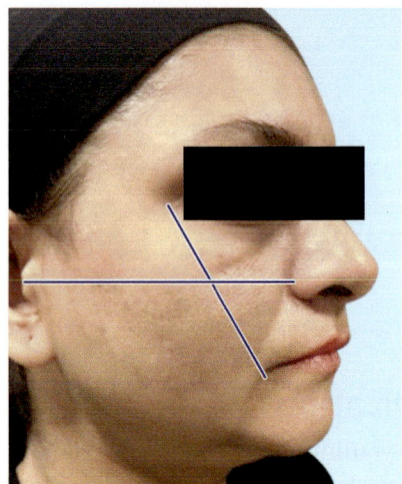

Fig. 2: Hinderer's lines.

eminence.[3] The midface can be divided into three regions by the Hinderer's lines namely superolateral, anteromedial, and inferolateral. The superolateral quadrant should receive the initial volume, feathering into the anteromedial and inferolateral.[4]

In author's opinion there is more simplified technique that works well for midface and beginners can use it comfortably in their practice. The cheek subunits must be divided as per the "the 5-point cheek reshape MD codes". Each cheek subunit is assigned a code as follows—Ck1 (zygomatic arch, lateral cheek); Ck2 (zygomatic eminence, anterior cheek); Ck3 (medial cheek); Ck4 (parotid area, lateral cheek); and Ck5 (submalar area) as seen in **Figure 3**. The midface sag lift and reshaping is done by creating structural support with Ck1 and Ck2 and then remaining volume loss is corrected with Ck3, Ck4, and Ck5. Optimum cheek architecture is obtained with these predefined MD codes. The plane of injection is supraperiosteal for Ck1 and Ck2 and the quantity of product is 0.1-0.2 mL for Ck1 and 0.2-0.4 mL for Ck2 as small bolus

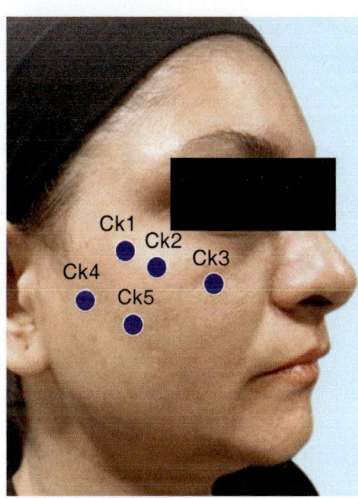

Fig. 3: MD codes for cheek and midface augmentation.

injections. Voluma is the best option for these two codes due to its lifting capacity to combat sagginess. Voluma is unique and a versatile, highly cohesive filler as it can be injected both into subcutaneous and supraperiosteal level, it is easy to mold, and its effects can be reversed. Place the noninjecting finger to prevent displacement of filler to the temporal area and the lower eyelid while treating Ck1 and Ck2, respectively. For Ck3, i.e. medial cheek, the plane of injection is supraperiosteal or subcutaneous and about 0.3–0.5 mL of the product can be injected by small bolus injections. The injections must be placed lateral to the midpupillary line. Ck4 and Ck5 are injected in the subcutaneous plane and 0.2–0.5 mL of the filler can be injected. The injections are placed as bolus doses in 4–5 areas or it can be deposited with a 25-gauge microcannula using a fanning technique to cover the area. The Ck5 code is optional and used mainly to correct submalar deficient areas. Avoid placing filler in Ck5 when the face is already having excess fat or fullness in the submalar area. Voluma, Volift, or Juvéderm Ultraplus is recommended for Ck3, Ck4, and Ck5. Overcorrection can be avoided by injecting in the deeper plane first followed by subsequent injections in the superficial plane and working from superior to inferior site on face. Injections of the filler in the medial malar region to correct the lateral infraorbital hollow and inferiorly to reposition the central part of midface yield natural results.

It is important to keep in mind that injecting cheeks randomly or single bolus dose to anchor the cheek is not adequate and will give unnatural results. An abnormal appearance is seen in the infraorbital region and medial cheek especially on animation when excessive quantity of filler is placed high in the tear trough or medial area of cheek. All injections must be slow, small amounts of product as bolus or through a constantly moving needle and aspirate before injecting every code. Aspirating during needle insertion ensures blood vessels are not penetrated and thus injected directly. It is important to remember that very hollow, empty face will require a lot of filler and more than one session and this must be discussed with the patient in detail before commencing the treatment. Patients with excessive elastosis of surface skin may also require large quantity of filler to appreciate satisfactory result. Gentle massage for molding the filler postinjection can help disperse the filler, especially with gels such as HA. Pre and post photographs of patients treated for midface with Juvéderm range of fillers by the author is shown in **Figure 4**.

PRECAUTIONS

With proper injection technique and patient selection, complications are rare. Bruising is transient and can be minimized by instructing patients to discontinue

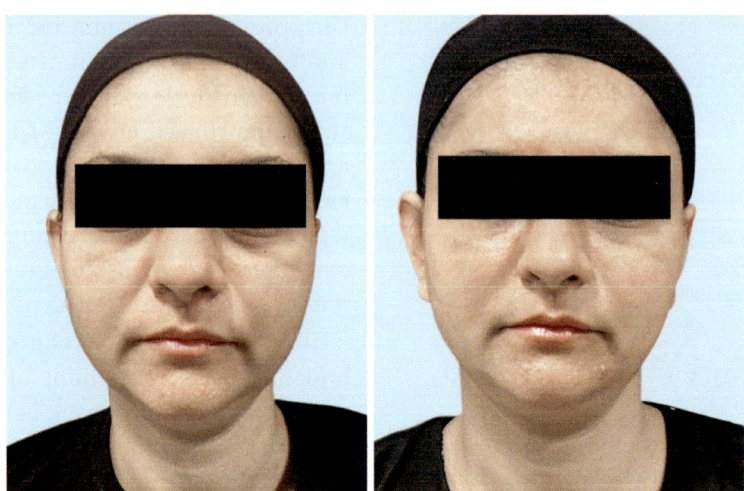

Fig. 4: Pre and post photographs of patient treated for midface with Juvéderm range of fillers.

nonsteroidal anti-inflammatory and blood-thinning supplements 7–14 days prior to plan injection.

Swelling typically occurs with volumizing injections although is temporary. Pain can be minimized with topical anesthetics and use of lidocaine mixed with the injectable.

The angular artery in the region of the medial maxilla and alar crease and the infraorbital artery inferior to the mid infraorbital rim are at risk with injectables in midface. If injected, microemboli can be transmitted to the orbit or brain leading to blindness. The infraorbital foramen lies in the midpupillary line about 1 cm inferior to the infraorbital margin. The branches of angular artery (facial or external carotid) and branch of internal carotid artery that arises through the infraorbital foramen, together with vein and the sensory neural system of the infraorbital nerve supply the malar region. In this region there is a thick layer of subcutaneous tissue and fat. The midsubcutaneous plane—which marks the transition between its looser and its denser part—makes the injection of fillers safe, as the neural structures are located at deeper levels and the main vessels go along the lateral line of the nasal region.[5] Avoid the angular and infraorbital arteries and veins, and ensure that injections are made below the orbital rim in the anteromedial cheek region. The eye and infraorbital foramen is protected by using index and middle fingers while injecting slowly. When the filler is injected medial to the midpupillary line and close to nose, a 25-gauge blunt microcannula is suggested in place of needle taking into consideration that it is an area of risk for severe vascular damage. While injecting the lateral and anterior cheek, mark the zygomatic facial vessels and nerves. In lateral cheek and submalar area, injectors need to be alert to avoid the facial artery and vein and the parotid duct, and to be careful near the buccal branches of the facial nerve. Injectors should be alert to avoid the transverse facial artery and vein too therefore subcutaneous injection is mandatory.[6]

Late complications can involve lumps that persist beyond the first couple of weeks. Subcutaneous nodules have been reported with fillers. Most nodules respond to time and massage.

POSTINJECTION INSTRUCTIONS

Postprocedure care plays a vital role in the achievement of optimal results and hence it is essential to educate patients on this aspect. Patients are advised to avoid exposure to direct sunlight, excessive cold weather and outdoor activities for a couple of days. Avoid extremes of temperatures like sauna and skiing for a week and massaging the area of filler injection for 2 weeks. Other treatments like peels, microdermabrasion can be done after a week while photofacial and laser hair reduction can be done after 2 weeks. Ask client to undergo dental work only after 2 weeks. No alcohol should be consumed on the day of treatment. The patient should also avoid vitamin E, omega-3 fatty acid, aspirin, and nonsteroidal anti-inflammatory drug (NSAID) ingestion for 3 days after treatment.

Client can be called for a follow-up for touch up after 4–5 days.

USEFUL TIPS

- Volumizing the upper midface before improving the nasolabial fold and marionette lines is generally more effective in restoring youthful balance than starting in the folds.
- Injection plane in cheeks should be supraperiosteal and subcutaneous. Avoid superficial injections in dermis as it will create an unnatural bulge.
- There is crucial vasculature in the cheeks, so it is mandatory to mark these no-go areas and then start the injections.
- The technique of injection is dependent upon condition of skin. When skin needs improved texture along with some volume correction, fanning with microcannula is advisable.
- When skin is in good condition, multiple small bolus injections in supraperiosteal plane. Reassess for desired 3D contour correction and projection. In case it is not achieved; additional fanning subcutaneous injections can be performed.

REFERENCES

1. Shaw RB Jr, Katzel EB, Koltz PF, et al. Facial bone density: effects of aging and impact on facial rejuvenation. Aesthet Surg J. 2012;32(8):937-42.
2. Kahn DM, Shaw RB. Overview of current thoughts on facial volume and aging. Facial Plast Surg. 2010;26(5):350-5.
3. Rohrich RJ, Pessa JE. The fat compartments of the face: anatomy and clinical implications for cosmetic surgery. Plast Reconstr Surg. 2007;119(7): 2219-27.
4. Jones D, Murphy DK. Volumizing hyaluronic acid filler for midface volume deficit: 2-year results from a pivotal single-blind randomized controlled study. Dermatol Surg. 2013;39(11): 1602-12.
5. Funt DK. Avoiding malar edema during midface/cheek augmentation with dermal fillers. J Clin Aesthet Dermatol. 2011;4(12):32-6.
6. de Maio M, DeBoulle K, Braz A, et al. Facial assessment and injection guide for botulinum toxin and injectable hyaluronic acid fillers focus on the midface. Plast Reconstr Surg. 2017;140(4):540e-50e.

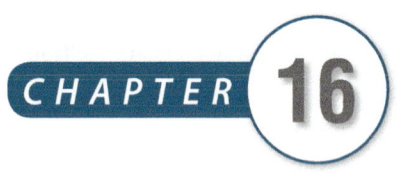
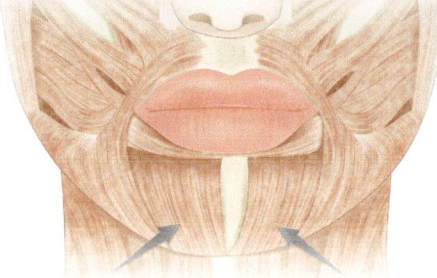

Fillers for Midface—Tear-Trough and Nose

Vanravi Vachatimanont, Rungsima Wanitphakdeedecha

MIDFACE AND TEAR-TROUGH

Indications

Malar projection and plump cheeks are desirable features that symbolize beauty and youthfulness, especially among Asians. In contrast, the appearance of flattened cheeks portrays aging. The aging process involves multilayer aspects such as elastosis, fat atrophy, and bone resorption, and loosening of the ligaments that aggravate the midface ptosis that occurs in conjunction with the appearance of prominent lines, from tear trough to nasolabial fold and down to jowls in the lower face.[1] Midface augmentation not only enhances volumization, but also helps to reshape the face by harmonizing the upper face and lower face.[2]

In addition, eyes are considered as the window to the heart. They are one of the first areas that capture another person's attention. Hence, often signs of aging are first noticed around the eyes, presenting as wrinkles, prominent tear troughs, under eye hollowness, and eye bags.[3] Periorbital aging signs such as the tear trough deformity are caused by loosening of the orbicularis retaining ligament on the medial side, and palpebromalar groove as it deepens on the lateral side due to bone resorption and fat loss. Moreover, loosening of the orbicularis ligament allows the septal fat to protrude downward causing a pseudoherniation of the intraorbital fat on the lower eyelid that is eventually presented as eye bags.

Anatomic Considerations

In general, Asians tend to have higher cheekbones as compared to other ethnicities, due to the pronounced zygomatic arch.[4,5] With aging depression of the cheeks results from the atrophy of the cheek fat and the resorption of the underlying bone. This deterioration dimensionally alters the face's features. It emphasizes the protrusion of the malar prominence and accentuates maxillary elongation. In addition, Asians also have a broad mandibular angle, which gives an overall appearance of a skeleton-like look.[2]

Midface plays an important role in supporting a strong framework of fascial extension of the superficial musculoaponeurotic system (SMAS) that connects the lower face to the midface.[1] Hence, correcting the midface will also improve the ptosis in the lower face as well as alleviating the appearance of tear trough deformity. As a result, correction of the midface, i.e. volumization of the cheeks, is usually one of the primary areas to improve aging appearance in the midface area.[2,6]

Fat is another important component of the face, as aging and gravity have shown a great impact on inferior displacement

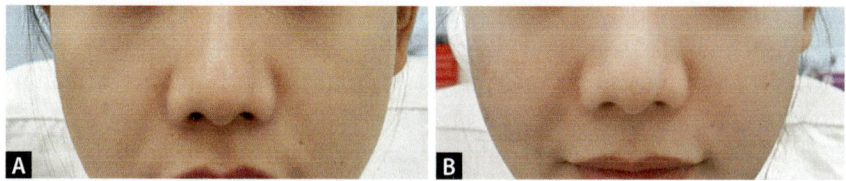

Figs. 1A and B: Midface augmentation. (A) Before photo, showing flat midface, which reflects an aging appearance; (B) After photo, filler augmentation produces more youthful appearance and also improves the prominent nasolabial folds.

of the superficial nasolabial and jowl fat compartments.[1,7] The medial and lateral cheek fat compartments do not, however, show significant inferior displacement.[1] This may be due to strong ligamentous support to the overlying fat compartment in that region, e.g. the medial cheek fat compartment attachment to the orbicularis retaining ligament. Similarly, in the lateral cheek compartment the fat lies above the mid-facial SMAS, cohering closely with the lateral orbital thickening, the inferior temporal septum, and the zygomaticocutaneous ligament on the zygomatic arch and extended inferiorly to the parotideomasseteric fascia.[1] For this reason, injection either to one or both of the superficial medial cheek compartment and the lateral cheek compartment will not only restore the volume of the cheek fat and increase the projection of the cheeks, but also create a lifting mobilization of the midface and lower face **(Fig. 1A and B)**.

Injection Techniques

Younger patients often require only correction of the depression of the cheeks, which can be done by augmentation of the anteromedial cheeks. It is advised to use mid-viscosity filler for volumization.[6] There are two techniques, either using sharp needles or with a blunt cannula. It is most convenient to use sharp needle injection, and a needle of 27 G is appropriate. The plane of injection is deep to the bone where the deep medial cheek fat lies; a bolus injection of approximately 0.2–0.3 cc may be required per injection site. For sharp injection in male patients, draw a line from the lateral canthus down to the cheek (1–2 cm), then inject a bolus injection on the bone with a volume of approximately 0.2–0.3 cc. However, for female patients, inject slightly more medially, close to the lateral limbus line with a similar technique. It is important to always aspirate before injecting and keep a steady hand to avoid misplacing the filler. Alternatively, a cannula of 25 G can be used, making an entry from the crossover point between a vertical line down the lateral canthus and horizontal line from the end of the nose. The cannula should be inserted deep and glide along the maxilla. Aspirate and slowly place filler to volumize the deep medial cheek fat pad, approximately 0.3–0.5 cc, using a fanning technique.

However, older patients tend to require more than just restoring the loss of volume, but also require lifting enhancement on the midface and lower face due to fat ptosis. In respect to the aging process, one should restore the bone resorption around the orbit and replace the lateral suborbicularis oculi fat pad (SOOF) for the lifting effect and strengthening the orbicularis retaining ligament (ORL) and zygomaticocutaneous ligament (ZL). Hassan Galadari and Wolfgang Redka-Swoboda have suggested the Redka-Galadari point (RG point) as a single and anatomically safe point to restore the midcheek deflation and correct the tear trough deformity from a single point of injection.[8] The RG point can be found by drawing a vertical line from the lateral canthus down to 1–2 cm below the orbital rim.[8] In addition, it could be useful to palpate for the infraorbital foramen first to decrease the chance of intravascular injection.

Consequently, one may use either a sharp needle (27 G) or a cannula of 25 G or less, or use mid- to hard viscosity filler[6] and inject a small bolus at the RG point on the bone with a volume of approximately 0.1–0.2 cc. Again, one should not forget to aspirate before injecting. Moreover, in aging patients, it can be beneficial to also replace the lateral part of the medial cheek fat to create a smooth and harmonized curvature from the midcheek to the lower face. This volume can be added by drawing a vertical line from the lateral canthus to approximately 3 cm down to the cheek and inject deep to the bone with a small volume of approximately 0.2–0.3 cc.

Lastly, if aging appearance has not improved after correction of the midface then you should aim to correct the tear trough deformity. Due to it being a highly vascularized area, it is advised to use a cannula of 25G or less, using the same entry as prior injection for the midface, at the crossover point between a vertical line down the lateral canthus and horizontal line from the end of the nose. Opt for soft to medium viscosity filler,[6] deposit 0.2–0.3 cc (on each side) on the supraperiosteal plane for volumization of the medial SOOF on the prezygomatic space. It is also possible to minimally deposit at the subcutaneous plane for contouring, if needed.

Precautions

The important anatomic structure to beware of at this area is the neurovascular bundle that comes out through the infraorbital foramen, which is located approximately at the mid-pupillary line, around 8–10 mm from the infraorbital margin, and 30 mm from the facial midline.[9] It consists of the infraorbital artery, vein, and nerve. The infraorbital artery originates from the maxillary artery and also gives rise to the inferior palpebral branch, nasal branch, and superior labial branch. It anastomoses with the facial artery and the dorsal nasal branch of the ophthalmic artery. Hence, injection into this artery may cause local skin necrosis and also blindness **(Fig. 2)**.

In addition, according to the study of Kim et al. on 31 cadaveric hemi-faces, there are four patterns of angular artery.[10] In type I (11%), the angular artery branches off from the lateral nasal artery at the ala of the nose and courses superiorly to the forehead. In

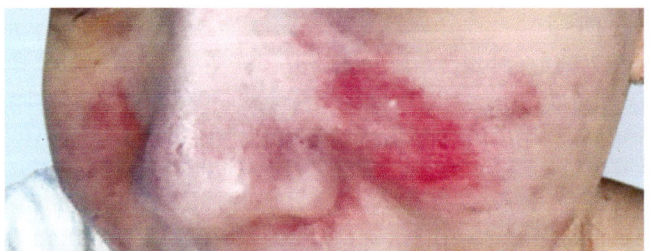

Fig. 2: Intravascular complication. Intravascular injection may initially present as blanching and redness, and eventually, skin necrosis.

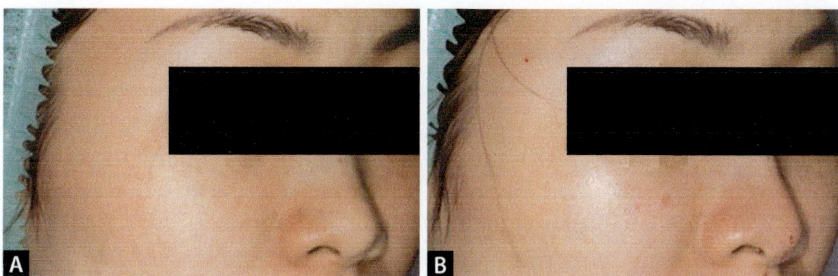

Figs. 3A and B: Nose augmentation. Filler augmentation can act as an initial trial option prior to a surgical treatment. Filler can help to correct the undesirable features of Asian noses [wide dorsum and flat tip of nose as shown (A)]. (B) After treatment photo.

type II (18%), close to the modiolus, the facial artery gives rise to the lateral nasal artery that runs medially to the nose, it then continues as the angular artery, passing superiorly to the infraorbital area through the tear trough. In type III (22.8%), the angular artery derives from the ophthalmic artery, where it courses inferiorly down the medial canthus and along the tear trough. In type IV (26.3%), the angular artery is not present as the facial artery discontinues as a lateral nasal artery. Therefore, these variations must be taken into consideration when injecting around the midface and periorbital area.

Postinjection Instructions

There may be some palpable nodules, therefore massage and mold the filler immediately after injecting. This will ensure a good distribution of the filler. However, advise the patient not to massage the area after the treatment is done. Minimal bruising and swelling may occur, reassure the patient that it should subside within a couple of days.

NOSE

Indications

The nose is another important facial feature as it is located at the center of the face. A beautiful nose brings harmony to the face's symmetry and enhances the face's attractiveness. Common characteristics of Asian noses are a broad and flat nasal bridge with poor projection due to a poorly defined cartilaginous structure of the nose.[4] Hence, rhinoplasty has become very popular amongst Asians to provide a tall and slender nose similar to Caucasians. Nevertheless, some may not wish for an invasive procedure with a permanent change, but rather prefer a nonsurgical procedure, i.e. filler injection with little to no downtime. Additionally, a dimple can be straightened and a flat tip can be raised without the need for invasive intervention **(Figs. 3A and B)**.

Anatomic Considerations

The nose is a dynamic structure consisting of different layers of soft tissues, skin, adipose tissues, and perichondrium. Since it is a highly vascularized structure with variable vascular anatomy, a level of expertise in anatomy is required. Therefore, the use of a cannula is advised to mitigate vascular sequelae.

The main arterial blood supply of the nose is the lateral nasal artery and dorsal nasal artery. The lateral nasal artery arises from the facial artery, where it branches off to supply the alar region. The dorsal nasal artery arises from the ophthalmic artery and supplies the dorsum of the nose. The dorsal nasal artery lies deep in between the fibromuscular layer and the deep fatty layer running down along the side of the nasal dorsum. The lateral nasal artery eventually runs medially from the nasal ala giving off small branches and ultimately anastomosing with the dorsal nasal artery descending from above.[5] Hence, an intravascular injection into either the lateral nasal artery or the dorsal nasal artery can cause the filler to embolize into the ophthalmic artery and cause blindness.[5] Lastly, the superior labial artery gives rise to the columella branches where they mainly supply the tip of the nose.

INJECTION TECHNIQUES

Dorsum of the Nose

The nose is one of the most dangerous and highly vascularized areas, therefore it is advised to use a blunt cannula. The desirable plane of injection is at the level of the supraperichondrial and supraperiosteal layer. An entry can be made at the infratip of the nose. Use a cannula of 22 G–25 G with a retrograde injection technique. Filler of choice is medium to hard viscosity with high G'.[6] The advantage of using a cannula is that you can correct many areas while making only one entry. One may correct the dorsum of the nose at the deep end and retrograde down to straighten or heighten the bridge of the nose down to the tip.[9]

Nasolabial Angle

Filling the nasolabial angle can provide a lifted support to the nasal spine, thereby creating better nose projection. Using a sharp needle of 27 G with hard viscosity and high G' prime filler,[6] inject deep on to the nasal spine with an approximate volume of 0.1–0.3 mL. To elevate the tip of the nose, insert the needle from the tip of the nose down along the nasal septum, all the way down touching the nasal spine. Use the nondominant hand to pinch in between the nasal septum, then slowly inject retrograde upwardly to the tip.

Precautions

The main arterial blood supply of the nose is the lateral nasal artery and dorsal nasal artery. The lateral nasal artery supplies mainly around the tip of the nose, whereas the dorsal nasal artery supplies predominantly around the dorsum of the nose. In addition, other smaller arterial branches around the nose also anastomose with these two main arteries, which eventually anastomose with the ophthalmic artery. Hence, the reversed blood flow increases the risk of embolism during intravascular complication.

Filler injection around the nose should be avoided in patients who have had previous surgical procedures as the anatomy may be altered, and thus may be at increased risk of intravascular accident.

Postinjection Instructions

Some palpable nodules may be present, gently massage and mold the filler immediately after the injection.

USEFUL TIPS

- Injection at midface has a moderate risk of intravascular accident compared to other high-risk sites such as the nose and forehead, which are more highly vascularized. Therefore, using a sharp needle injection at midface would be a comparable technique to using a cannula.

- All precautions should be taken in both techniques, using sharp needles and cannulas as there is neither safest technique nor a safe zone in any injections.

REFERENCES

1. Schenck TL, Koban KC, Schlattau A, et al. The functional anatomy of the superficial fat compartments of the face: a detailed imaging study. Plast Reconstr Surg. 2018;141(6):1351-9.
2. Wu WT, Liew S, Chan HH, et al; Asian Facial Aesthetics Expert Consensus Group. Consensus on current injectable treatment strategies in the Asian face. Aesthetic Plast Surg. 2016;40(2):202-14.
3. Mojallal A, Cotofana S. Anatomy of lower eyelid and eyelid-cheek junction. Ann Chir Plast Esthet. 2017;62(5):365-74.
4. Tan KL, Jin HR. The changing face of aesthetic facial plastic surgery among East Asians. In: Hiscock TY (Ed). Aesthetic Plastic Surgery of the East Asian Face. New York: Thieme Medical Publishers; 2016. p. 6.
5. Kim HJ, Seo KK, Lee HK, et al. General anatomy of the face and neck. In: Kim HJ, Seo KK, Lee HK, Kim J, (Eds). Clinical Anatomy of the Face for Filler and Botulinum Toxin Injection. Seoul: Springer Nature; 2015. pp. 45-8.
6. Sundaram H, Liew S, Signorini M, et al. Global aesthetics consensus: hyaluronic acid fillers and botulinum toxin type A-recommendations for combined treatment and optimizing outcomes in diverse patient populations. Plast Reconstr Surg. 2016;137(5):1410-23.
7. Mendelson BC, Wong CH. Anatomy of the aging face. In Section I Aesthetic Surgery of the Face. Plast Reconstr Surg. 2012:78-92.
8. Galadari H, Redka-Swoboda W. Injection of filler for volume replacement of the whole face using a single-entry method. J Am Acad Dermatol. 2017;77(6):e163-4.
9. Ercikti N, Apaydin N, Kirici Y. Location of the infraorbital foramen with reference to soft tissue landmarks. Surg Radiol Anat. 2017;39(1):11-5.
10. Kim YS, Choi DY, Gil YC, et al. The anatomical origin and course of the angular artery regarding its clinical implications. Dermatol Surg. 2014;40(10):1070-6.

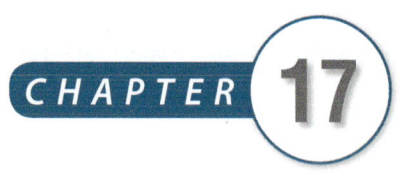
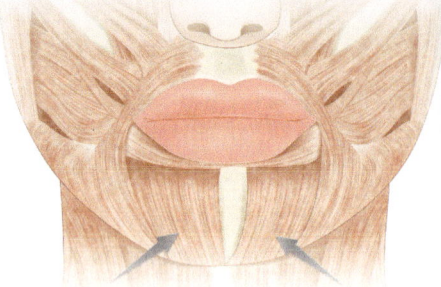

Fillers for Midface—Nasolabial Folds

Vivek Nair

INDICATIONS

The nasolabial folds (NLF) are probably the most common indication for which patients request dermal filler treatment. These lines are a visible sign of skin aging, though in some instances these can be present from a young age. As the facial skeleton and soft tissue ages, the scaffold for the superficial facial fat compartments fails to provide adequate support, resulting in mid-facial ptosis along either side of the nose—the visual manifestation of this being the NLF. Other names for the NLF are the melolabial fold, smile line, nasomandibular fold, and the nose-lip fold.

ANATOMIC CONSIDERATIONS

The NLF starts from the tip of the alae nasi and ends at the cheek adjacent to the corner of the mouth. The NLF can be classified as concave, straight, or convex.[1] There are numerous grading scales for assessing the severity of the NLF ranging from three point to 14-point stratification [e.g. Wrinkle Severity Rating Scale (WSRS), Lemperle Scale, Modified Fitzpatrick Wrinkle Scale]. These scales have been validated and used in numerous studies. Of these, the WSRS is elegant and simple to use clinically.[2] This is as follows: 1 = absent (no visible fold), 2 = mild (shallow fold), 3 = moderate (not visible when stretched), 4 = severe (prominent, long, and deep fold), and 5 = extreme (extremely deep and long folds detrimental to facial appearance).

INJECTION TECHNIQUES

Injection techniques for correction of the NLF have changed significantly over the last decade. The initial emphasis was on filling directly into the fold to improve the depression. As much as 0.8–1.0 cc of filler was often required per side and even then patients were frequently not satisfied with the final result. Higher volumes could fill out the folds effectively but created unnatural bulges, while smaller volumes often left too much of the folds uncorrected. The triangular area of the alar-facial groove was considered the area to put the most filler in. Some authors advocated filling the area above the upper lip and perioral complex to prevent sinking of the medial portion of the NLF.

In the author's opinion, the NLF should never be corrected in isolation unless it is very minor (Grade II). This can either be done through linear threading along the nasolabial fold or through a modified fanning technique injecting in the fold and medial to it (**Figs. 1 and 2**). Point A requires the maximum filler (0.2–0.3 cc). There are three

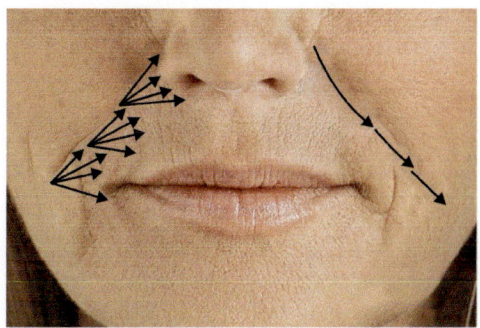

Fig. 1: Basic injection technique for filling the nasolabial fold. Linear threading as shown on the left is the most common technique. Medial fanning as shown on the right is done when there is significant volume loss in the area or a hypoplastic maxilla.

maxillary bone using a needle, near the pyriform aperture. In the first two injection techniques, the filler is placed in the lower dermis or immediate hypodermis **(Fig. 3)**. Mid-viscosity fillers are most suitable (e.g. Juvéderm Ultraplus, Perlane). The cannula is the preferred technique as the facial artery is perilously close to the NLF and has a variable course making intra-arterial injection a real danger. The third technique of injecting on the bone is the safest as this plain never has the facial artery. More filler (0.3–0.4 cc) is required however for appreciable benefit in the NLF. Too much filler will also affect the

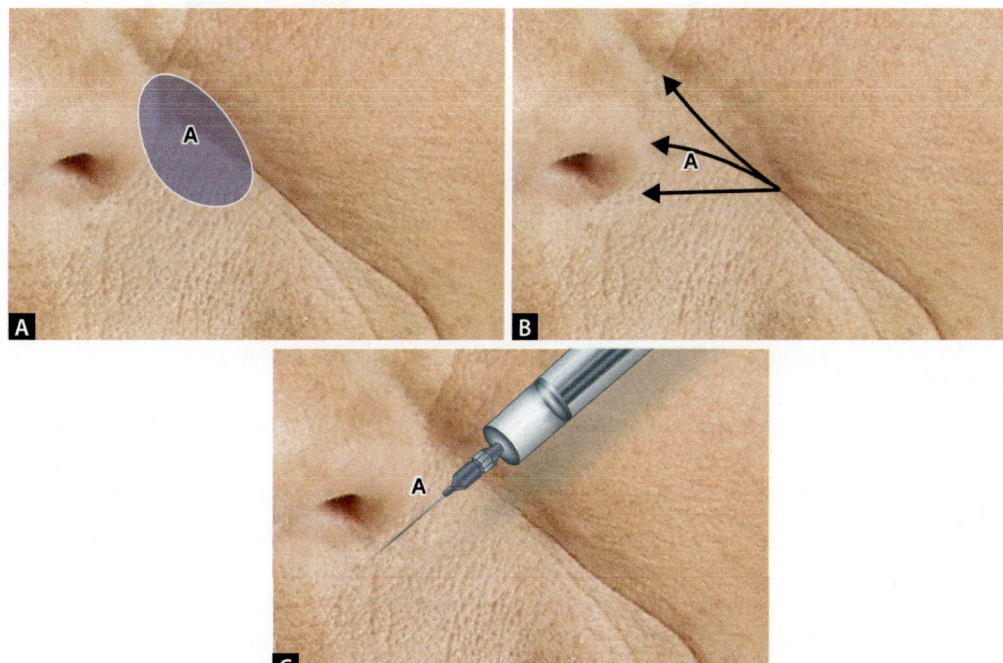

Figs. 2A to C: Point A in these diagrams refers the alar-facial groove. This is a very important point in NLF correction. (A) Simple placement of filler with a needle or cannula in the lower dermis; (B) V-shaped fanning in the groove for filling the area; and (C) Injection on the maxillary bone using a needle pointed toward the contralateral nasal ala. Aspiration before injection is an absolute must.

primary techniques of injection here—simple retrograde linear threading with a needle/cannula, a "V"-shaped injection technique or fanning in the alar-facial groove to fill it with a needle/cannula, or deep injection through the alar-facial groove onto the

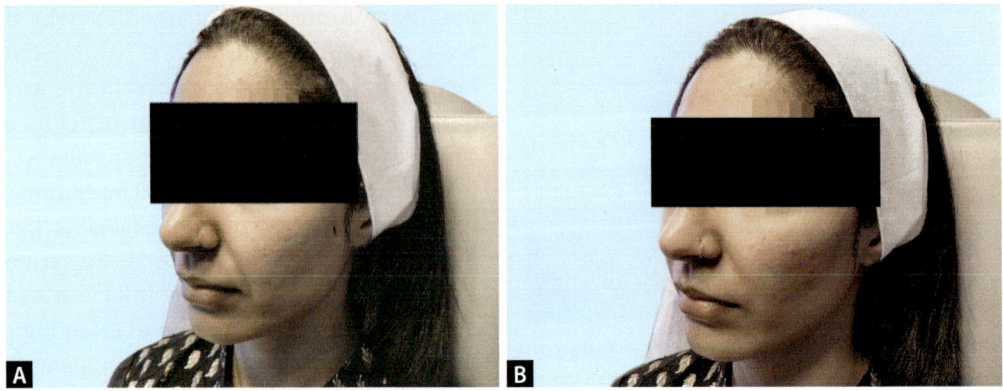

Fig. 3: Mild NLF Correction with 1 cc Filler—(A) Before (B) After.

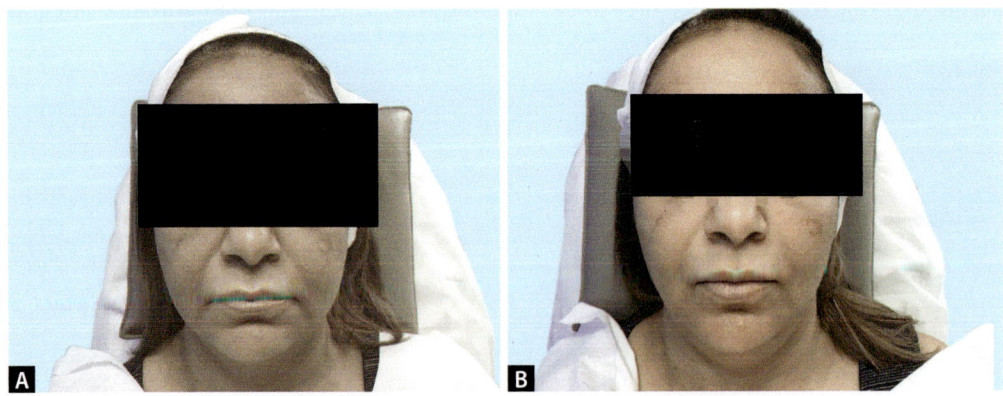

Fig. 4: Moderate NLF Correction with 2cc Filler—(A) Before (B) After.

nasal columella and upper lip. A high viscosity filler like Juvéderm Voluma can be used in this area and will last longer.

Moderate-to-severe NLF (Grade III, IV, V) always require correction of the midface deficit before direct injection into the fold itself **(Fig. 4 and 5)**. This usually leads to a significant improvement due to lateral lift. In particular, the zygomatic prominence and the anteromedial cheek provide the maximum lateral lift. Placing a finger on these areas and pulling laterally will show the points which lift the NLF the most; these should be pulled slightly laterally and then injected with vertical injection points on the bone. After this, the NLF can be injected as usual; lesser filler material will be required as compared to isolated NLF injection.

Very severe NLF will require surgical correction as the skin is usually fibrosed in the crease. Fillers can be used for further augmentation.

When using the needle, one must always aspirate before injecting. The plunger must be pulled back slowly and held for at least 5–10 seconds because it can take that long to see blood in the hub or syringe especially with narrow gauge needles (27 G and higher).[3] After that care must be taken to not move the needle before the filler is injected. The injection then proceeds retrograde as the needle is slowly withdrawn. Avoid injecting a large bolus in

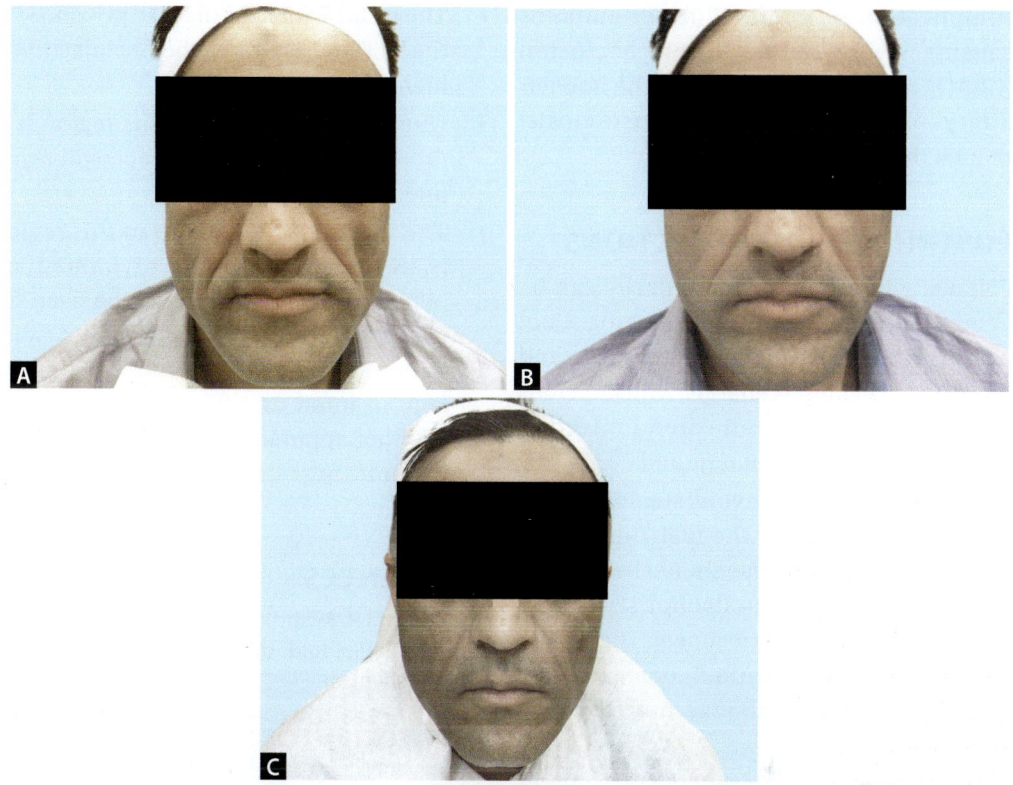

Figs. 3A to C: Severe NLF correction: (A) Baseline; (B) After first correction with 3 cc filler; (C) After second correction 5 years later with 3 cc Filler. No filler was used in the intervening period.

one place. Also avoid injecting with too much pressure. Care must be taken not to inject superficially at the point of entry of the needle as this will be visible as a superficial bleb and may cause a Tyndall effect.

PRECAUTIONS

The main concern with injecting in the NLF region is the proximity of the facial artery. The facial artery is very tortuous in the lower face after crossing the mandibular border along the anterior border of the masseter. Thereafter, it can have one of four possible courses but in over 90% of cases it lies in close vicinity to the NLF (within 5 mm of the NLF in 43% cases, and crossing the NLF in 34% cases). Recent studies of the cadaveric and in-vivo course of the facial artery have shown that in 49–74% the facial artery terminates between the upper lip and the nasal ala.[4,5] The classic cadaveric finding of the facial artery transitioning into the angular artery is only found in 19–24% of cases,[4,5] though some studies still cite this as the most common course of the facial artery with 51% frequency in one cadaveric study.[6] The facial artery and its branches lie in the subcutaneous layer on the surface of facial muscles between the upper lip and nasal ala in 85.2% cases.[7] Hence, it is best to inject in the dermal or immediate subdermal plane. Inadvertent injection into the facial artery can cause local skin necrosis as well as the dreaded complication of a retinal artery embolus causing central retinal artery occlusion (CRAO) and blindness through the angular artery—dorsal nasal artery anastomosis; though the latter is very rare.

POSTINJECTION INSTRUCTIONS

Following injection, any nodularity can be gently massaged in by the injector. Cool packs can be helpful in reducing swelling and bruising but in most scenarios, with judicious amount of filler use and careful injection technique, these are not required.

Ask the patient to avoid steam, sauna, and facial massage for the first 7 days after treatment. Heavy exercise should be avoided for at least 3 days. No alcohol should be consumed on the day of treatment. The patient should also avoid vitamin E, omega-3 fatty acid, aspirin, and NSAID ingestion for 3 days after treatment.

In the rare case requiring post-treatment analgesia, acetaminophen is the drug of choice. However, pain after filler injection is unusual and the patient should always be called back to the office to check for vascular compromise.

The patient must also be instructed to contact the treating physician immediately if there is significant bleeding, irregular swelling, dusky discoloration of the treated area, blurred vision, vision loss, or headache.

USEFUL TIPS

- The NLF is amongst the most common indications for which patients present to the cosmetic dermatologist.
- Injection techniques have shifted from direct filling of the fold to indirect correction via injection of the mid-face and zygomatic region.
- The facial artery lies in close proximity to the NLF and aspiration before injection is highly recommended.
- Due to the thick skin in this region it is rare to cause a Tyndall effect, still avoid injection too superficially.
- The ideal injection depth in this region is in the lower dermis or immediate hypodermis. A cannula can be used for additional safety as it is less likely to cause an intra-arterial injection but it must be kept in mind that this is not full proof. Another approach is to inject directly on the bone near the pyriform fossa using a needle.

REFERENCES

1. Rubin LR, Mishriki Y, Lee G. Anatomy of the nasolabial fold: the keystone of the smiling mechanism. Plast Reconstr Surg. 1989;83(1):1-10.
2. Day DJ, Littler CM, Swift RW, et al. The wrinkle severity rating scale: a validation study. Am J Clin Dermatol. 2004;5(1):49-52.
3. Carey W, Weinkle S. retraction of the plunger on a syringe of hyaluronic acid before injection: are we safe? Dermatol Surg. 2015;41(Suppl 1):S340-6.
4. Mathes DW, Furukawa M, Anzai Y. Evaluation of facial artery with computed tomographic angiography using 64-slice multidetector computed tomography: implications for facial reconstruction in plastic surgery. Plast Reconstr Surg. 2013;131(3):526-35.
5. Kim YS, Choi DY, Gil YC, et al. The anatomical origin and course of the angular artery regarding its clinical implications. Dermatol Surg. 2014;40(10):1070-6.
6. Yang HM, Lee JG, Hu KS, et al. New anatomical insights on the course and branching patterns of the facial artery: clinical implications of injectable treatments to the nasolabial fold and nasojugal groove. Plast Reconstr Surg. 2014;133(5):1077-82.
7. Lee JG, Yang HM, Choi YJ, et al. Facial arterial depth and relationship with facial muscular layer. Plast Reconstr Surg. 2015;135(2):437-44.

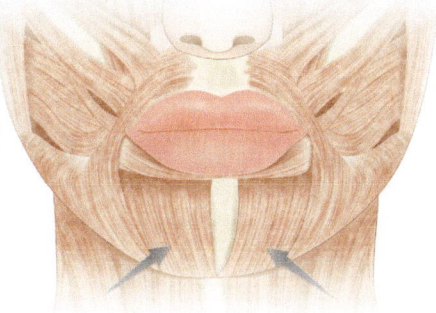

CHAPTER 18

Fillers for Lower Face—Marionette Lines

Richa Ojha Sharma

INDICATIONS

The central lower face, comprising the lips, chin, and mandible are the mobile structures of the face and have a significant contribution in overall facial expressions and appearance. Marionette lines are curvilinear creases beginning at the oral commissures and extending to the mandible. Also called melomental folds and sometimes mouth frown, they cause an appearance of drooping of the mouth leading to a sad or depressed look. This downturn of the oral commissures can be congenital, without any obvious anatomical abnormality, or it may be acquired.

ANATOMIC CONSIDERATIONS

Downturning of the angle of the mouth is often used for expressing emotions of sadness, dejection, dissatisfaction, and disgust **(Fig. 1)**. The muscle responsible for this downturn is the depressor anguli oris (DAO). It arises from the oblique line of the mandible and inserts in the modiolus of the mouth.[1] In younger individuals, frequent contraction of the DAO is the main cause of melomental folds.[2] It may be associated with malocclusion and hypognathia.[3]

Involution of almost all structures in the lower face occurs in the aging process that eventually leads to marionette lines.

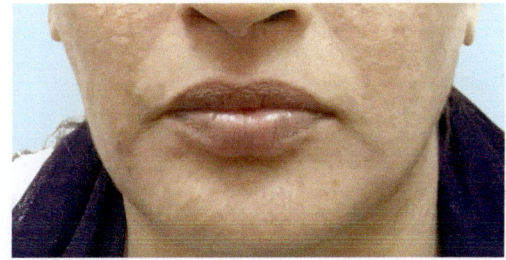

Fig. 1: Downturn of corner of mouth due to hyperactive DAO.
(DAO: depressor anguli oris)

There is atrophy of the submandibular fat compartments, along with dehiscence of the mandibular septum. This leads to a descent of the fat compartments toward the neck. This is further complicated by bone resorption and laxity of skin.[4]

The superficial musculoaponeurotic system, popularly known by the acronym SMAS, is located beneath the skin as a thin, yet strong, layer comprising of fibrous tissue. The SMAS begins just in front of and below the ear and extends downward to the neck where it merges with the platysma. The SMAS ensures that the muscles of facial expression of the midface work as a cohesive unit while emoting. The SMAS becomes lax with age causing sagging of the mid and lower face, resulting in changes such as prominent nasolabial and melomental folds, and jowl formation.[6]

Table 1: The marionette line grading scale.[6]

Grade	Features
0	No visible fold, continuous skin line
1	Shallow but visible fold with slight indentation
2	Moderately deep folds with clear feature at normal appearance but not when stretched
3	Very long and deep folds that are a prominent facial feature **(Fig. 2)**
4	Extremely long and deep folds that are detrimental to facial appearance

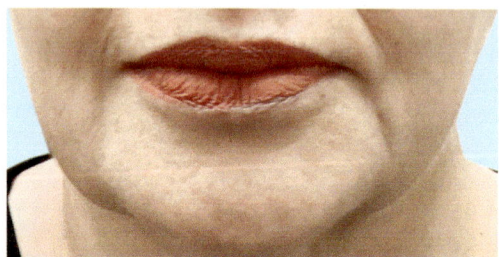

Fig. 2: Grade 2 marionette lines.

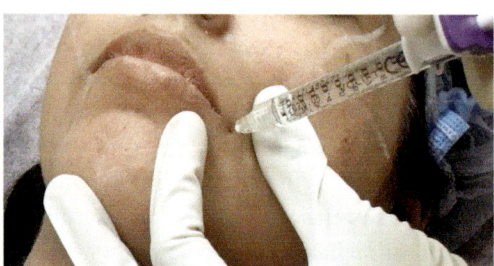

Fig. 3: Tower technique of filler injection into modiolus.

A five-point grading scale has been developed by Carruthers et al. This photonumeric scale was developed to quantify the severity of melomental folds and is summarized in **Table 1**.[6]

INJECTION TECHNIQUES

After understanding the etiology of marionette lines, it is clear that a multimodal approach works best for their treatment. A hyperactive DAO can first be relaxed with botulinum toxin so that the undue tug at the mouth corners while talking and emoting are reduced. This approach, though not essential, extends the longevity of the dermal filler in the region by reducing the muscular contraction that can accelerate hyaluronic acid (HA) absorption.[7] It has been found that treatment outcome and patient satisfaction are superior when botulinum toxin and HA filler injections are combined for perioral treatments.[8]

A high G′ and high viscosity HA filler will render a good lift and volume replacement in the area. Products used could be Restylane Lyft, Belotero Intense, Voluma, and Volift. A 30 G needle or 27 G cannula is used in this area.

The first step is to give support to the oral commissures and lower lip. For this two techniques are useful—(1) the needle is inserted just below the modiolus and filler is placed as a vertical column or tower, while withdrawing the needle. This gives support to the corner of the lip **(Fig. 3)**; (2) a horizontal line of filler is injected along the vermillon border of the lower lip in its lateral one-third.

Filler is then injected by a linear threading or serial puncture technique to fill the marionette line (slightly medial to the fold) **(Fig. 4)**. Sometimes cross hatching in the actual fold is done when there is substantial laxity of tissue.[9,10]

After this, the area medial to the fold is corrected. This can be done by cross hatching or fanning in the subcutaneous plane. This builds support, preventing overhang across the fold. Crosshatching is done by first inserting the needle from inferolateral part of the fold toward the lip and then perpendicularly, from the superolateral part of the fold toward the inferomedial area in the center of the chin.[3] For fanning, the entry point of the cannula is the lower end of the melomental fold and then moving the cannula in a V-shaped area out from the single entry point all over the medial area of the marionette fold.

Gentle massage is done to evenly spread the product. A volume of about 0.5–1.5 mL is needed for correction depending upon the deficit. Unlike in other areas such as the tear trough where undercorrection is aimed at in the first session, the aim of injection in the marionette fold is 100% correction and not over or undercorrection **(Figs. 5A and B)**. In many cases, injecting about 0.1–0.2 mL of filler into the lower lip to create subtle contouring goes a long way in creating an even and integrated look to the entire perioral area.

Midface fillers also indirectly improve marionette lines owing to lifting of the SMAS

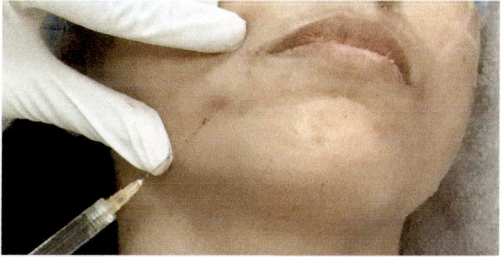

Fig. 4: Injection by linear threading into melomental fold.

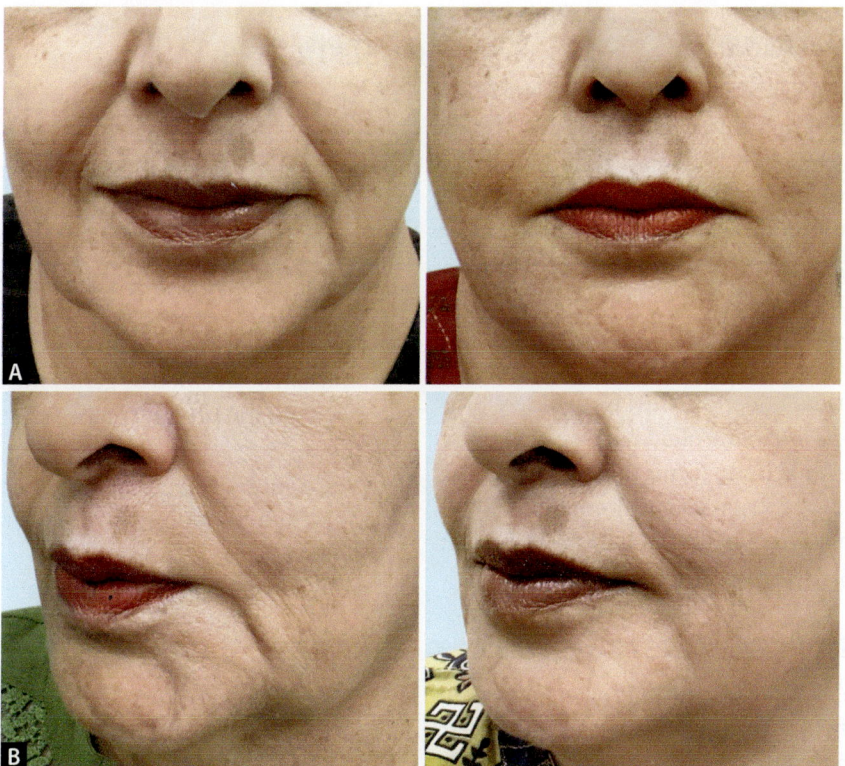

Figs. 5A and B: Improvement in marionette lines after filler injections in perioral area and midface.

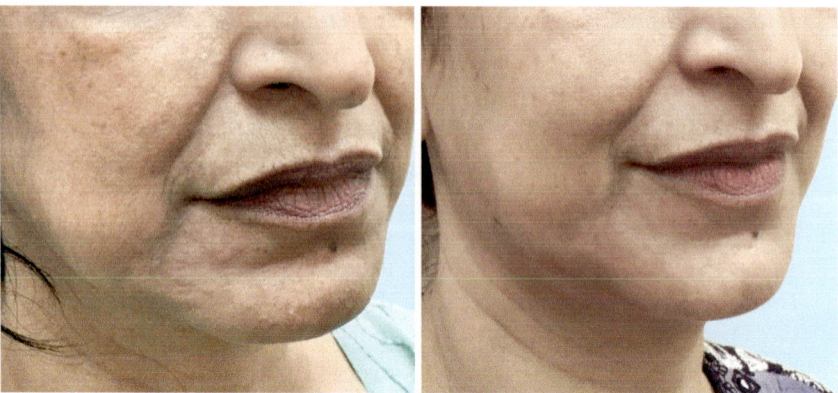

Fig. 6: Midface filler injections leading to lifting of SMAS causing improvement of marionette lines.
(SMAS: superficial musculoaponeurotic system)

(**Fig. 6**). Deep bolus filler placement with high G′ products in the malar area causes an indirect improvement in the depth of the marionette lines.[11]

PRECAUTIONS

The inferior labial and sublabial veins must be avoided in the area close to the modiolus. In the lower part of the fold mental artery, vein and nerve are to be avoided. Using cannulas minimizes bruising and more severe complications such as vaso-occlusive episodes. If bruising does appear, vitamin K, arnica, and bromelain may be used to alleviate it.[12] In order to prevent nodule and lump formation, intradermal injection must be avoided. Slow injections and controlled volume of product also prevents lump formation. If a nodule or lump is formed, massaging immediately helps, but sometimes hyaluronidase may be needed to dissolve the lump.

POSTINJECTION INSTRUCTIONS

An evaluation is done 1 week after the injection to assess the improvement, look for asymmetries and advise further treatment if needed. Standard postfiller precautions like avoiding facial steam, sauna, and massage for at least 7 days apply.

USEFUL TIPS

- Melomental folds are among the earliest signs of aging and are a cause for concern as they lead to a persistent sad appearance.
- The labial and mental arteries and veins must be avoided. This area is among the most prone to bruising after filler injections.[13]
- Nodulation and lumpiness are frequent and can be avoided by gently massaging to even out the product in the subcutaneous plane.
- The plane of injection for the modiolus is deep subcutaneous, while for the marionette fold it is subdermal or superficial subcutaneous.
- Midface volumization with deep bolus injections of high G′ fillers leads to an indirect improvement in the melomental folds due to an upward pull.

REFERENCES

1. Shimada K, Gasser RF. Variations in the facial muscles at the angle of the mouth. Clin Anat. 1989;2:129-34.
2. Choi YJ, Kim JS, Gil YC, et al. Anatomical considerations regarding the location and boundary of the depressor anguli oris muscle with reference to botulinum toxin injection. Plast Reconstr Surg. 2014;134(5):917-21.
3. Bae GY, Na JI, Park KC, et al. Nonsurgical correction of drooping mouth corners using monophasic hyaluronic acid and incobotulinumtoxinA. Cosmet Dermatol. 2019. [Epub ahead of print].
4. Braz A, Humphrey S, Weinkle S, et al. Lower face: Clinical anatomy and regional approaches with injectable fillers. Plast Reconstr Surg. 2015 Nov;136(Suppl 5):235S-57S.
5. Okuda I, Yoshioka N, Shirakabe Y, et al. Basic analysis of facial ageing: The relationship between the superficial musculoaponeurotic system and age. Exp Dermatol. 2019;28(Suppl 1):38-42.
6. Carruthers A, Carruthers J, Hardas B, et al. A validated grading scale for marionette lines. Dermatol Surg. 2008;34(Suppl 2):S167-72.
7. Carruthers J, Carruthers A. A multimodal approach to rejuvenation of the lower face. Dermatol Surg. 2016;42(Suppl 2):S89-93.
8. Carruthers A, Carruthers J, Monheit GD, et al. Multicenter, randomized, parallel-group study of the safety and effectiveness of onabotulinumtoxinA and hyaluronic acid dermal fillers (24-mg/ml smooth, cohesive gel) alone and in combination for lower facial rejuvenation. Dermatol Surg. 2010;36(Suppl 4):2121-34.
9. de Maio M, Wu WTL, Goodman GJ, et al. Facial assessment and injection guide for botulinum toxin and injectable hyaluronic acid fillers: Focus on the lower face. Plast Reconstr Surg. 2017;140(3):393e-404e.
10. Wollina U. Perioral rejuvenation: restoration of attractiveness in aging females by minimally invasive procedures. Clin Interv Aging. 2013;8:1149-55.
11. Wollina U. Facial rejuvenation starts in the midface: three-dimensional volumetric facial rejuvenation has beneficial effects on nontreated neighboring esthetic units. J Cosmet Dermatol. 2016;15(1):82-8.
12. Ho D, Jagdeo J, Waldorf HA. Is there a role for Arnica and Bromelain in prevention of post-procedure ecchymosis or edema? A systematic review of the literature. Dermatol Surg. 2016;42(4):445-63.
13. Alam, M, Tung R. Injection technique in neurotoxins and fillers: Indications, products, and outcomes. J Am Acad Dermatol. 2018;79(3):423-35.

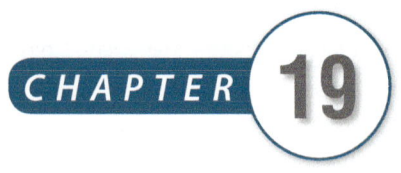
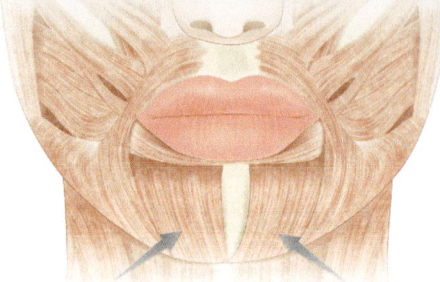

CHAPTER 19

Fillers for Lower Face—Chin

Gillian Ruth Britto, Rashmi Sarkar

INDICATIONS

The chin is unique to human beings and we have long speculated the reasons for its existence. Researchers have shown that due to evolution when our faces became smaller, it made the bone at the lower tip of the face more prominent. The chin aids in mastication by providing extra support to the jaw and protecting against mechanical stresses. Other possible uses of the chin could be assistance in speech and as a way to measure attractiveness when seeking a partner. A male chin is generally squarer while a female chin is more pointed and elongated.

Surgical correction was the gold standard method for treating chin asymmetry.[1] In recent times, filler injections have gained popularity as an efficient way of treating the retruded chin, square chin, a short chin or a double chin. The undesirable contour can also be treated with fillers.

ANATOMIC CONSIDERATIONS

The most centrally projecting aspect of the chin is the pogonion, whereas the menton is the most inferior component of the chin. The chin consists of the mentalis muscle. The muscle is cone shaped with its apex arising from the incisive fossa of the mandible. Its medial fibers descends anteromedially and cross together forming a dome-shaped pattern creating a V-shaped triangle which contains deep fat in the medial portion and connects laterally with the depressor labii inferioris (DLI). A contraction of the mentalis muscle produces wrinkling of the skin of the mentum **(Figs. 1 and 2)**.[2]

The chin should be assessed along with the lips, nose, and teeth at rest and in animation. The activity of the mentalis muscle and the surrounding soft tissue support should also be assessed. Photographs should be taken in all dimensions—anteroposterior, superoinferior, transversely, and obliquely.

Dr Robert Ricketts, an orthodontist, developed an assessment tool called the Rickett's esthetic line to assess proper balance from the lateral profile. To have a pleasing profile, if an imaginary line is drawn from the tip of the nose to the tip of the chin, the upper lip would be 4 mm and the lower lip 2 mm behind the line.[3] This assessment tool may determine if the chin needs to be augmented and provide the proper proportions **(Fig. 3)**.

Chin augmentation should take into consideration both the projection and elongation of the chin. The mandible may be small or positioned more posteriorly (retrognathia), or the chin itself may be small (microgenia), in the vertical or horizontal dimension. The lower face profile can be

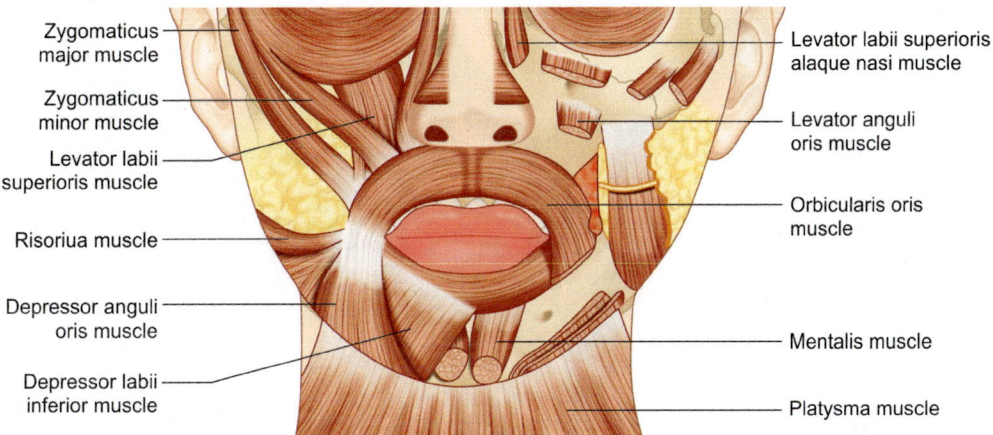

Fig. 1: Muscles of the face.

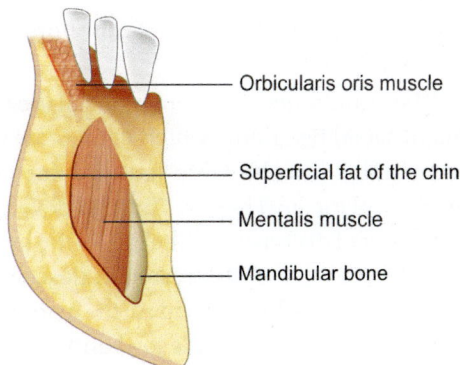

Fig. 2: Sagittal section of the chin.

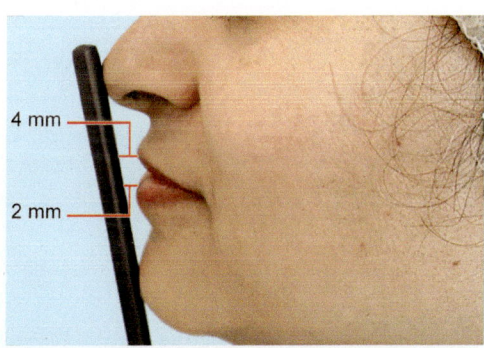

Fig. 3: Rickett's esthetic line to assess proper balance from the lateral profile, the upper lip would be 4 mm and the lower lip 2 mm behind the line.

classified into three types: Class 1, 2, and 3 as per Angle's classification **(Fig. 4)**.[4]

Class 1: Facial profile is usually balanced.

Class 2: Facial profile is usually convex (Retrognathia appears "chinless"; upper lip is far too forward from the lower lip).

Class 3: Facial profile is usually concave (Mandibular prognathism).

With respect to the mandible it was found in a study by Shaw et al. that the mandibular length and height decreased significantly in both sexes with aging.[5] The chin becomes more anterior, oblique, and shorter, which is significant when analyzing the face and planning appropriate treatment.[6] The protrusion of the chin further reduces by approximately 3–4 mm by the age of 60 in males and females.[7]

Hypertrophy of the mentalis muscle often leads to cobblestone appearance of the skin on the chin. Filler injection alone is often insufficient to bring about a significant improvement of shape due to strong contraction of the mentalis muscle. Therefore, treatment of this may require the combined use of botulinum toxin and fillers **(Fig. 5)**.

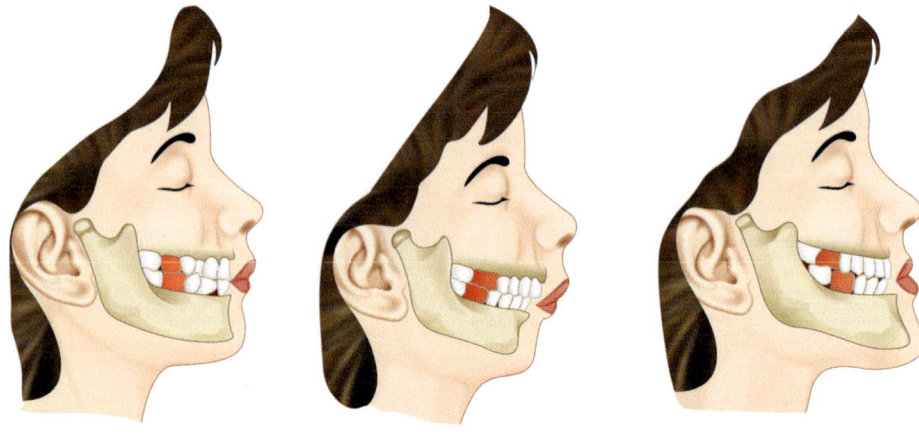

Fig. 4: Types of facial profiles based on the position of the lower jaw.

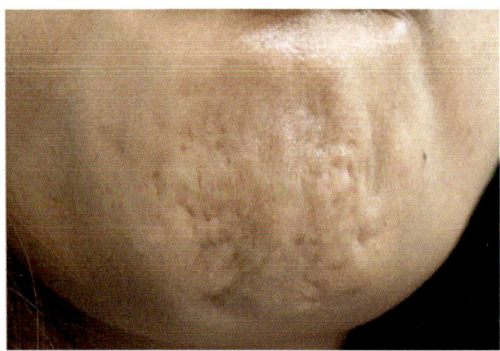

Fig. 5: Cobblestone appearance of the skin on the chin.

The chin is supplied by the submental artery which is the largest branch of cervical part of facial artery, given off when the artery separates from the submandibular gland. It ascends upwards running over the mylohyoid muscle, passes over the mandible, and terminates by dividing into superficial and deep branches. It anastomoses with the branches of sublingual and inferior alveolar artery and supplies the chin and the lower lip. The mental artery which is the branch of the inferior alveolar artery along with the mental nerve exits the mental foramen (located at the longitudinal axis of the 2nd premolar tooth, a finger's breadth above the inferior border of the mandible).[2]

The mandibular ligament is one of the two major facial ligaments which demarcate the transition from the labio mandibular fold above and the jowl below. The jowl develops as a result of distension of the roof of the lower premasseter space with resultant descent of the soft tissues below the body of the mandible. The more pronounced the jowl appears, the more apparent is the dimpling or tethering of the mandibular ligament. It is important to recognize this as it may affect the esthetic appearance of the chin. The dimpling and tethering effect cannot be effaced with dermal fillers or botulinum toxin and may only be corrected surgically.[2]

INJECTION TECHNIQUES

A needle of 27G with HA of a high G prime is used. In case of females, where a more pointed or triangular chin is desired, we mark two injection points on the chin, drawn by two vertical lines from the ala of the nose to the anterior aspect of the chin **(Figs. 6, 7A and C)**.

In case of males, where a squarer chin is desired, the injection points correspond to two vertical lines drawn from the angles of the mouth to the anterior aspect of the chin (**Figs. 6 and 7B**).

About 0.1–0.5 mL per injection site is administered. The injection is at an angle of 90° and the plane is periosteal.

For elongation of the chin, the needle is directed vertically upwards at an angle of 90° at the mentum. **Table 1** summarizes these points.

Chin correction can be combined with the following to improve results:
- *Combination treatment of chin with toxins*: Due to repeated contractions of the mentalis muscles, dimpling of the skin over the chin maybe seen. This leads to a flattened chin and a deep mental crease. Therefore, combining dermal filler augmentation with botulinum toxin injection for the mentalis muscle can improve the desired outcome.

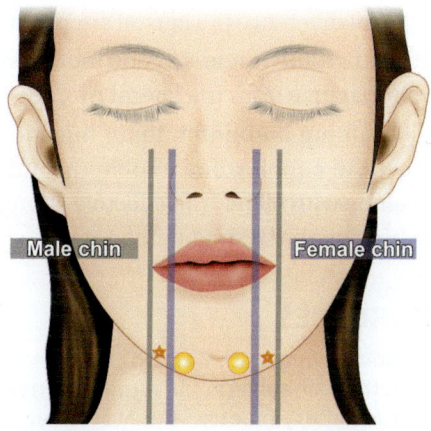

Fig. 6: Landmarks for administering the filler.

Table 1: Aims: Lengthening, protrusion or narrowing. The same technique applies for needle and cannula.

Type/criteria	Parameters/technique
Cannula type	25 G/27 G–38 mm
Needle type	27 G
HA (hyaluronic acid) concentration	24–25 mg +
Landmarks	Front side of chin—two injection sites as shown in picture
Angle of insertion	90° (periosteal)
Quantity	0.5–0.1 mL per injection site

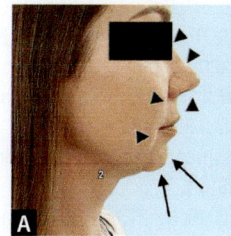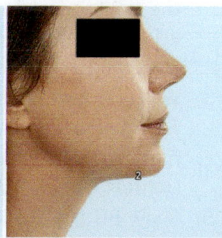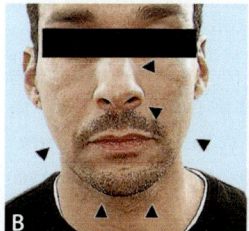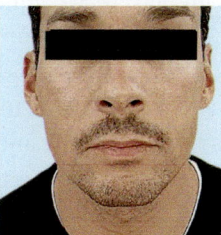

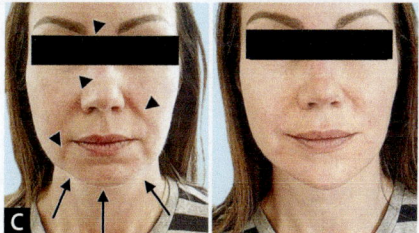

Figs. 7A to C: Before and after clinical pictures.
(*Courtesy*: Dr Zack Ally)

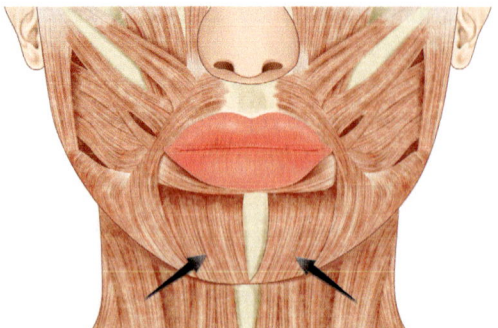

Fig. 8: Points of injection for botulinum toxin.

- *Procedure and method of injection*: Two injections sites 1 cm apart at the center of the chin is marked out. 2.5 units of Botox© at each injection site is given. Dilution is 2 mL 0.9% saline in 100 units of Botox©—5 units per 0.1 mL.
- The muscle is grabbed between the thumb and the index finger and the needle is directed at 90° angle **(Fig. 8)**.

- *Dermal filler in the mental crease*: The mental crease is the area between the lower lip and chin. Contraction of the mentalis muscle elevates the lower lip and contributes to the mental crease. Concurrent treatment with chin augmentation can enhance results.
  - *Procedure and method of injection*: Filler is injected at multiple levels in the dermis and subdermal subcutaneous tissue to elevate the crease. A combination of linear threading both parallel and perpendicular to the crease can be used.

SIDE EFFECTS AND COMPLICATIONS

Hyaluronic acid dermal fillers are becoming popular all over the world. However, complications arising due to vascular compromise are becoming more common. Therefore, a thorough knowledge about the blood vessels in the face is imperative to avoiding such complications. The chin is a relatively safe area for filler injections especially due to the fact that the injections are periosteal. However, the usage of needle can lead to severe bruising and care should be taken to avoid this.

USEFUL TIPS

A subtle correction of the chin can make a significant difference to a person's appearance.

Rickett's esthetic line is a good tool to assess proper balance from the lateral profile.

Combining botulinum toxin injection to correct the cobblestone appearance of the chin along with fillers is an effective approach to achieving the desired outcome.

REFERENCES

1. Christou T, Kau CH, Waite PD, et al. Modified method of analysis for surgical correction of facial asymmetry. Ann Maxillofac Surg. 2013;3(2):185-91.
2. Standring S, Borley NR, Gray H. Gray's anatomy: the anatomical basis of clinical practice. 40th ed., anniversary ed. [Edinburgh]: Churchill Livingstone/Elsevier. 2008.
3. Ward J, Podda S, Garri JL, et al. Chin deformities. J Craniofac Surg. 2007;18(4):887-94.
4. Angle EH (1899). Classification of malocclusion. Dental Cosmos. 4:248-64.
5. Shaw RB Jr, Katzel EB, Koltz PF, et al. Aging of the facial skeleton: aesthetic implications and rejuvenation strategies. Plast Reconstr Surg. 2011;127(1):374-83.
6. Pessa JE, Slice DE, Hanz KR, et al. Aging and the shape of the mandible. Plast Reconstr Surg. 2008;121(1):196-200.
7. Sykes JM, Fitzgerald R. Choosing the best procedure to augment the chin: is anything better than an implant? Facial Plast Surg. 2016;32(5):507-12.

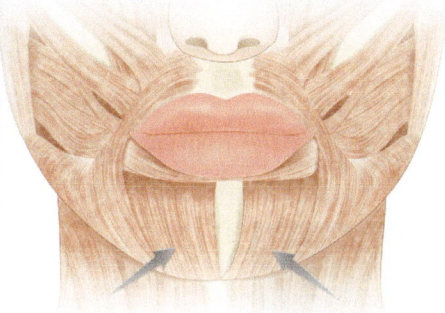

CHAPTER 20

Fillers for Lower Face—Jawline

Hema Pant, Gillian Ruth Britto, Vivek Nair

INDICATIONS

Facial aging often presents with a loss of continuity that comes with a straight, youthful jawline. This occurs due to fat atrophy and volume loss from bone resorption and tissue decent. Facial jowling can be worsened by the attenuation of the mandibular septum leading to the descent of the superior and inferior jowl fat compartments. Fillers of the lower face are mainly indicated at the meliomental folds, jawline (including the angle of the mandible), and chin. An ideal jawline demonstrates relatively sharp and angular transitions to the neck, as a sharp jawline frames the lower third of the face.

ANATOMIC CONSIDERATIONS

The mandible bone forms the jawline and consists of the ramus that projects with two processes called the coronoid process, to which the temporal muscle attaches, and the neck and condyle process, which is topped by the articular surface, forming the mandibular part of the temporomandibular joint. Between these two processes of the ramus is the mandibular notch. The large masseter muscle attaches to almost the entire surface of the ramus of the mandible. There are two important foraminae, one each side, transmitting the inferior alveolar branches of the mandibular branch of the trigeminal nerve **(Fig. 1)**.[1]

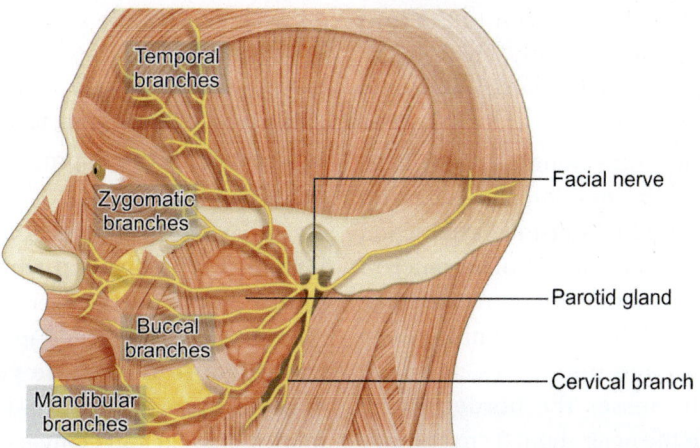

Fig. 1: Anatomy of the face.

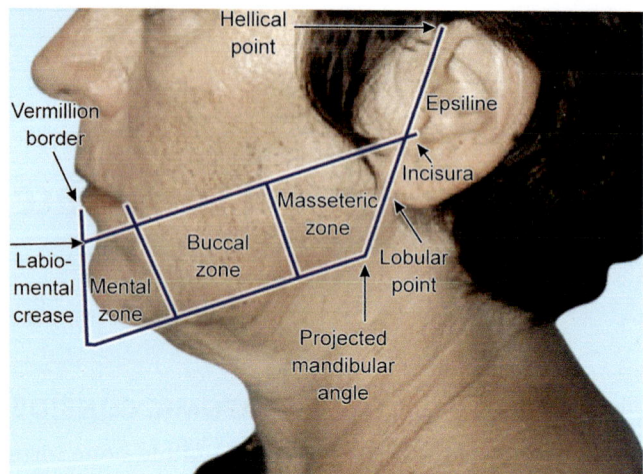

Fig. 2: Zones in the lower jaw.
(*Source*: Moradi A, Shirazi A, David R. Nonsurgical Chin and Jawline Augmentation Using Calcium Hydroxylapatite and Hyaluronic Acid Fillers. Facial Plastic Surgery. 2019; 35:140-8)

Superficial fat pads are an important consideration when it comes to injectables. The superior and inferior jowl (or mandibular) fat pads lie anteriorly over the anterolateral surface of the body of the mandible. They are separated by ligaments which give rise to the aging appearance of the lower face. The mandibular septum, which separates the jowl fat pads from the neck fat and is adherent to the anterior surface of the body of the mandible, and the mandibular cutaneous ligament, which tethers the skin anterior to the jowl fat pads to the bone anteriorly, creating the groove seen anterior to the jowl with descent of the fat pads with age **(Fig. 2)**.[2]

The facial artery runs along the deep plane, just anterior to the masseter muscle and further upward in a superior-medial direction **(Fig. 3)**. The marginal mandibular branch of the facial nerve is another important structure to be aware of when injecting. Running deep to the platysma and the depressor anguli oris (DAO), it crosses the border of the mandible from the neck about 3 cm anterior to the angle of the mandible, always superficial to the facial artery and anterior facial vein, and provides motor supply to the depressor labii inferioris, DAO, and mentalis, and communicates with the inferior alveolar nerve.[3]

The jawline in males are much larger stronger and heavier with more definition at the angle and ramus of the mandible. They have a higher muscle bulk generally. The bigonial width is wider and approximates the bimalar width giving a squarer appearance. In the profile view, the male jaw at the gonial angle appears to be squarer with an angle of 90°. The jawbone visually appears to be a stabilizing a supportive platform to the upper and midface. The chin is wider and more square and should approximate the corners of the mouth.[4]

The jawline in females is more slender and V-shaped. The bigonial width is narrower, thus accentuating the overriding cheekbone prominences. The jawline appears curvilinear and lifted. In the profile view, the gonial angle measures about 110–120°. The chin is more V-shaped and elongated and the width approximates the interalar distance of the nose.[4]

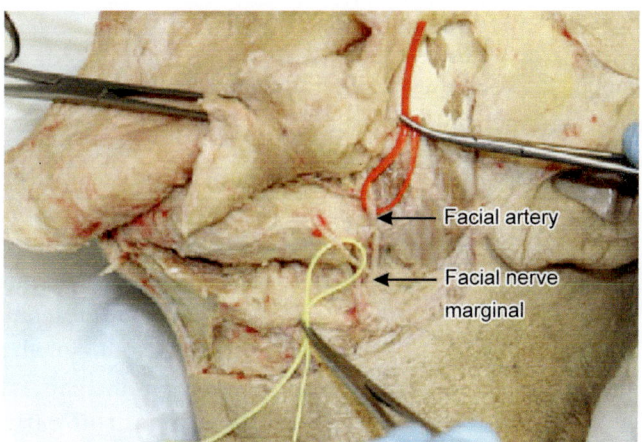

Fig. 3: Anatomical location of facial artery and facial nerve.
(*Source*: Moradi A, Shirazi A, David R. Nonsurgical Chin and Jawline Augmentation Using Calcium Hydroxylapatite and Hyaluronic Acid Fillers. Facial Plastic Surgery. 2019;35:140-8)

INJECTION TECHNIQUES

It is important to correct the midface region before working on the lower face since the former automatically improves the latter to a certain degree by pulling up the face.

Fillers with a high G-prime are used as fillers in the jaw area, since these are subject to a number of deforming forces. Depth of injections is supraperiosteal for thicker molecules. Prejowl and mandible body can be injected with 21 G cannula for better cosmetic outcome. Cannulas also ensure minimal bruising and are safer with respect to avoiding the facial artery as it crosses the mandible.

When planning correction of the jawline, one must assess both the dynamic and static factors leading to a loss of the ideal smooth and sharply defined contour of the area. Dynamic factors are the pull of the platysma on an aging face as well as the pull of the DAO muscle in the chin. These should be ideally addressed with botulinum toxin before planning fillers. If skin tightening is planned then again it should be done a few months before doing fillers—this decreases filler requirement and improves esthetic outcomes.

While injecting the mandible, it is important to mark out the facial artery crossing the mandible, this occurs at the anterior border of the masseter and then to inject on either side of it; avoid crossing the artery with either a needle or cannula. A slow retrograde technique with the cannula making sure it is as deep as possible is safe. With a needle small supraperiosteal boluses can be placed and gently massaged linearly. Following this another layer of the filler can be injected on top for smoothening out the contour.

A bolus injection near the angle of the mandible can serve a tethering function to pull the jawline and make it more defined. While doing this, avoid injecting too high up on the face to avoid the parotid gland. Also avoid squaring up the jaw in a female patient.

If the chin area needs work then it is best to correct it along with the jawline. This, as well as marionette line correction, is addressed elsewhere in the book.

PRECAUTIONS

As long as the facial artery is avoided while injecting the jawline, this part of the face is among the safer zones to inject filler in. The fact that the facial artery can be exactly palpated is a big advantage—this is unlike most other areas of the face where the presence of vasculature must be inferred by demographic patterns.

That said the jawline is very sensitive to asymmetry and so it is important to balance both sides while injecting and to avoid superficial injections which are visible as lumps under the skin. Such lumps can usually be easily massaged into the skin if they occur inadvertently.

POSTINJECTION INSTRUCTIONS

Following injection, any nodularity can be gently massaged in by the injector. Cool packs can be helpful in reducing swelling and bruising but in most scenarios, with judicious amount of filler use and careful injection technique, these are not required. Avoid pillow pressure for 48–72 hours.

Ask the patient to avoid steam, sauna, and facial massage for the first 7 days after treatment. Heavy exercise should be avoided for at least 3 days. No alcohol should be consumed on the day of treatment. The patient should also avoid vitamin E, omega-3 fatty acid, aspirin, and nonsteroidal anti-inflammatory drug (NSAID) ingestion for 3 days after treatment.

In the rare case, requiring post-treatment analgesia acetaminophen is the drug of choice. However, pain after filler injection is unusual and the patient should always be called back to the office to check for vascular compromise.

The patient must also be instructed to contact the treating physician immediately, if there is significant bleeding, irregular swelling, or dusky discoloration of the treated area.

USEFUL TIPS

- Do not treat the jawline in isolation. Always try and correct the midface before working on the lower face.
- The jawline is shaped by both dynamic factors (platysmal and DAO action) and static factors [superficial musculoaponeurotic system (SMAS) descent, fat pad descent, mandibular resorption]. Hence, correction should account for all of these.
- The size of the chin is also an important determinant of early jowl formation; smaller chins are more prone to lead to the appearance of jowling with even mild facial descent. Correcting the chin can improve jowl appearance without even injecting the jawline in such cases.
- The jawline is a particularly product hungry area and it is not uncommon to require 1–2 mL of filler on each side for adequate correction.
- It is very important to mark the facial artery as it crosses the mandible and to avoid crossing it with either a needle or cannula while injecting.

REFERENCES

1. Hur MS, Hu KS, Cho JY, Kwak HH, Song WC, Koh KS et al. Topography and location of the depressor anguli oris muscle with a reference to the mental foramen. Surg Radiol Anat. 2008; 30(5):403-7.
2. Reece EM, Pessa JE, Rohrich RJ. The mandibular septum: anatomical observations of the jowls in aging-implications for facial rejuvenation. Plast Reconstr Surg. 2008;121(4):1414-20.
3. Alghoul M, Codner MA; Retaining ligaments of the face: review of anatomy and clinical applications. Aesthetic Surg J, 2013;33(6): 769-82.
4. Mommaerts MY. The ideal male jaw angle—An Internet survey. J Craniomaxillofac Surg. 2016; 44(4):381-91.

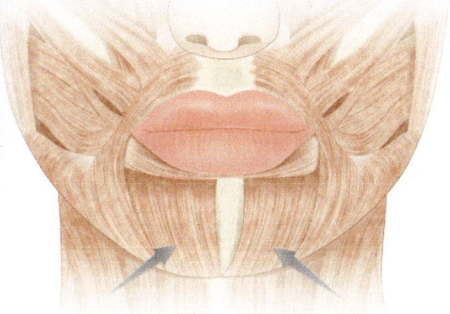

CHAPTER 21

Fillers for Lower Face—Lip Augmentation

Gillian Ruth Britto

INTRODUCTION

For centuries, luscious and voluminous lips have been considered as a sign of beauty. As far back as the ancient Egyptians, Queen Cleopatra used red lip paint to highlight her lips. Currently, lip augmentation procedures are being performed as frequently as every 20 minutes worldwide. The American Society of Plastic Surgeons' reported a 50% increase of lip treatments between 2000 and 2017. In the last years, more than 27,000 lip procedures were performed in 1 year alone in the US.[1]

Lips come in various shapes and sizes, which follow a racial predisposition, e.g. individuals of African descent have genetically voluminous lips, which are well known. Visually attractive lips usually follow the Da Vinci's golden ratio, where the upper lip to lower lip ratio is 1 to 1.618 and was a proportion that many Renaissance artists considered perfect in relation to the human profile. However, these anthropometric measurements refer to Caucasians, and need not necessarily be considered while treating patients of other ethnicities. Moreover, ideal lips for any person would depend upon the skills of the medical practitioner and the patient's expectations.

LIP ASSESSMENT

Lip augmentation procedures involve elaborate, intricate, and varied treatments. Patients may present with lip asymmetry, lack of vermillion volume, vertical lip lines due to a strong orbicularis oris muscle, down turned mouth corners, and/or elongated upper lip due to normal aging process.

Lips should be assessed from the frontal view, at rest and in animation to determine any asymmetries. The lips should be seen from the lateral profile to determine proper balance by using the Ricketts esthetic line, an assessment tool developed by Dr Robert Ricketts in 1950. The assessment examines the relationship of the upper and lower lips by drawing an imaginary line from the tip of the nose to the tip of the chin. To have a pleasing facial profile, in an average Caucasian face the lower lip should be 2 mm behind the line and the upper lip 4 mm behind the line, with variations being normal for patients of different ethnic backgrounds, but with some commonalities applying to all patients **(Fig. 1)**. The assessment tool may determine, if the chin needs to be augmented and will provide the proper proportions.

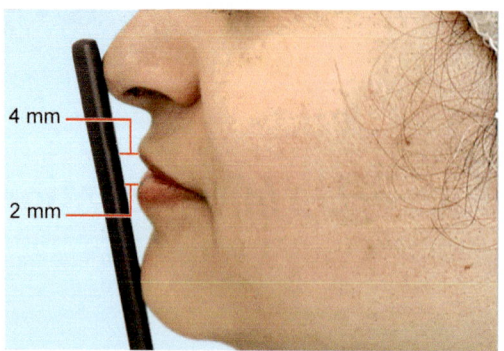

Fig. 1: Ricketts' esthetic line to assess proper balance from the lateral profile, the upper lip would be 4 mm and the lower lip 2 mm behind the line.

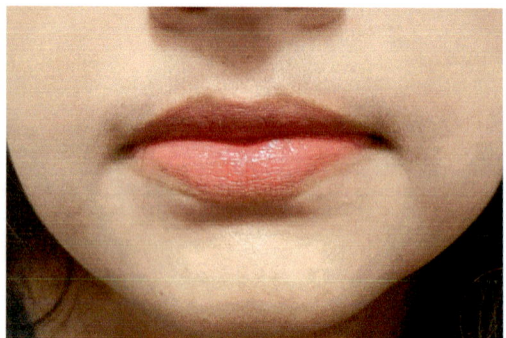

Fig. 3: Ideal lip proportions.

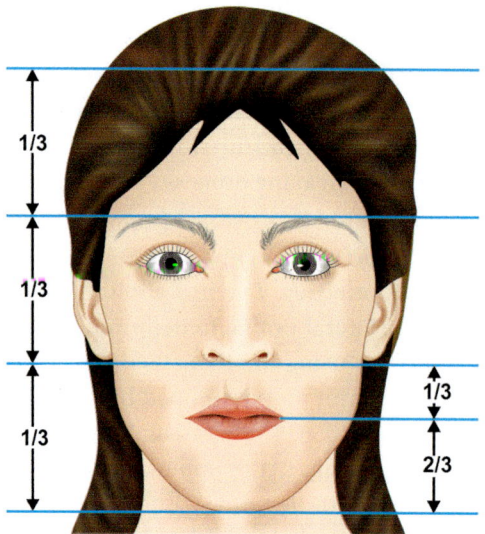

Fig. 2: Face proportions—frontal view.

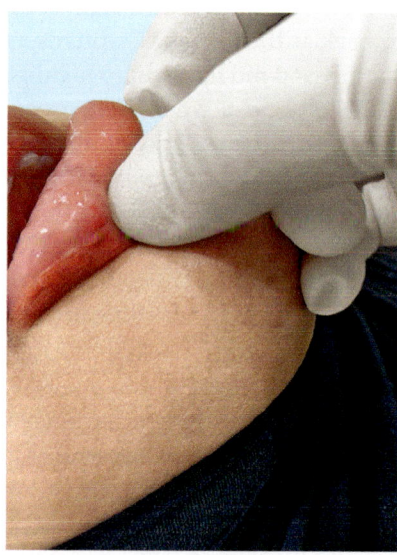

Fig. 4: Lumps caused by hyaluronic acid filler.

In the frontal view, the facial analysis commonly divides into three equal horizontal thirds **(Fig. 2)**. The lower third of the face consists of the portion from the subnasale to the menton. The lower lip (lower vermillion border to the menton) is twice the height of the upper lip complex (from the upper vermillion to the subnasale).

To also achieve natural lip symmetry, the upper lip should be 70–80% the volume of the lower lip **(Fig. 3)**.[2]

Before the treatment, the injector should carry out an examination by looking, feeling, and moving the lips.
- *Look at:* Size, shape, volume, cupid's bow, oral commissures, asymmetry, scars, lumps dryness, and profile balancing
- *Feel for:* Lumps, bumps, scar tissue, old filler
- *Movement:* Ask patient to smile and flip their lips to view the inside and the mucosa in case they have had fillers before which may have left old lumps **(Fig. 4)**.

ANATOMY OF THE LIP

The upper lip consists of three sub units; the central philtrum and the two lateral subunits and the lower lip a single subunit. The esthetic upper lip has a flattened "M" configuration at the vermillion—cutaneous junction, commonly referred to as "cupid's bow". At the border of the cutaneous portion to the mucosa, the vermillion border is a raised area of skin of variable prominence known as the "white roll", which is a defining outline and the result of light reflection from this area. The vermillion is red due to the absence of keratin and the closely underlying rich vascular plexus. The most superficial layer of the lips is the epidermis, followed by the subcutaneous tissue orbicularis oris muscle fibers and the mucosa. The orbicularis oris is the primary muscle of the oral commissure responsible for lip animation. It is comprised of two components superficial and deep. The superficial component is responsible for closing the lips and lip protrusion. The deep component helps in pressing the lips against the teeth.[3]

The orbicularis oris muscle inserts and fuses with the depressor anguli oris (DAO) and risorius muscles at the oral commissure known as the modiolus **(Figs. 5 to 7)**.

PERIORAL MUSCLES AND THEIR ACTIONS

Perioral muscles and their actions have been given in **Table 1**.

BLOOD AND NERVE SUPPLY

Muscles of the lips receive motor nerve innervation from the facial nerve and sensory innervation from the maxillary and mandibular branches of the trigeminal nerve. Blood supply to both the lips is via the superior and inferior labial arteries. These branches of the facial artery are located deep to the mucosa and the orbicularis oris muscle. The arteries run about 5 mm deep along the upper and lower lip between the muscle and mucosa. Therefore, superficial injections to the vermillion border are usually considered safe.

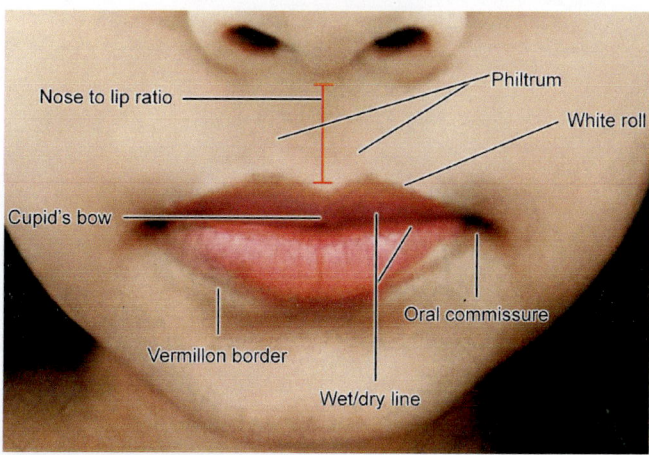

Fig. 5: Anatomy of the lip.

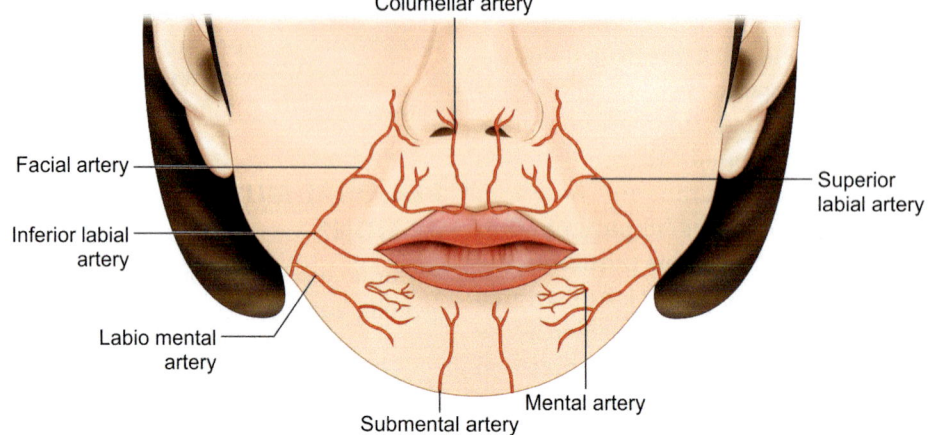

Fig. 6: Perioral blood vasculature.

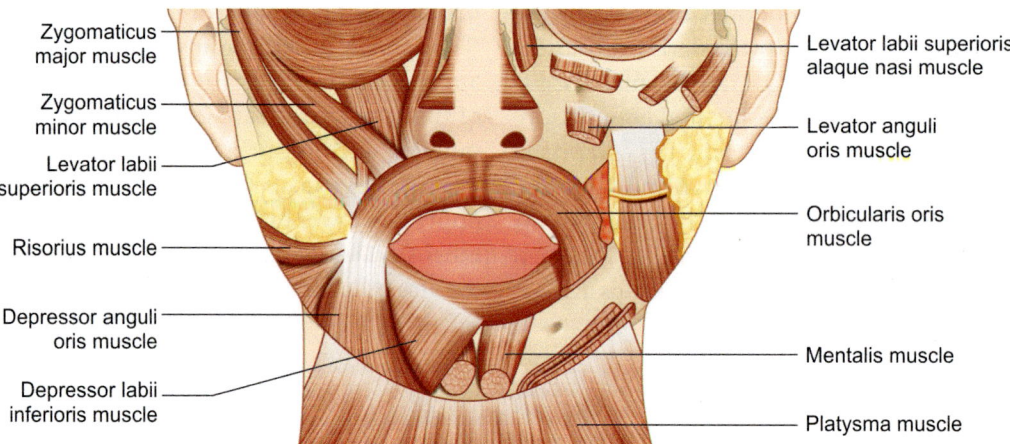

Fig. 7: Perioral muscles.

Table 1: Perioral muscles and their actions.	
Muscle	Action
Orbicularis oris	Fine/sphincteric movements
Levator labii superioris	Pulls upper lip upward
Zygomaticus major/minor, risorius, and buccinator	Pull corners laterally
Depressor anguli oris	Pull corners downward
Depressor labii inferioris	Depresses lower lip
Mentalis	Pushes lower lip upward

AGE-RELATED CHANGES

The perioral area with its abundant blood supply and frequent movements ages more rapidly than other areas of the face. With advancing age, the lips lose their shape, volume and moisture, looking dry and thin with downturned corners, and barcodes (smoker's lines) forming. The mental crease (horizontal line under the lower lip) can deepen, and nasolabial folds, marionette lines, and jowls become deeper and descend. It is important to take the whole perioral area into consideration when treating lips in middle aged and older patients. Very often, a combination of treatments provides an infinitely more esthetically pleasing outcome **(Fig. 8)**.

PROCEDURE

Informed consent should be obtained from the patient. Photographs must be taken both from the frontal and lateral view **(Figs. 9 to 11)**. The majority of patients receive a combination of topical, local, and regional anesthesia. Topical anesthetic creams such as eutectic mixture of local anesthesia (EMLA) and benzocaine are applied 15–30 minutes prior to the procedure. Regional anesthesia includes infraorbital and mental nerve blocks with 1% lidocaine and 1:200,000 epinephrine.

Another option is to use a cold ice pack, which can help relieve swelling as well as temporarily numbing the area. Vibration devices such as the Vibrata act as a distraction during injections and can be helpful for some anxious patients **(Fig. 12)**. In some cases, patients either prefer not to have any anesthesia or cannot have it due to previous hypersensitivity reactions. For the latter group, a dermal filler without local anesthesia is recommended.

PRODUCT CHOICE

Various factors to be considered while choosing the ideal lip filler would depend on:
- Personal choice of the patient and injector
- Experience with certain products
- Cost of the product
- Longevity.

It is recommended that nonpermanent fillers consisting of hyaluronic acid (HA) are used for lip augmentation as they are linked to fewer side effects and long-term complications. They are also the only dermal

25 years old   35 years old   45 years old

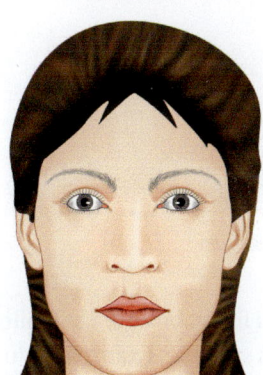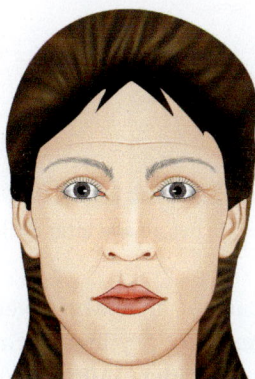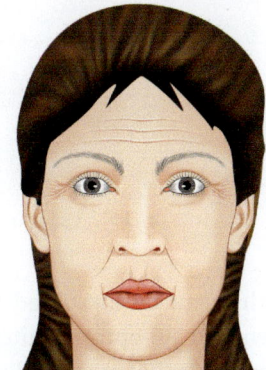

Fig. 8: Aging facial changes.

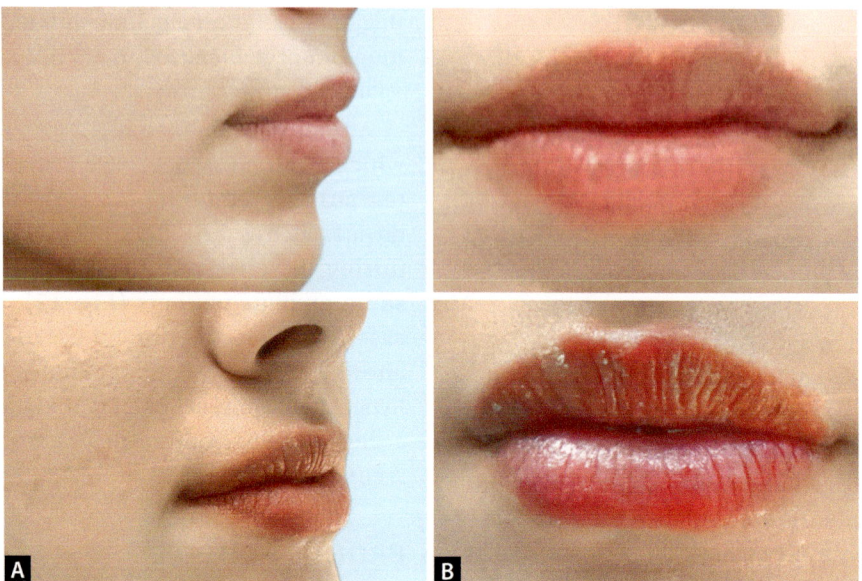

Figs. 9A and B: Before and after clinical pictures.

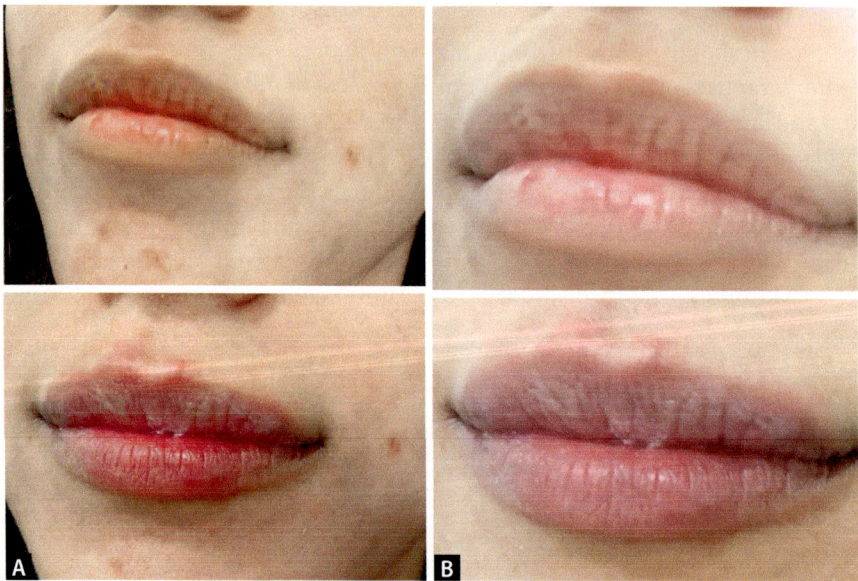

Figs. 10A and B: Before and after clinical pictures.

fillers that can be dissolved in case of an emergency or suboptimal outcome.

For patients that are middle aged or older and want a very subtle change, and for those who never had fillers before, a soft filler with a low G-prime is suitable. Examples—Juvéderm Ultra smile, Volbella, Teosyal RHA 2, and Intraline 1.

Chapter 21: Fillers for Lower Face—Lip Augmentation

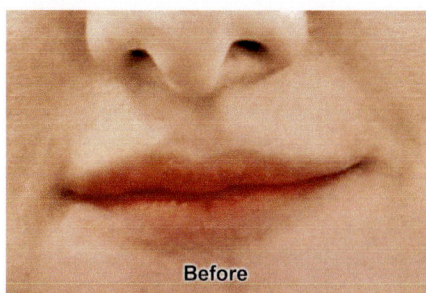
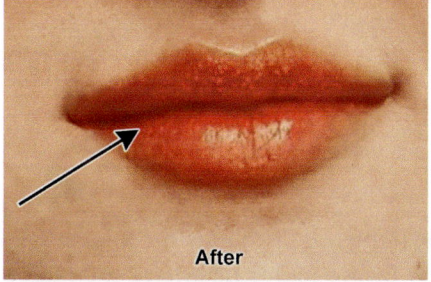

Fig. 11: Before and after clinical pictures (Black arrow).
(*Courtesy:* Dr Zack Ally)

For patients who want a noticeable and lasting result, a medium thickness filler is a good choice. Examples—Juvéderm 3, Intraline 2, and Teosyal RHA 3.

Some clients are looking for a drastic change with plenty of volume, protrusion, and plumpness. They often require multiple treatments over time to achieve the desired look. Suitable products would be a thick and long-lasting filler, which attracts more fluid to the lips. Examples–Juvéderm Volift and Teosyal Kiss.

INJECTION TECHNIQUES

Vermillion Border

Injecting the vermillion border gives a subtle volume but mainly enhances the shape **(Fig. 13)**.

Technique

- Insert the whole needle superficially at 10–20° angle in the pink part of the border
- Retrograde injection with small amount of filler 0.05–0.1 mL
- Continue around the whole lip contour.

Plumping and Volumization

Linear threading can be used inside the body of the lip with a similar technique as above to achieve volumization **(Fig. 14)**.

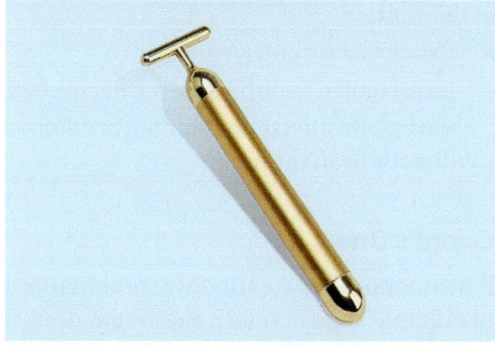

Fig. 12: Vibrata was introduced by Simon Ourian, MD for pain management during cosmetic procedures.

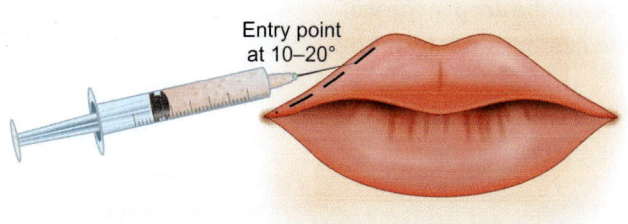

Fig. 13: Technique for vermillion border enhancement.

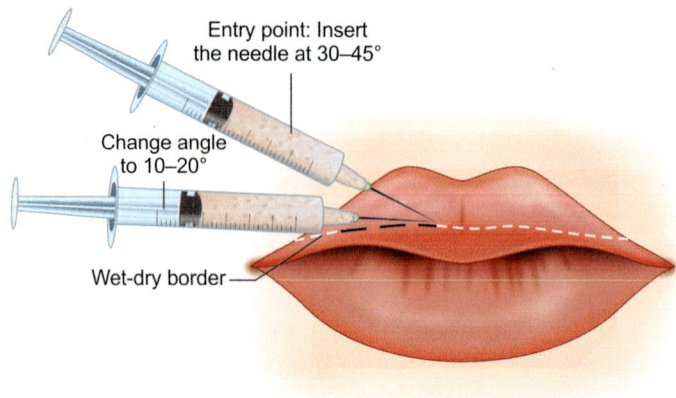

Fig. 14: Technique for plumping and volumizing the lip.

Technique
- Insert half the needle deep in the wet-dry border of the lip at 30-45° angle.
- Change angle/flatten and insert the whole needle before retrograde injection with small amount of filler 0.05-0.1 mL—stop injecting while one-third of the needle is still in the lip tissue to avoid creating superficial lumps.
- Can be done in the upper and lower lips.

Bolus Injections Technique
This is excellent for central volumization, where the patients request extra plumpness in the middle of their lips, particularly the lower lip.
- Pinch the lower lip between your fingers and insert half the needle deep in the wet-dry border at the center of the lower lip at 90°.
- Hold the needle still and inject a bolus of 0.05-0.1 mL of filler, massage gently.

Vectoring/Vertical Fanning
With this technique, only one entry point is used, with fanning in different directions via linear threads. It helps with lifting the cupid's bow in the upper lip where the injections are placed at the "peaks" on each side of the cupid's bow. The same technique can be used in the lower lip to help creating a "drop effect" at the center.
- Use the same entry/exit point.
- Insert half to two-thirds of the needle with retrograde injections, fanning in different directions in the area.

Cupid's Bow Lift
For this popular treatment, combinations of different injection techniques are used to enhance the cupid's bow in order to make it more peaked and prominent **(Fig. 15)**.
- Starting from the "peaks" of the upper lip, insert the needle superficially and inward at 10-20° angle, stopping when reaching the center point.
- At this point, rotate the syringe upward to 90° until it touches the side of the nostril, and inject as you come out. Repeat on the opposite side.
- To further enhance the cupid's bow, inject two little punctures at the top of the "peaks" on each side.

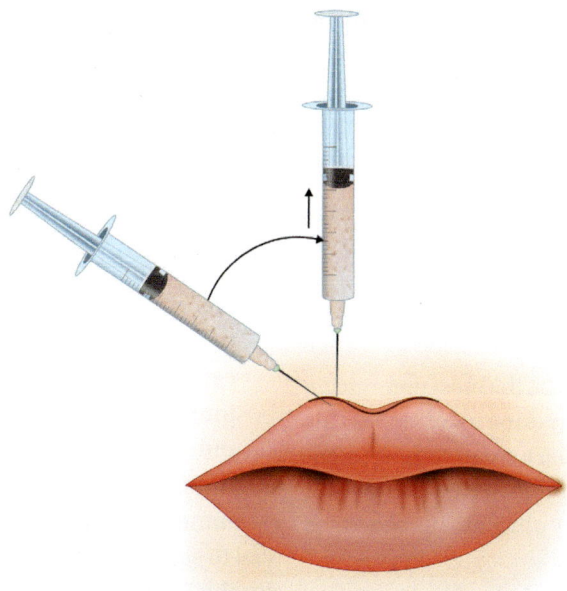

Fig. 15: Technique for cupid bow's enhancement.

Enhance the Philtrum Columns

Pinch each philtrum column, insert the whole needle at 10–20°, starting at the peak going upward toward the nasal septum, and inject a thin retrograde linear thread.

Lip Contouring

This is very similar to vermillion border injections with the difference of adding a twisting motion during injecting. The technique allows the injector to reshape the lip borders and making them rounder. The aim is to define rather than enlarge.
- Insert the whole needle superficially at 10–20° angle at the pink part of the vermillion border.
- Retrograde linear threads are injected while moving the wrist in a twisting motion.

Upturned Mouth Corners

Depending on severity, downturned mouth corners can be corrected using both botulinum toxin and dermal fillers. This treatment is different from filler in the marionette lines and intended to correct minor descent.
- Insert the needle from above the oral commissure, retrograde injection while curving the needle upward at the corners.
- Place a small bolus of filler in the oral commissure at 90° angle.

Tenting Technique

Tenting can seem very painful as a large number of injections are inserted from the border of the lips toward the wet-dry border in the center, with just a few mm between each injection point. It is always advisable to start filling the vermillion border first to allow the area to become numb before moving on to tenting. Small microdroplets of 0.025–0.05 mL of filler is used for each injection which minimizes the risk of lumpiness occurring.
- Insert the needle starting at the vermillion border, toward the wet-dry border at the center of the lip.

- Be careful not to insert the needle too deep as this can leave lumps of filler in the wet-dry border.
- Retrograde injections of tiny amounts of filler around the whole lip, upper, and lower.
- Varying depth according to lip shape.

SIDE EFFECTS AND COMPLICATIONS

Unfortunately, lips can be the most unforgiving area, if the treatment is done incorrectly. This is due to the space being a small compartment with fairly superficial injections. Lumps and asymmetry can be very obvious, and the tissue is extremely sensitive.

Complications can be classified based on onset.

Early (Minutes–Days)

- Redness—occurs with most lip fillers but usually subsides within the same day.
- Swelling—extremely common side effect, which could last for a few days up to a few weeks.
- Bruising—may or may not occur but can sometimes be prolonged lasting for weeks. Advise patient to use OTC Arnica tablets or creams.
- Tyndall effect—happens if the filler is injected too superficially. Usually, this is seen in the lip border, appearing like a bluish discoloration.
- Lumpiness—can happen with any filler treatment and may either be massaged with heat compression or dissolved if it bothers the patient.
- Asymmetry—can sometimes be very distressing for patients. It is important to point out any natural asymmetry to the patient if observed before the treatment.
- Allergic reaction—not very common but can happen. No treatment should ever be carried out without a first aid kit being available for use in case of an emergency.
- Infection/abscess formation—happens when aseptic technique has not been used.
- Avascular necrosis—this is a medical emergency, which cuts the blood supply to the tissue via blockage of an artery. It can occur either through direct injection into the vessel causing embolization, or indirectly via compression of the vessel from the outside with filler.

Immediate use of a dissolving agent is crucial to save the tissue from necrosis. Look out for the 5-P signs (pain, pallor, pulselessness, paresthesia, and perishingly cold).

Late (Days–Weeks)

- Product leakage—happens when too thick a filler has been used which attracts fluid to the lips, or when the filler has been injected in the white part of the vermillion border rather than the pink. The filler forms a swollen ring-like appearance around the lips. This often needs to be corrected via dissolving the product.
- Irregularity—can occur if the filler breaks down at different rates within the lip tissue. This can be corrected via retreatment.
- Granuloma—this is an immune reaction to the filler by the body, where a "capsule" forms around the filler with giant cells and macrophages infiltrating the tissue. Granulomas feel like hard lumps and need to be surgically excised as a last resort. They occur more frequently with permanent filler, sometimes even years after the treatment.

HYALURONIDASE

Hyaluronidase also called as Hyalase is an enzyme that can degrade HA, which is stabilized with animal protein. It comes in the form of a sterile, freeze-dried powder and each ampoule contains 1,500 international units of hyaluronidase. There is a risk of allergy, which could cause life-threatening anaphylaxis (allergy rate 1:1,000).

In urgent situations (such as vascular emergency), guidelines suggest administering the Hyalase via flushing the area, as the priority is saving the tissue from necrosis. Other possible temporary side effects of Hyalase administration include pain on injection, bleeding, bruising, redness and swelling, and blurred vision.

COMBINATION TREATMENT WITH LIPS—TOXINS

Orbicularis Oris

In middle aged/older patients or smokers, barcode lines can form which may extend into the lips. Treating this area can achieve an overall more esthetically pleasing result.

Inject a small amount of Botox (max 4 units) superficially into the muscle to soften the "barcode" lines and curve the upper lip slightly **(Fig. 16)**.

Depressor Anguli Oris

The DAO is a muscle responsible for pulling the corners of the mouth downward. A small amount of Botox can relax the muscle to allow the zygomaticus to lift the corners.

Inject a small amount of Botox (2.5–5 units) into the muscles on each side to subtly turn the mouth corners upward **(Fig. 17)**.

Levator Labii Superioris Alaeque Nasi

This treatment is also called gummy smile Botox. A hyperactive muscle can pull the upper lip too high and reveal too much of the patient's gum which can make them self-conscious when they smile. Botox can relax the muscle and also correct an asymmetric smile.

Inject 2.5–5 units of Botox on each side to evenly relax and drop the upper lip and conceal the gums. For correction of asymmetry, Botox

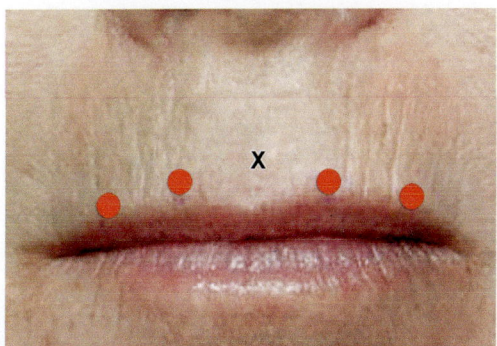

Fig. 16: Perioral lines treatment with botulinum toxin.

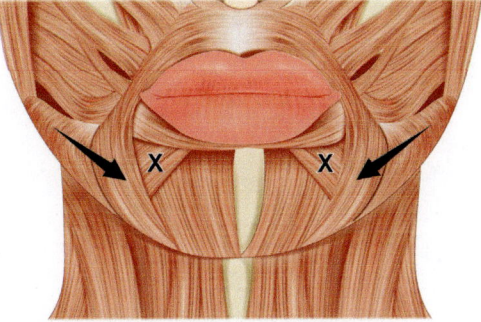

Fig. 17: Botulinum toxin injection of depressor anguli oris.

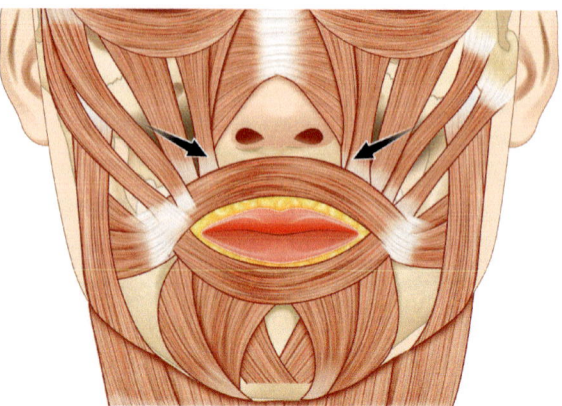

Fig. 18: Botulinum toxin injection for gummy smile.

will be injected on the affected side only **(Fig. 18)**.

CONCLUSION

Lip augmentation has become the most sought after procedure. The rise of social media has contributed to its popularity. It is imperative that patients choose a well-trained injector while seeking such treatments. A thorough knowledge of anatomy can prevent any complications.

REFERENCES

1. American Society of Plastic Surgeons (2017). Plastic Surgery Report 2017. [online] Available from: https://www.plasticsurgery.org/documents/News/Statistics/2017/plastic-surgery-statistics-full-report-2017.pdf [last accessed on December, 2019].
2. Hotta T. Lip enhancement: physical assessment, injection techniques, and potential adverse events. Plast Surg Nurs. 2018;38(1):7-16.
3. Standring S. Gray's Anatomy, 40th edition. London: Churchill Livingstone; 2008.

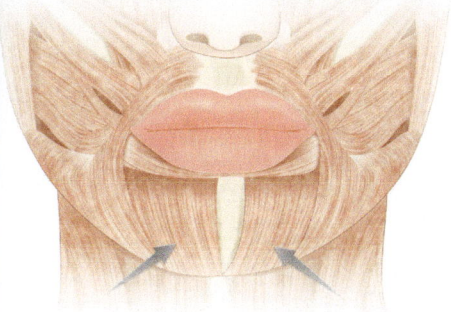

CHAPTER 22

Fillers for Nonfacial Areas and Scars

Madhuri Agarwal

INDICATION

With speedy growth in facial esthetic procedures, there has also been a parallel growing intervention in nonfacial areas due to the obvious contrast between the younger and revitalized face and rest of body such as earlobes and décolletage (chest). The hands are also one of the most conspicuous parts of the body and often show aging in a noticeable way.

ANATOMIC CONSIDERATIONS

Age-related changes and ultraviolet radiations evoke dermal thinning and lipoatrophy which manifest into visibility of muscles and rhytids along with signs of photodamage such as lentigines, telangiectasia, and dyschromia in décolletage.[1-3] Sun exposure, friction, temperature variations, use of chemical agents (e.g. soaps, detergents, household cleaners, etc.) thinning of dermis, and loss of elasticity affect the hands.[3] As a result, back of the hands exhibit laxity pronounced muscles, tendons, prominent bones, large intermetacarpal spaces, and bulging reticular veins. The nonfacial areas also show increase in skin roughness and hyperpigmentation. Congenital small ear lobes, asymmetrical bilateral earlobes, caved in appearance due to scar tissue and thin sagging ear skin with wrinkles are common considerations for ear lobe fillers. Dermal and subcutaneous fillers have shown significant improvement in scarring. Fillers raise the scar deficit to the level of the surrounding skin; thereby, working to even out skin texture and enhance overall contour.

INJECTION TECHNIQUES

Technique for Hand Fillers (Fig. 1)

Hand fillers can be injected by various techniques such as serial fanning, bolus depots, and linear threading. The filler selection depends on the expected results. A low G prime filler with low cohesivity and elements of noncross-linked hyaluronic acid (HA) is preferred for hydration and improvement of the skin quality in hands. This filler is ideally injected in the superficial dermis and dermoepidermal junction of the skin. In cases of moderate volume loss, a high G prime filler with high cohesivity is recommended to be injected in the mid to deep dermis and subcutaneously above the muscles and tendons. Avoid injections in the fingers due to the bony tissues and terminal vasculature.

The author endorses different techniques for both the indications. For hydration, the filler can be injected in bolus depots over the

150 Section 1: Dermal Fillers

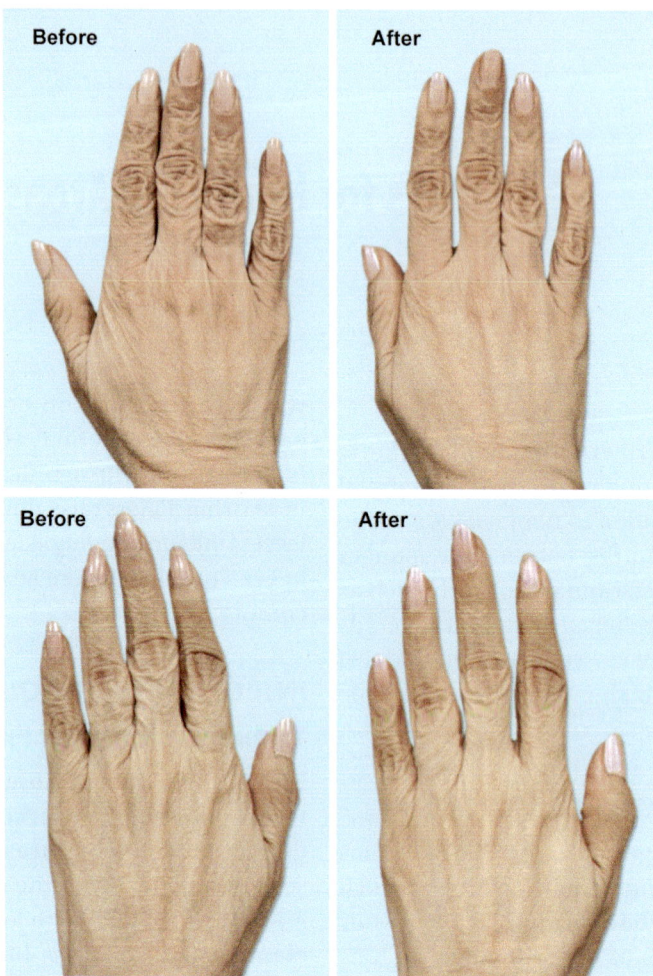

Fig. 1: Before and after 1 month results of dermal fillers for hands aging and rejuvenation. The volume loss is corrected in a single session using 18 G needle and 2 mL Voluma hyaluronic acid filler.

surface of dorsum of hand taking care to avoid the veins. Beginners can draw a grid on the dorsum and then the filler can be injected in each grid superficially concentrating on the areas of fine lines, dry, dehydrated patches. The filler quantity used is around 1 mL for each hand. The injections should be repeated every 4 weeks after the first session at least twice (total of three sessions with 6 mL of filler) for long lasting results. In cases of volume loss, use an 18-G cannula to inject the entire dorsum of each hand. An entry point is made with 18-no needle at the base of hand. Then using the 18-G cannula, the filler is injected in a retrograde fanning manner in the subcutaneous plane. The hand is massaged vigorously after the filler injection to disperse it equally and properly. A total of 2–4 mL filler can be used in a single session for both hands to achieve complete correction. Patients are advised to follow the

"5-5-5" rule of massaging: Massage the treated area for 5 minutes 5 times a day for 5 days.

Technique for Décolleté

For treatment of chest wrinkles and furrows, fillers can be injected using a threading technique in the chest with a cannula. Another technique is using either a 30- or 32-gauge needle, a serial puncture or retrograde linear threading technique is utilized to inject the product. The injection plane should be the superficial dermis for a low G prime filler and deep dermis for a higher G prime filler, giving the patient an even, smoother cosmetic appearance without Tyndall effect.

Technique for Earlobe Repair

Earlobe repair involves the use of HA fillers for the vertical rhytids immediately anterior to the ear and filling of sagging earlobes to rejuvenate appearance. The filler used is moderate G prime and around 0.5–1 mL can be injected in each lobule depending on the correction required. The earlobes are palpated to ascertain the site of filler injection and filler is injected using a 27–30 G needle. The depth of injection is intradermal or subcutaneous plane. Start by injecting the filler in the lateral edge of the earlobe, then angle the needle toward the tragus and inject the filler into the subcutaneous plane. A bolus injection of filler is adequate for small deficiencies of the earlobe. In case of major correction, bolus injection technique is done primarily with additional filler deposited with serial fanning technique in the subcutaneous plane for complete correction. In author's opinion, this approach helps to deliver optimum shaping and achieve a natural transition between the injection filling edge regions. To reduce the diameter of ear piercing and tighten the earhole, the filler can be injected in a circular pattern around the ear hole using micro bolus technique.

Technique for Scars

Scars are amenable to filler provided the appropriate type of scar is selected. Atrophic scars respond well to filler treatment as there is a volume loss and deficit that can be corrected with dermal fillers. Box scar, rolling, and iceprick are the kind of atrophic scars that show good results. The choice of filler is essential for optimum results. Choose a dermal filler that can be molded easily in the scars and has adequate solidity to lift the scars. Scar correction technique with fillers is a combination approach. The author recommends that subcision is done, with a Nokor needle or a tri-beveled needle (18 or 20 gauge), a week prior to filler injection for a smooth placement of filler. The filler is injected in individual scars after defining the treatment area. The filler is injected in the pitted or depressed area with the bevel of the needle facing up. Immediate lifting out of the area is observed. Some scars have tortuous tissue lying underneath which displaces the filler when the needle is withdrawn. In that case, massage the filler in such a way that is not visible. Then subsize the scar tissue with a needle breaking down few of them and then try to massage the filler back in the same location. All scars in the affected areas are injected in a similar manner. Massage the scar area, where required, after filler injection. As the filler treatment progresses, local swelling will increase making it difficult to separate individual scars, hence work systematically. Once the local edema increases to a point where it makes further procedure difficult, discontinue the process. The patient is then called back for future sessions to achieve a complete result.

PRECAUTIONS

Hands and décolletage are relatively safe areas for filler injections. Care must be taken to avoid injecting in large veins to prevent embolism. In earlobes, complication that can occur is the retrograde migration of HA filler to the superficial temporal artery (STA) and other branches of the external carotid. Experts recommend use of thicker needles and low flow volume, aspiration and physical blocking of adjacent vasculature with fingers as a precaution to avoid these complications.[4,5] Aseptic measures should be adopted to prevent any kind of infection and earlobes should be palpated to identify any nodules (such as sebaceous cyst).

POSTINJECTION INSTRUCTIONS

The common side effects that occur and are transient are edema, bruising, and pain. Nodule formation can be decreased by not overcorrecting, not injecting intra dermally, avoiding excess quantities of product for injecting, sessions to be conducted with a gap of more than 4 weeks and post-treatment massage. Poly lactic acid fillers when used in hands can cause pain, transient erythema, ecchymoses, edema, pruritus, and hematomas, but the best-known complication is nodule formation.[6] Ears have extensive capillary network and are rich in blood supply, thus making them less prone to serious complications such as necrosis or ischemia. However, bleeding and bruising can occur easily after injection. Use of sharper needle and application of pressure on injection site immediately with sterile cotton or gauze and application of ice intermittently both immediately and up to 24 hours after injection is recommended. Local swelling is also common due to the absorption of water by the HA filler material which usually subsides in 3–4 days postinjection. For sun-exposed skin (décolletage, and hands), use broad-spectrum, mineral-based UV protection of at least 30 SPF daily for all areas of the body, add a moisturizing agent with restorative additives for improvements in skin quality and appearance.

USEFUL TIPS

- Rejuvenation of the décolletage, creates a seamless transition between the face and nonfacial skin and contributes greatly to an overall more youthful appearance.
- The skin in the décolletage area has thin epidermis, variable distribution of subcutaneous fat, and decreased pilosebaceous unit as compared to facial skin. This leads to slower healing and higher risk of complications such as scarring with chemical peels or ablative techniques. Thus, it is safer to address concerns with fillers and nonablative techniques.
- Formulate a detailed, individualized treatment plan based on a thorough assessment of anatomy and signs of aging and/or photodamage.
- Discuss follow-up and maintenance sessions (if necessary) to maintain or prolong esthetic results.
- Low-viscosity HA filler with or without lidocaine has also been shown to reduce the appearance of rhytids, noticeable veins,

bony prominence, and dermal atrophy for 6–9 months in hands.

REFERENCES

1. Peterson JD, Goldman MP. Rejuvenation of the aging chest: a review and our experience. Dermatol Surg. 2011;37:555-71.
2. Dayan SH, Arkins JP, Chaudhry R. Minimally invasive neck lifts: have they replaced neck lift surgery? Facial Plast Surg Clin North Am. 2013;21(2):265-70.
3. Fabi SG, Burgess C, Carruthers A, et al. Consensus recommendations for combined aesthetic interventions using Botulinum toxin, fillers, and microfocused ultrasound in the neck, décolletage, hands, and other areas of the body. Dermatol Surg. 2016;42(10):1199-208.
4. Rho NK, Chang YY, Chao YY, et al. Consensus recommendations for optimal augmentation of the Asian face with hyaluronic acid and calcium hydroxylapatite fillers. Plast Reconstr Surg. 2015;136(5):940-56.
5. Qian W, Zhang YK, Coa Q, et al. Clinical application of earlobe augmentation with hyaluronic acid filler in the Chinese population. Aesthetic Plast Surg. 2017;41(1):185-90.
6. Vanaman M. Décolletage regional approaches with injectable fillers. Plast Reconstr Surg. 2015;136(Suppl 5):276S-81S.

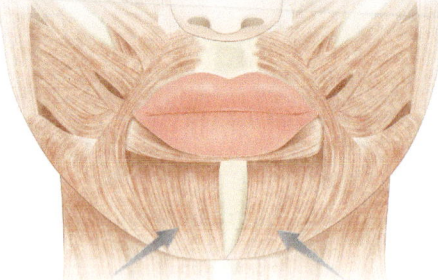

CHAPTER 23

Complications of Fillers and their Treatment

Mukta Sachdeva, Ayushi Khandelwal

INTRODUCTION

Perception of beauty among present generation is changing due to rapid globalization and increase in the exposure to social media. There is increasing demand for facial rejuvenation procedures especially with less invasive procedures, like fillers and botulinum toxins, due to fast actualization of results and minimal morbidity. Dermal fillers rank second among the top five nonsurgical cosmetic procedures, behind botulinum toxin injections.[1] According to American Society for Dermatologic Surgery survey, interest in cosmetic procedures continues to rise and these procedures continue to grow with demand, and that there has been a significant (58%) increase in the hyaluronic acid (HA) filler since 2014.[2] Because of the favorable safety record and versatility of the fillers, the popularity will continue to increase further. There is an alarming trend of increasing numbers of nonmedical professionals using these products; therefore one needs to be prepared to tackle these complications even if one is not the injector.

A thorough knowledge of anatomy, the different properties of the available filler substances and injection techniques are essential to prevent complications of the filler. It is also necessary to detect complications early and manage them effectively to minimize adverse effects and improve patient outcomes.

All dermal fillers and filler procedures can lead to complications, which may be related to one of the following 3P's **(Table 1)**.[3]

Hence, it is important to be aware of all the above considerations to avoid or minimize complications.

Table 1: Dermal fillers can lead to one of the following complication, which may be related to the following 3P's.[3]

Product-related	Permanent nonresorbable products and antigenic nature of the material
Physician-related	Lack of knowledge and insufficient experience
Patient (host)-related	Altered host defense mechanism

COMPLICATIONS (FIGURES 1 TO 5)

The classification of filler complications can be divided according to severity (mild, moderate, or severe); nature (ischemic complications and nonischemic); or by the time of the onset as—immediate onset (up to 24 hours after procedure); early onset (24 h–4 weeks); and late onset (more than 4 weeks).[4] Complications with fillers can range from simple bruising, erythema, and edema to asymmetry of the face, permanent scarring. In general, the type

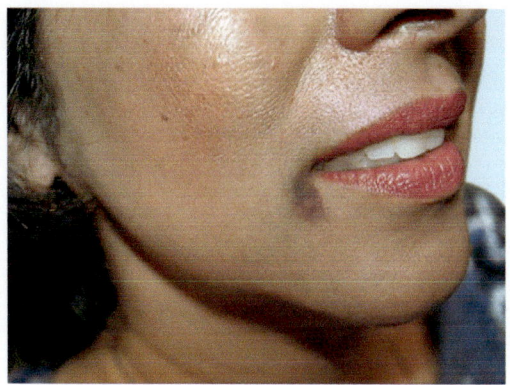

Fig. 1: Bruise seen on the injection site.

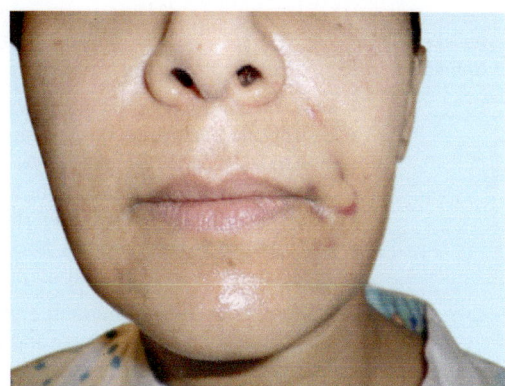

Fig. 4: Post inflammatory hyperpigmentation on the injection site.

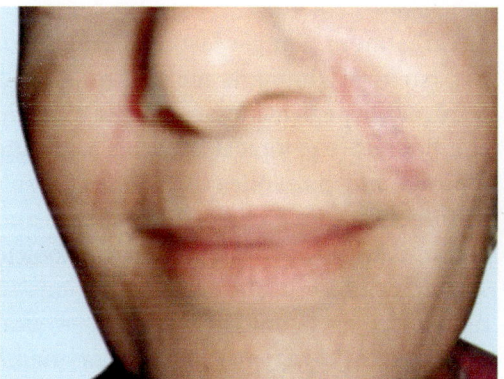

Fig. 2: Bilateral granuloma seen as a complication of nasolabial filler.

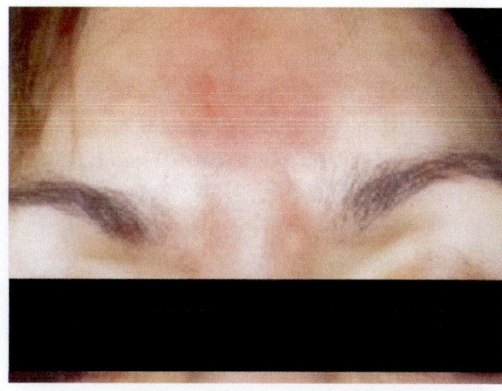

Fig. 5: Skin blanching seen on the forehead due to possible vascular occlusion.

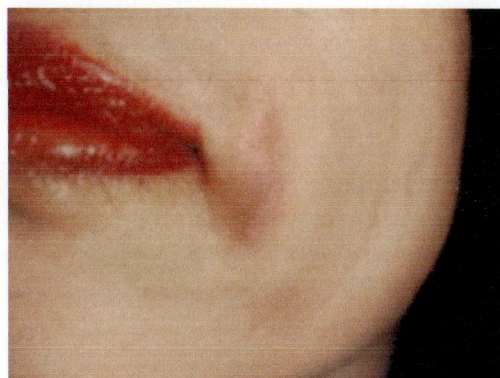

Fig. 3: Inflammatory nodule seen on the left angle of mouth.

of the filler used, the skill of the practicing doctor, the inherent type of the patient's skin, and the indication for which the filler is being used determine the outcome of the procedure. Permanent and semipermanent fillers have potentially more adverse effects than temporary fillers.[5] Hence it would be more cautious to use temporary filler, initially. For beginners, it is prudent to start with HA fillers to gain confidence and experience. Variability in individual results must be stressed upon to patients.

Complications are classified in **Table 2**.

Table 2: Classification of filler complications.

Immediate	Pain, hypersensitivity, and anaphylaxis
Early	• *Injection site reactions:* Erythema, edema, ecchymosis, pruritus, and tenderness • *Skin discoloration:* Erythema, cyanosis, blue appearing papules (Tyndall effect of superficially placed fillers), and blanching of skin. • *Infection:* Erythema, edema, pain, and fluctuant mass • *Tissue necrosis* and venous congestion secondary to vascular compromise • *Nodules:* Due to inappropriate placement of filler • *Vascular compromise:* Blurred vision and tissue necrosis
Late	• *HSV activation:* Itching, burning, erythema, edema, vesicles, and pustules • *Granuloma formation:* Palpable and visible nodules • Clumping and migration of filler • Aseptic abscess or biofilm reaction
Permanent	Scarring, persistent discoloration, and hyperpigmentation,

(HSU: herpes simplex virus)

Pain

Mild pain from needle puncture is a common event in most filler procedures. This can be minimized with topical anesthesia use. Pain can be further minimized by making sure the needle stays sharp during injection—change it as many times as required since touching the bone during injection dulls needles. Smooth quick movement and tactile distraction by rubbing or gentle pinching of neighboring skin significantly decrease needle pain. Use of long needles to reduce needle pricks, ice anesthesia, and warming up the filler to body temperature also minimize pain. Some manufacturers incorporate an anesthetic agent in the product formulations itself. Certain anatomical regions are more sensitive to pain, e.g. periorbital and perioral regions. If the pain is severe then the filler injection must immediately be terminated and the patient should be checked for any signs of vascular compromise like tissue blanching.

Erythema

Transient erythema is common after fillers and usually disappears in 30-60 minutes without any treatment. Longer lasting erythema or persistent erythema is more commonly a result of a hypersensitive reaction to different compounds (e.g. topical anesthesia, aseptic topicals, and antibiotic cream) or as a result of infection. So a careful evaluation and appropriate treatment are necessary.[6] Topical steroids can be used for short periods to reduce the erythema. In severe cases, oral propranolol (20 mg) may make the erythema less evident.[3]

Edema

Edema may occur immediately after the injection because of manipulation and rarely persists for more than a couple of days. This can be effectively managed by gentle pressure and ice packs. Because dermal fillers are essentially foreign bodies, some patients may develop hypersensitivity which is an IgE-mediated immune reaction. This may occur as an angioedema at the site of injection or at distant sites with or without urticarial reaction over the body.[7] This is treated with antihistamines and systemic steroids over a period of several weeks. Delayed hypersensitivity, which occurs days to months after the injection can result in facial edema. Delayed hypersensitivity reaction is nonresponsive to antihistamines. It usually responds to oral steroids. The last and the best option is to remove the causative filler material.

Papulopustular Lesions

Sterile folliculitis lesions occur because of occlusion of sebaceous or sweat gland openings and mimic bacterial infections or acneiform eruptions. If the filler is injected too superficially into the papillary dermis, it can be extruded through the sebaceous glands and appear like acne. Firm massaging soon after the injection may prevent the occurrence of these lesions. Topical treatment with astringents will help in clearing these papulopustular lesions.

Bruising, Hematoma, and Ecchymosis

Bruising, hematomas, and ecchymoses may occur because of needle pricks and bleed from these points. It is more commonly seen in patients on anticoagulants or alcohol intake. This can be minimized by cold compresses before and after the procedure. Stopping the intake of anticoagulants as well as supplements like ginkgo biloba, green tea, vitamin E, and omega-3 fatty acids 1 week before the procedure. Use of arnica, topical vitamin K, or bromelain has also been helpful to decrease the incidence of ecchymosis.

Infection

Infections can be prevented with standard aseptic precautions and treated with appropriate antibiotics or antiviral agents. Contaminated filler product is another concern. Fillers must be bought from credible sources and not shared among patients. Avoid storing and reusing the filler even in the same patient as filler contaminated with bacteria can function like a culture medium. Pigmentation at the site of infection, especially in skin of color, is a major concern.

Biofilm

Biofilm reaction[7] is defined as, an aggregate of microorganisms in which cells are stuck to each other and/or to a surface, embedded within a self-secreted extracellular protective and adhesive matrix of an extracellular polymeric substance (EPS). The biofilm may be active or dormant (persister) based on the external causative factor. The colony is resistant to antibiotics and is also difficult to culture in media. Trauma, injection, and manipulation provoke the activation of the biofilm resulting in local low-grade infection, abscess, sinuses, local lumps, foreign body granuloma, nodule, or systemic infection; delayed reactions are also possible.[8] The reactions, even though uncommon may persist for weeks to months. Most of these manifestations resolve with the use of broad-spectrum bactericidal antimicrobials for 2–3 weeks. Thorough cleansing of the area prior to the injection, aseptic precautions while injecting, and application of topical antibiotic after injection of fillers, patients should be counseled to report any tenderness developing after injection in the treated area, which should be promptly treated with broad spectrum antibiotics, help a great deal to prevent the development of biofilms. The role of prophylactic antibiotics is controversial.

Scar Formation

Scar formation is relatively a rare occurrence with dermal fillers. When they do occur, they are managed with intralesional steroids. Silicone gels and tight bandaging help to a certain extent.

Overcorrection

Overcorrection may appear as bumps, nodules, or irregularities, especially when too much of the material is injected. Appropriate volume and depth of placing the filler product will prevent the formation of lumps and bumps. Technique corrections prevent this. Simple digital pressure, drainage, aspiration, or incision and drainage in case of persistent nodules may salvage the situation. HA products may be easily resolved using hyaluronidase. In case of non-HA, a simple puncture with a wide bore needle and drainage of the excess product may suffice. Intralesional triamcinolone is used for persistent bumps.

Skin Discoloration

A bluish discoloration also known as the Tyndall effect may occur if an excessive amount of HA is placed superficially under the skin, and this can be treated by injecting hyaluronidase.

Vascular Complication

The devastating complication of necrosis is avoidable by having a sound knowledge of regional anatomy. Inadvertent placing of filler material in a vessel or depositing too much volume around a vessel may lead to vascular compromise and skin necrosis. This may manifest as immediate discoloration and possibly blindness and stroke depending on the site of injection.[9] Although the first symptom of intravascular placement is often described as pain, the common addition of local anesthetics to filler formulations may obviate this sign. Vigilant observation of skin color change, which may be remote from the injection point, is mandatory. Although usually immediate, the onset has been reported to be delayed up to 24 hours. Any suspicion of inappropriate pain, skin blanching, or mottled discoloration warrants immediate cessation of injection with the application of warm compresses, injection of hyaluronidase, and massage of the affected area. The patient should be given two tablets (650 mg) of aspirin to chew and swallow. High-dose hyaluronidase (500–1,000 IU) mixed with lidocaine in repeated hourly doses for 3 hours forms the backbone of the emergent therapy.[10-11] It is advisable to use a large bore cannula for instillation of the hyaluronidase in the subdermal plane to avoid bruising, which would confound the visual feedback of improving skin color.

Aspirating the syringe before injecting, slow and cautious injecting technique with smaller volumes progressively increased over multiple sessions help reduce the chances of vascular complications. Blunt cannulas reduce but do not eliminate the risk.

CONCLUSION

Dermal fillers continue to rise in popularity and it is important to be aware of all potential complications and be prepared to treat them effectively.

Being well aware with prevention, recognition, and early and effective management of complications is the key to a successful and safe filler practice.

In general, most complications are avoidable if factors such as:

- Detailed understanding of facial anatomy
- Appropriate patient and product selection for a particular anatomical site
- Preparation and injection techniques determine the outcome.

REFERENCES

1. American Society of Plastic Surgeons (2014). 2014 Plastic surgery statistics report. [online] Available from: http://www.plasticsurgery.org/Documents/news-resources/statistics/2014-statistics/plasticsurgery-statistics-full-report.pdf [Last accessed on December, 2019].
2. American Society for Aesthetic Plastic Surgery (2016). 2016 Cosmetic surgery national databank statistics. [online] Available from: http://www.surgery.org/sites/default/files/ASAPS-2016-Stats.pdf [Last accessed on December, 2019].
3. Vedamurthy M. Beware what you inject: Complications of injectables—dermal fillers. J Cutan Aesthet Surg. 2018;11(2):60-6.
4. Rohrich RJ, Nguyen AT, Kenkel JM. Lexicon for soft tissue implants. Dermatol Surg. 2009;35(Suppl 2):1605-11.
5. Duffy DM. Liquid silicone for soft tissue augmentation: histological, clinical and molecular perspectives. In: Klein AW (Ed). Tissue Augmentation in Clinical Practice, 2nd edition. New York: Taylor & Francis; 2006. pp. 141-238.
6. King M. Management of edema. J Clin Aesthetic Dermatol. 2017;13:E1-4.
7. Van Dyke S, Hays GP, Caglia AE, et al. Severe acute local reactions to a hyaluronic acid-derived dermal filler. J Clin Aesthet Dermatol. 2010;3(5):32-5.
8. Sadashivaiah AB, Mysore V. Biofilms: Their role in dermal fillers. J Cutan Aesthet Surg. 2010;3:20-2.
9. Sachdev M, Anantheswar Y, Ashok B, et al. Facial granulomas secondary to injection of semi-permanent cosmetic dermal filler containing acrylic hydrogel particles. J Cutan Aesthet Surg. 2010;3(3):162-6.
10. Chiang YZ, Pierone G, Al-Niaimi F. Dermal fillers: pathophysiology, prevention and treatment of complications. J Eur Acad Dermatol Venereol. 2017;31(3):405-13.
11. Urdiales-Gálvez F, Delgado NE, Figueiredo V, et al. Treatment of soft tissue filler complication: expert consensus recommendations. Aesth Plast Surg. 2018;42(2):498-510.

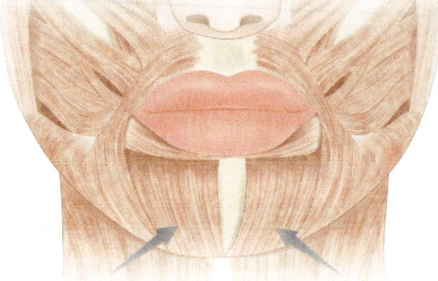

Combination Therapies with Fillers

Ishad Aggarwal

INTRODUCTION

Fillers are commonly used to treat signs of aging such as volume loss, to fill important lines and creases on the face and to provide structural support to sagging skin and to enhance contours and projections on the face. But cosmetic enhancement of a face would be incomplete, if all aspects of cosmetic deterioration are not taken care of. For example, a patient presenting with dyspigmentation and textural changes in epidermis along with signs of aging may feel disappointed, if he or she is treated with fillers alone. Thus a thorough global assessment of a patient's face is the most vital step in preparing a road map of treatments a patient would need to look better. The factors that affect a face are manifold and can afflict all the structures on the face, from bone to epidermis. Therefore more often than not, various modalities of treatments are used in combination with fillers to achieve cosmetically gratifying results.

RELEVANT ANATOMY

A thorough understanding of the anatomy of various layers of face and the factors affecting them is essential for an esthetic physician. **Table 1** summarizes the various layers of the face, factors affecting them and the resultant changes that happen on the face due to them.[1]

A review of applied anatomy makes it clear that hyaluronic acid (HA) fillers can help in cosmetic correction of the face by addressing different components.[2-4] The most common use of fillers is to address deflation of the facial fat pads such as a deep malar fat pads and the canine fossa. Fillers can also give structural support to lax ligaments such as zygomatico-cutaneous ligament and the mandibular ligament. Fillers help in restoring youthful appearance to face by filling lines, enhancing contours, providing a structural support in areas of bony resorption, and by improving overall suppleness of skin by retaining water and keeping the skin hydrated. However, fillers come with their own limitations. They do not work on dyspigmentation and dyschromias. Also, while they can give structural support to the ligaments, they have a major limitation in repositioning of lax ligaments and generation of collagen. Fillers do not address facial adiposity and do not give as predictable myomodulation as does botulinum toxin.

To address these limitations of fillers, an esthetic physician has to choose from other modalities of cosmetic enhancement to improve patient outcomes and satisfaction. Almost all modalities of cosmetic correction can be used with fillers; however, following factors must be thought through:

Table 1: Various layers of the face.

S. no.	Anatomical structure	Factor affecting	Resultant change of the face
1.	Epidermis	Sun damage, xerosis, decreased turnover of cells, and hyperkeratosis	Dyspigmentation, skin roughness, loss of smoothness of skin, dullness, seborrheic keratosis, and sun spots
2.	Dermis	Loss of collagen, elastin loss, elastosis, pigment incontinence, follicular occlusion, and loss of glycosaminoglycans	Loss of suppleness of skin, dryness, static and dynamic rhytides, thinning of skin, acne and acneiform eruptions, postinflammatory hyperpigmentation, dyspigmentation, and dyschromias
3.	Superficial fat compartment	This layer of the face is predominantly affected by hypertrophy and displacement	Inversion of the triangle of beauty making the face bottom heavy, prominent nasolabial folds, loss of contours of the face
4.	Fibrous retinacular cutis ligaments	They bind the dermis to the underlying superficial musculoaponeurotic system (SMAS). Loss of collagen and elastin weakens the ligaments over time	Loosening and sagging of the skin
5.	SMAS	This is an important layer of the face. It envelops the muscles of facial expressions and platysma, weakening of SMAS due to loss of collagen and elastin happens with age	Formation of jowls, sagging of skin, marionette lines, obscuring of transition between neck and face, and decreased sharpening of the jawline
6.	Muscles of facial expressions	They undergo hypertrophy or atrophy with age	Dynamic and static wrinkles, downturning of corners of the lips, and perioral aging
7.	Deep fat pads	They are generally fixed and undergo depletion with age	Periorbital hollowness and cheek deflation
8.	Retaining ligaments	They anchor the bone to the skin, creating support to various compartments of the face. Weakening of the retaining ligaments happens because of loss of collagen and elastin	Infraorbital hollowness, tear troughs, nasojugal grooves, marionette lines, and jowls
9.	Bone	The bony structure gets eroded with age causing lack of structural support to soft tissue	Deep canine fossa, mandibular erosion leading to poor jawline contours, midfacial bony erosion could lead to cheek deflation

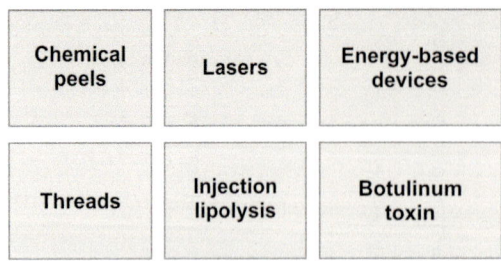

Fig. 1: Combination of modalities with the fillers.

- Time gap between different modalities and fillers
- Sequence of different modalities and fillers
- Interaction of other modalities with fillers
- Financial considerations of the patient.

In the following text, the author shall discuss the combination of following modalities with the fillers **(Fig. 1)**.

Chemical Peels with Fillers

A lot of our patients who present to us for fillers have a variety of textural issues such as pigmentation, dyschromias, acne vulgaris, rosacea, open pores, and photodamage. Correction of deeper signs of aging may not give a satisfactory change to such patients, because of the issues in the overlying epidermis and dermis. Chemical peels have been in use for many years for treating skin conditions such as tanning, dyschromias, acne vulgaris, postinflammatory hyperpigmentation, photodamage, and open pores.[5-7] Chemical peels can be done before fillers to improve above mentioned textural changes, and they can also be done postfillers to maintain the overall skin texture.

Although most of the chemical peels commonly used in practice are superficial to medium depth peels and in most cases do not interfere with the plane of fillers, it can become important if noncross-linked HA injections have been planned to be placed in dermis to increase skin hydration and turgor.

It is recommended to defer the filler injections if on presentation, the patient has visible exfoliation, erythema, persistent erythema, and open wounds due to chemical peels. Also there are theoretical risks of biofilm formation, if there is not sufficient gaps between deep peels and filler injections.

Combination of Lasers with Fillers

Injectable HA fillers and laser/light procedures have become increasingly popular for nonsurgical facial rejuvenation. There are no human studies to demonstrate the effect of lasers on the dermal fillers; however, a study conducted in porcine skin examined the effect of laser/light treatments on HA fillers. In the study,[8] the abdomen of six Yorkshire pigs were injected with three different brands of cross-linked HA fillers and then treated with lasers 2 weeks after the injections. The lasers used were, intense pulsed laser 560 nm (Sciton, Palo Alto, CA), Sciton Nd:YAG, Lux 1540, Sciton 2940 Er:YAG laser, and Active FxCO$_2$ fractional (Lumenis, Israel). The study concluded that injected HA fillers were unaffected by the nonablative laser/light and superficial ablative treatments. However, the deep ablative lasers like CO$_2$ fractional and Er-YAG 2940 nm can affect the longevity of the fillers and efficacy of the treatment.

In absence of any guidelines and literature, the author recommends a gap of at least 2 weeks with nonablative lasers and a gap of 4 weeks with ablative lasers such as CO$_2$ fractional and Er-YAG 2940 lasers after the filler injections. The lasers should ideally be planned before filler injections. After doing the laser session, a gap of at least 1 week is recommended after nonablative lasers and 2 weeks after ablative lasers or until complete reepithelialization has happened.

Lasers should be avoided in areas where the filler has been placed superficially due to the danger of exaggerated or persistent edema on account of the hygroscopic action of filler material interacting with the postlaser inflammatory cascade. This effect can even be seen 1 month later (personal observation). Therefore in cases of periorbital rejuvenation, filler injections should be the last treatment after the area has been treated with multiple sessions of peels and lasers.

COMBINATION OF ENERGY-BASED DEVICES WITH LASERS

Aging is a complex process that involves an interplay of various factors that involve the different layers of skin. A lot of patients present with laxity of skin owing to degeneration of the dermis and the superficial musculo aponeurotic system (SMAS). Combining esthetic interventions and targeting different layers give much better outcomes than single modality treatments.

Nonsurgical skin tightening devices work on the principle of neocollagenesis in the dermis and subdermal layers. Many sophisticated devices are now available and have been approved for these indications. Majority of them are based upon either the RF or the focused ultrasound beam.

Most of the RF-based devices cause diffuse heating of the dermis and cause collagen production in upper and mid reticular dermis, while focused ultrasound-based devices cause focused microinjuries in upper, mid reticular, deep reticular dermis, and SMAS. Treatments can be customized by adjusting the energy and focal depth of the ultrasound.

In an ideal scenario, a RF or focused ultrasound-based skin tightening procedures should be done before the dermal fillers. It would be even prudent to wait for the full effect of the skin tightening procedure to manifest before fillers are injected. However, patients demand lesser waiting periods because of lack of time and a need to see faster results. Therefore the question arises as to what happens to the dermal fillers if skin tightening is done over them. Several reviews have addressed this question for RF-based devices; however, there is not much literature for the same for focused ultrasound-based devices.

The first study was done by England et al.[9] They used a pig model to study the effect of monopolar RF on five different types of fillers. They observed no change in dermal fillers after doing monopolar RF treatments. Similar results were also observed in a second similar study done on pig model by Shumaker et al.[10] Alam et al.[11] conducted a similar study in humans in which monopolar RF was done 2 weeks after the injection of either HA or calcium hydroxyapatite fillers. No difference was seen in subjects with filler compared to controls even on histological examination. These results were further validated by a study conducted by Goldman et al.[12] Energy-based devices like 1320-nm Nd:YAG laser, 1450-nm diode laser, monopolar RF, and intense pulsed light (IPL) were used on one nasolabial fold while the other served as control. Twenty-one out of these 36 subjects had HA injected into the nasolabial folds. No statistical differences were observed on histological evaluation in all the test subjects.

While there is literature on synergistic usage of monopolar RF over fillers, there is no published literature on effects of focused ultrasound beam on fillers. Theoretically, the focused ultrasound-based therapies raise the temperature of the SMAS to as much as 65°C, but fillers are mostly sterilized at higher temperatures than that, therefore there is not a theoretical risk of filler degeneration due to the beam. But most users of ultrasound-based devices such as ulthera or high-intensity focused ultrasound (HIFU) avoid doing these treatments over fillers. In authors' experience, superficially placed filler, such as in the infraorbital region tends to get dispersed after doing HIFU over it. Most patients who have taken ultrasound-based skin tightening procedures immediately or within a week of doing fillers, often complain of loss of contour previously created by the fillers. In authors' experience, treatments like HIFU or ulthera are best done before fillers.

Combination of Threads of Fillers

Thread lifting is a cosmetic procedure that lifts and realigns sagging tissue, while adding definition to facial contours by using threads that are manufactured from the same materials used in surgery to close wounds.[13-14]

When placed under skin, the threads can be used to tighten the tissue, add volume and reposition the soft tissue.

Most commonly used threads are absorbable threads and are of the following types **(Table 2)**:

The aim of the thread insertion is to generate collagen in the dermis and to reposition lax soft tissue such as ligaments and SMAS. Therefore correct assessment plays a vital tool in choosing the type of threads for a particular patient. The depth of insertion of most monofilament threads is deep dermal while that of Cog threads is in the plane of the SMAS layer.

Thread lift is commonly combined with fillers in esthetic practice; however, there is not much published literature on the effects of threads on fillers. In a typical setting, the questions most pertinently asked are about the sequence of combining the two procedures and possible complications in such a setting. Most esthetic practitioners prefer to do the thread lift before fillers. The reason for this approach being that once the soft tissue repositioning has been achieved with the threads, fillers use can be best optimized. Although the plane of insertion of threads is more superficial to that of fillers, it is not advisable to do threads over the fillers to prevent filler manipulation by the traction of soft tissue achieved with the threads. The author recommends a gap of 3-4 weeks between the two procedures and ideally if the patient could wait, fillers should be done after 2-3 months of the thread lift, because it takes about 8-12 weeks for the final outcome of thread lift to manifest on the face.

Injection Lipolysis[15,16]

Phosphatidylcholine and deoxycholate (PC-DC) injections have been used as nonsurgical alternatives to liposuction over the last decade. However, the results are most optimal when the excess fat is less than 500 mL in volume and in small fat pockets. Results are more encouraging, if the fat is uniform and easily compressible. In esthetic practice, patients often come looking for improvement in their jawline definitions and reduction of submental fat excess. While fillers can be used

Table 2: Types of nonbarbed threads and barbed threads.	
Nonbarbed threads	**Barbed threads**
Plain or monofilament threads	Cog threads
Corkscrew or spiral threads	Unidirectional threads
	Bidirectional threads

to enhance the jawline by chin augmentation and by supporting the mandibular ligament and premasseteric fascia, injection lipolysis can be effectively combined with fillers to reduce submental fat excess. The combination synergistically gives more gratifying results.

Phosphatidylcholine and deoxycholate injections are given in the subcutaneous plane and often multiple sessions are needed to achieve the desired outcome. Although the procedure can be done simultaneously or after the filler injections on the lower face, in the authors' opinion, injection lipolysis should be done before filler injections. The logic behind this approach being that once the fat dissolution has occurred from the submental area, fillers can be optimized in quantity to improve jawline contour and definition. Further PC-DC causes an inflammatory response, which takes few days to settle and can cause breakdown of filler if injected during this time. Fillers take 2-4 weeks for tissue reconstitution before which time they are susceptible to displacement and dissolution; hence injection lipolysis should be deferred to beyond this interval if done after fillers for any reason.

COMBINATION OF BOTULINUM TOXIN WITH FILLERS[17,18]

Botulinum toxin is one the most commonly used treatments in esthetic rejuvenation of the face. Botulinum toxin works by chemodenervation of muscles in which it is injected, thereby giving a temporary improvement in dynamic wrinkles. However, advanced injectors also use botulinum toxin for improving jawline tautness by relaxing the platysma, to cause facial slimming by injecting the toxin in hypertrophic masseters, to improve arching of the eye brows, to lift the corners of the lips by selectively injecting the depressor angularis oris muscles, to improve gummy smile by selective injection in the levator labii alaeque nasi muscle, and many more of such indications. Recently, techniques have been developed where diluted botulinum toxin in smaller boluses is delivered to reduce open pores. Needless to say that a very thorough understanding of the facial musculature is essential to use botulinum toxin in such a wide variety of indications.

Combination of botulinum toxin with the fillers is one of the most favored esthetic treatment combinations all across the globe. Since there is no interference of the toxin with the filler, in either the plane of injection or the mechanism of action, these two procedures can be simultaneously done in the same sitting. However, it is advisable that botulinum toxin be done before fillers in perioral rejuvenation and jawline contouring. Of late there is a new interest in myomodulation of the muscles of facial expression by fillers and this is very commonly seen in the perioral region. Therefore, if a combination of toxin and fillers is planned for this indication, toxin could be done at least 2 weeks prior to the fillers, to ensure proper utilization of the product. Three other indications—masseter injection should be done 6-8 weeks before fillers since there may be mild facial laxity after which can be address with either threads or fillers, temple filler injection should be done before toxin since the former itself causes some lateral brow elevation, forehead filler injections should be done after toxin to see which areas have not been corrected by the toxin and address those. *These are our preferences—if your preferences are different please feel free to change the recommendations with an adequate explanation in the text. At any cost we feel that these three points should be included in this section.*

Formulating a Treatment Plan with Combination of Esthetic Procedures

There has been a significant shift toward a multilayered, 3-dimensional approach toward pan facial global improvement of face and this commonly involves combining one or more esthetic treatments in patients requesting cosmetic enhancement of the face. In this section, the author shall discuss treatment planning and strategies while combining treatments such as botulinum toxin, threads, and skin tightening energy-based devices with HA fillers.

For the sake of this chapter and easier understanding, the face can be divided into these treatment areas:

- *Upper face:* This includes the forehead lines, glabellar complex, temple hollowness, and crows' feet.
- *Midface:* This includes the tear trough, volume loss in cheek, and nasolabial region.
- *Lower face:* This includes the chin, jawline, perioral region, lips marionette lines, jowls, and submental fat excess.

Sequence of Esthetic Procedures in a Stepwise Manner

Carruthers et al.[19] came up with expert consensus recommendations for a stepwise approach using botulinum toxin, energy-based devices and HA fillers. According to this consensus, they recommend using neuromodulators first, followed by soft tissue fillers and then skin tightening treatments with a gap of 1–2 weeks, which allows local side effects such as bruising, swelling to reduce, and permits better assessment. However, due to time constraints or scheduling issues or patients' demands, multiple procedures are also performed on the same day. In such a setting, they recommend, doing skin tightening procedures first, followed by neuromodulators, and then the fillers.

The author differs in his approach when combining multiple esthetic procedures spanning over a few weeks. He prefers to first do the neuromodulators, then the energy-based device and threads, and fillers in the end. However, he agrees and follows the same principles as the recommendation, if all treatments have to be combined on the same day.

Treatment Recommendations for Upper Face[20-22]

Upper Face Concerns

The upper face aging is evident by hollowness in the forehead, ptosis of the brow, dynamic and static wrinkles, and deflation in the temples. The treatment plan for upper face aims at addressing the above mentioned concerns. The dynamic wrinkles can be improved by injecting the botulinum toxin and fillers, the hollowness of forehead and static wrinkling can be corrected by fillers, brow repositioning can be done with fillers, threads, and the botulinum toxin and temple hollowness is filled with the fillers. Collagen induction with energy-based devices can also aid in brow lifting in a noninvasive manner.

Treatment Plan for Upper Face

In upper face, the brow dictates most of the treatment protocols. Botulinum toxin can be used to improve eyebrow arching and give a subtle lift. Forehead lines, glabellar lines, and crows' feet are easily amenable to toxin injections. However, to improve the lift of the brow, ultrasound-based devices and threads can be used. Forehead and temple filling with the fillers are an advanced indication. The vascular anatomy should be borne in mind before attempting injections in this region. Temple filling improved the brow lift and also gives symmetry and proportion to the face. Forehead fillers improve the overall projection of the upper face and make it more youthful and feminine.

Treatment for the Midface[23-26]

Midface Concerns

Aging in the midface is usually heralded by loss of deep fat pads causing cheek deflation, hypertrophy, and displacement of superficial fat pads causing prominent nasolabial folds, lack of support in the zygomatic and buccal retaining ligaments and bony recession in maxilla exaggerating the deflation and nasolabial lines.

Sequence of Treatments in Midface

The first treatment would be to induce collagen and strengthening of the retaining ligaments and should be done with energy-based devices. The author prefers to use HIFU in such cases. The second treatment would be to reposition the displaced anatomical structures and soft tissue, which can be done with the threads. The choice of threads should be dictated by the severity of tissue displacement and need for collagen induction. The author favors the barbed cog threads. The third treatment should be to augment deflated fat pads and should be done with the HA fillers, starting on the zygomatic arch and moving anteriorly to the deep malar fat pads and then to the tear trough and nasolabial folds. Nose defects can be corrected with fillers and bunny lines can be corrected with the toxin.

Treatment Plan for Lower Face[27-31]

Bony and soft tissue structures in lower face undergo significant attrition with age, there is a significant displacement and hypertrophy of the fat compartments and laxity of the retaining ligaments, giving rise to overhanging soft tissue over the mandible causing formation of jowls and marionette lines. The perioral areas contribute significantly to the aging look. It is dominated by thinning of lips and structural support to the lips, causing drooping corners giving the patient a sad appearance. Also the perioral region is marked by static and dynamic lines which become more pronounced on animating, such as during pouting. Lack of support from the chin could be either due to bony erosion or due to congenitally retruded or hypoplastic chin. Along with submental excess, these factors cause obliteration of jawline making it more obscure.

Sequence of Treatments in Lower Face

The first thing to be addressed in the lower face would be the laxity of SMAS and the retaining ligament, which can be done with energy-based devices such as HIFU. Botulinum toxin can be used to improve the downward pull of the platysma and to improve the pull of the mentalis muscle in the chin. The botulinum toxin injections on the mentalis muscle also improve the longevity of the filler to be placed on the chin. Careful and selective superficial injection of the depressor anguli oris muscle with the toxin can improve the lip corners. Perioral rhytides can also be corrected with superficial toxin injections into the orbicularis oris. The SMAS tightening can also be achieved by cog thread lift in the lower face, and is authors' third preferred treatment in this sequence. Finally, fillers can be strategically injected on the chin to improve the jawline and making the face more vertically proportionate. Fillers are also used to fill the marionette lines, to augment thinned out lips and to improve perioral rhytides. Recently, fillers have also been used to give support to SMAS and to improve the sharpness of the jawline when injected linearly across the mandible in subcutaneous plane. Sharpness of angle of the mandible can further be enhanced by injecting fillers in the angle of the mandible.

ILLUSTRATED EXAMPLES OF COMBINATION OF ESTHETIC PROCEDURES WITH FILLERS

Case 1 (Fig. 2)

The patient came for improvement of signs of aging. She was injected with 2 mL of Juvéderm Voluma in midface and 2 mL of Juvéderm Volift in nasolabial folds and marionette lines. She also underwent thread lift with 4 cog threads on each side to reposition her lax ligaments in midface and in lower face. Although she showed improvement in signs of aging, but her overall results were unsatisfactory because textural improvement of her skin was required. She needed improvement in her pigmentation and roughness of skin. This is an example to show how a pan facial multifactorial approach is needed to target all the layers of skin to give gratifying results.

Case 2 (Fig. 3)

This patient came for cosmetic improvement of her face. She was bothered about sagging of her skin and her face being very broad in lower half. As we can see, she presented with laxity of SMAS, poor chin support, displacement of superficial fat pads due to gravity making her lower face look heavy and bulky. Sequential treatments were planned for her. Initially, she underwent thread lift with 90-

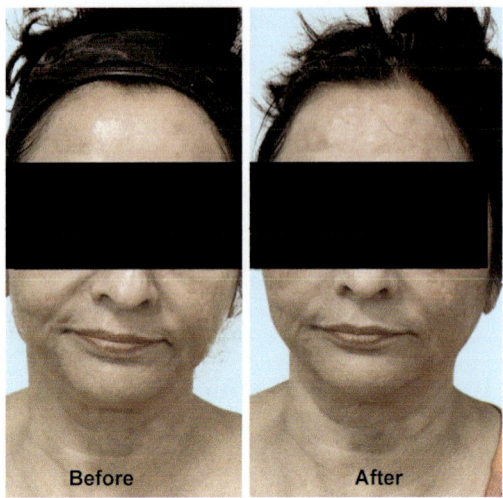

Fig. 2: Improvement in the signs of aging after the procedure (2 mL Juvéderm Voluma, 2 mL Juvéderm Volift and 4 cog threads on each side).

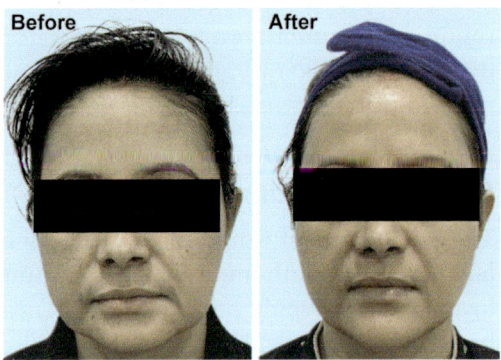

Fig. 3: Overall cosmetic improvement in the patient after sequential treatments.

mm cog threads to reposition lax SMAS and ligaments, 4 on each side. In the same session, she was injected with botulinum toxin (Botox, Allergan) in the glabellar complex, forehead, crows' feet, and in the platysmal bands. Two weeks later she was injected with HA fillers. 2 mL Juvéderm Voluma in the midface to augment the depleted cheek fat pads, 1 mL of Juvéderm Volift in the nasolabial folds, 2 mL of Juvéderm Voluma in the chin. The after result is 2 months after the filler injections were done.

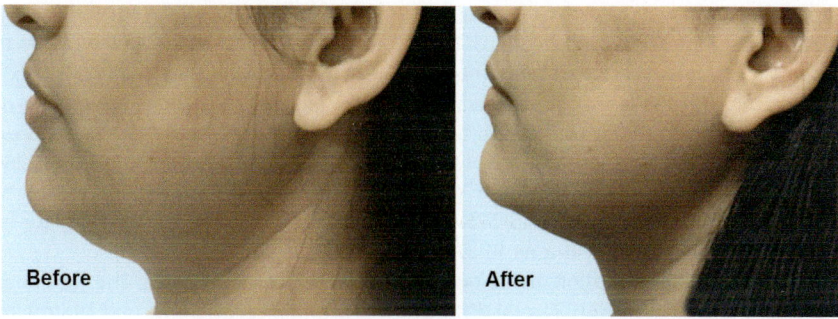

Fig. 4: Improvement of jawline contour.

Case 3 (Fig. 4)

This patient is a 40-year-old female who wanted to improve her jawline contour. She has submental fat excess and mild laxity of the skin. She first underwent HIFU on the lower face, 400 shots with 4.5-mm probe (Doublo). Three sessions of injection lipolysis were done with PC-DC injections in the submental fat 6 weeks apart. Finally 1 mL of Juvéderm Voluma was used to enhance her chin.

CONCLUSION

Better understanding of the complex interplay of various factors, across all the layers of skin, has facilitated a 3-dimensional, multimodality approach to improve facial aging. However, appropriate selection of these treatments is the most important thing while addressing the concerns of the patients. Understanding the tissue, interactions of these modalities give the esthetic practitioners better tools to combine with fillers, and enable them to successfully deliver more satisfying outcomes.

REFERENCES

1. Kurban RS, Bhawan J. Histologic changes in skin associated with aging. J Dermatol Surg Oncol. 1990;16(10):908-14.
2. Beer KR. Combined treatment for skin rejuvenation and soft-tissue augmentation of the aging face. J Drugs Dermatol. 2011;10:125-32.
3. Borrell M, Leslie DB, Tezel A. Lift capabilities of hyaluronic acid fillers. J Cosmet Laser Ther. 2011;13(1):21-7.
4. Sundaram H, Cassuto D. Biophysical characteristics of hyaluronic acid soft-tissue fillers and their relevance to aesthetic applications. Plast Reconstr Surg. 2013;132(4 Suppl 2):5S-21S.
5. Soleymani T, Lanoue J, Rahman Z. A practical approach to chemical peels: A review of fundamentals and step-by-step algorithmic protocol for treatment. J Clin Aesthet Dermatol. 2018;11(8):21-8.
6. Sarkar R, Bansal S, Garg VK. Chemical peels for melasma in dark-skinned patients. J Cutan Aesthet Surg. 2012;5(4):247-53.
7. Castillo DE, Keri JE. Chemical peels in the treatment of acne: patient selection and perspectives. Clin Cosmet Investig Dermatol. 2018;11:365-72.
8. Farkas JP, Richardson JA, Brown S, et al. Effects of common laser treatments on hyaluronic acid fillers in a porcine model. Aesthet Surg J. 2008;28(5):503-11.
9. England LJ, Tan MH, Shumaker PR, et al. Effects of monopolar radiofrequency treatment over soft-tissue fillers in an animal model. Lasers Surg Med. 2005;37(5):356-65.
10. Shumaker PR, England LJ, Dover JS, et al. Effect of monopolar radiofrequency treatment over soft-tissue fillers in an animal model: part 2. Lasers Surg Med. 2006;38(3):211-7.
11. Alam M, Levy R, Pajvani U, et al. Safety of radiofrequency treatment over human skin previously injected with medium-term injectable

soft-tissue augmentation materials: a controlled pilot trial. Lasers Surg Med. 2006;38(3):205-10.
12. Goldman MP, Alster TS, Weiss R. A randomized trial to determine the influence of laser therapy, monopolar radiofrequency treatment, and intense pulsed light therapy administered immediately after hyaluronic acid gel implantation. Dermatol Surg. 2007;33(5):535-42.
13. Abraham RF, DeFatta RJ, Williams EF 3rd. Thread-lift for facial rejuvenation: assessment of long-term results. Arch Facial Plast Surg. 2009;11(3):178-83.
14. Gülbitti HA, Colebunders B, Pirayesh A, et al. Thread-lift sutures: Still in the lift? A systematic review of the literature. Plast Reconstr Surg. 2018;141(3):341e-7.
15. Thomas MK, D'Silva JA, Borole AJ. Injection lipolysis: A systematic review of literature and our experience with a combination of phosphatidylcholine and deoxycholate over a period of 14 years in 1269 patients of Indian and South East Asian Origin. J Cutan Aesthet Surg. 2018;11(4):222-8.
16. Môle B. A five years experience of subcutaneous chemical lipolysis with phosphatidylcholine injections. Ann Chir Plast Esthet. 2011;56(2):112-9.
17. Carruthers J, Fournier N, Kerscher M, et al. The convergence of medicine and neurotoxins: a focus on botulinum toxin type A and its application in aesthetic medicine–a global, evidence-based botulinum toxin consensus education initiative: part II: Incorporating botulinum toxin into aesthetic clinical practice. Dermatol Surg. 2013;39(3 Pt 2):510-25.
18. Pavicic T, Few JW, Huber-Vorländer J. A novel, multistep, combination facial rejuvenation procedure for treatment of the whole face with incobotulinumtoxinA, and two dermal fillers-calcium hydroxylapatite and a monophasic, polydensified hyaluronic acid filler. J Drugs Dermatol. 2013;12:978-84.
19. Carruthers J, Burgess C, Day D, et al. Consensus recommendations for combined aesthetic interventions in the face using botulinum toxin, fillers, and energy-based devices. Dermatol Surg. 2016;42(5):586-97.
20. Presti P, Yalamanchili H, Honrado CP. Rejuvenation of the aging. Upper third of the face. Facial Plast Surg. 2006;22:91-6.
21. Coleman SR, Grover R. The anatomy of the aging face: volume loss and changes in 3-dimensional topography. Aesthet Surg J. 2006;26:S4-9.
22. Carruthers A, Carruthers J. Eyebrow height after botulinum toxin type A to the glabella. Dermatol Surg. 2007;33:S26-31.
23. Rohrich RJ, Pessa JE. The fat compartments of the face: anatomy and clinical implications for cosmetic surgery. Plast Reconstr Surg. 2007;119:2219-27.
24. Rohrich RJ, Pessa JE, Ristow B. The youthful cheek and the deep medial fat compartment. Plast Reconstr Surg. 2008;121:2107-12.
25. Sulc AE, Sharma P, Czyz CN. The anatomic basis of midfacial aging. In: Hurstein ME, Wulc AE, Holck DE (Eds). Midfacial Rejuvenation. New York, NY: Springer; 2012; pp. 15-28.
26. Pessa JE, Zadoo VP, Mutimer KL, et al. Relative maxillary retrusion as a natural consequence of aging: combining skeletal and soft-tissue changes into an integrated model of midfacial aging. Plast Reconstr Surg. 1998;102:205-12.
27. Carruthers J, Carruthers A. Botulinum toxin A in the mid and lower face and neck. Dermatol Clin. 2004;22:151-8.
28. Vleggaar D, Fitzgerald R. Dermatological implications of skeletal aging: a focus on supraperiosteal volumization for perioral rejuvenation. J Drugs Dermatol. 2008;7:209-20.
29. Levy PM. The "Nefertiti lift": a new technique for specific re-contouring of the jawline. J Cosmet Laser Ther. 2007;9:249-52.
30. Rho NK, Jeong CW, Lee DP, et al. Long-term efficacy and safety of micro-focused ultrasound for skin tightening and lifting: results in 183 Korean subjects. Lasers Surg Med. 2011;43 (Suppl 23):937-8.
31. Cuerda-Galindo E, Palomar-Gallego MA, Linares-Garciavaldecasas R. Are combined same-day treatments the future for photorejuvenation? Review of the literature on combined treatments with lasers, intense pulsed light, radiofrequency, botulinum toxin, and fillers for rejuvenation. J Cosmet Laser Ther. 2015;17:49-54.

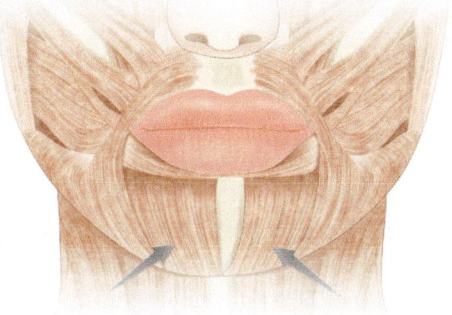

CHAPTER 25

Fractional Laser-assisted Botulinum Toxin Delivery

Weeranut Phothong, Woraphong Manuskiatti

INTRODUCTION

Botulinum toxin (BTX) has been well-known for its esthetic uses of targeting small facial muscles and minimizes their contractions. Another useful indication which results in a significant change in patients' quality of life is hyperhidrosis. By interfering acetylcholine release, intradermal injection is a common treatment modality regarding sweat gland anatomy. United States Food and Drug Administration (FDA) has approved BTX use of primary axillary hyperhidrosis treatment since 2004.[1] Thereafter, dermatologists expand its application for patients with palmoplantar hyperhidrosis. Unlike cosmetic indications which involve few injection spots into small facial muscles, hyperhidrosis treatment requires extensive multiple injections and superficially placed toxin according to dermosubcutaneous location of sweat glands. Patients reported moderate pain, almost 6 from 10 visual analog scale in one study.[1] Insufficient pain management can prevent patients from treatment adherence especially when injecting toxin in to highly innervated palms and soles.[2] Too deep toxin placement also results in hand muscle weakness.[3] Other therapeutic scenarios for superficial and extensive area of toxin injections include full-face rejuvenation and facial enlarge pores.[4,5] Neck rejuvenation also requires multiple injections into broad muscular layer and too deep placement of toxin can cause significant complications. Authors have reported dysphagia caused by toxin effect on deeper muscles.[6] Filler, on the other hand, has not yet been established for extensive and superficial injection technique. Placing filler superficially has been reported to improve acne scar appearance.[7]

Ablative laser has been firstly demonstrated to enhance transdermal drug delivery in 1987.[8] Stratum corneum, the major barrier to most hydrophilic compounds, has been full-field removed by ablative laser and increased transdermal absorption was evident. To preserve an ability of stratum corneum removal but lessen downtime and wound severity, Manstein et al. firstly reported the novel concept of ablative fractional laser (AFXL).[9] Multiple microablative columns serve as epidermal bypass for applied drugs while unaffected healthy skin columns serve as reservoirs for rapid wound healing. *In vivo* studies also showed an evidence of increased drug penetration after AFXL as well as clinical significance of AFXL pretreatments for skin-cancer photodynamic therapy.[10,11] Thus, a number of studies focusing on laser-assisted drug delivery have risen significantly in the last 10 years as an attempt to maximize advantages by combining two in-hands technology.[12] For those indications requiring extensive toxin and filler injections into the dermis, AFXL facilitates a fast, less painful, and predictable ablative depth mode of delivery. This chapter will cover the concept of AFXL-assisted injectables delivery into skin. BTX for hyperhidrosis treatment will be the main focus. Other possible benefits from different injectables will be discussed briefly as well.

ANATOMY CONSIDERATION

The anatomical section of palmoplantar skin can be vertically simplified as shown in **Figure 1**. Sweat glands located in the deep dermis next to subcutaneous layer are the primary targets of hyperhidrosis treatments. The aim is to assist toxin to reach this level and perform a blockage of neurotransmission in the sweat glands. Palmar skin thickness, defined by the distance of skin surface to dermosubcutaneous junction, varies according to gender, age, and concurrent systemic disorders. Using ultrasonography, Nedelec et al. showed palmar skin tended to increase thickness in male, compared to female and in elderly, compared to young adult. At 20–29-year age group, male subjects showed 1.37-mm palmar thickness versus 1.14 mm of female subjects. Older age group (70–85 years) showed the similar trend with 1.41 versus 1.34 mm, in male and female group, respectively.[13] To determine the depth of ablative columns is challenging due to the fact that BTX solution has diffusive property which depends on types of toxin, degrees of dilution, and injection techniques. Unlike intradermal injection, an evidence of diffusion through fractional laser channels has not yet elucidated. It is worth to be taken into account that toxin can cause an undesirable effect on intrinsic hand muscles resulting in hand

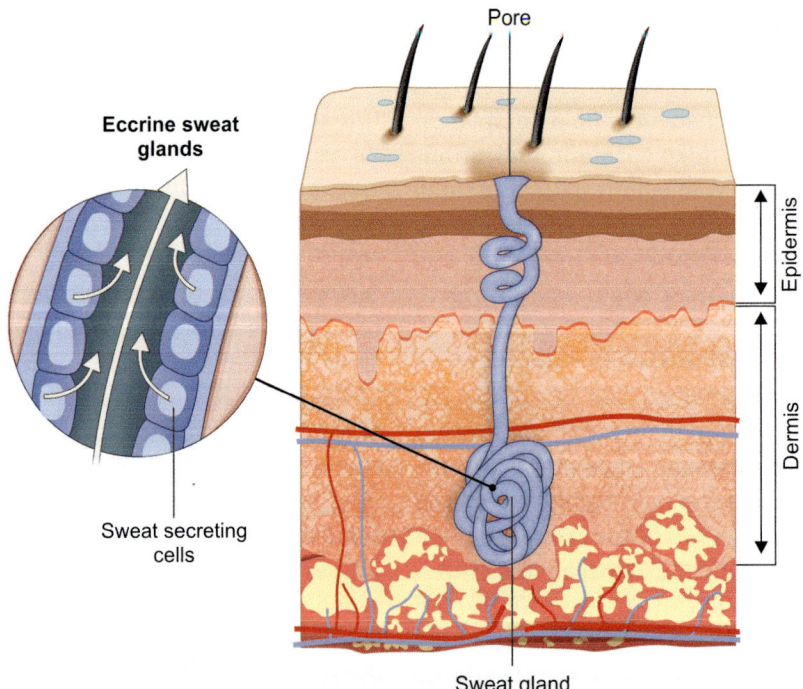

Fig. 1: An illustration showing sweat glands located at deep dermis and dermosubcutaneous junction.

weakness when diffusing too deep. Thus, the dermosubcutaneous junction is not a suitable depth for AFXL due to aforementioned diffusion. Moreover, higher energy of laser can cause more pain and delayed wound healing. Authors recommend superficial to mid dermis depth of ablation for effective therapeutic result, feasible procedure, less pain, and less healing time.

Facial skin also demonstrates different thickness at varying anatomical locations. It is practical to recall facial skin thickness as anatomical subunits. The thinnest portion is upper eyelids, followed by nasal bridge, lower eyelids, and lips.[14] The thickest portion is the nose tip.

TREATMENT TECHNIQUE

Patients with palmar hyperhidrosis should be free from topical treatments for at least 1 week prior to a procedural visit and the skin of the area to be treated should be healthy. Minors' iodine starch test serves as a guidance of treatment area when feasible. Authors recommend 2.5%-lidocaine and 2.5%-prilocaine cream application under occlusion for 1 hour before laser treatment. A recent study reported a superior pain alleviation effect by ice application during toxin injection treatment.[15] Thus, a cooling device can be applied in AFXL-BTX treatment on palms when needed as well. Fractional carbon dioxide laser is an AFXL of choice due to its desired penetration depth and hemostasis property. Higher energy setting showed broader and deeper ablative columns in micron-range **(Fig. 2)**. Since this technique employs the concept of transdermal drug delivery, molecular weight should be taken into consideration. A previous study also showed superior transdermal penetration of smaller molecules such as imiquimod (240.3

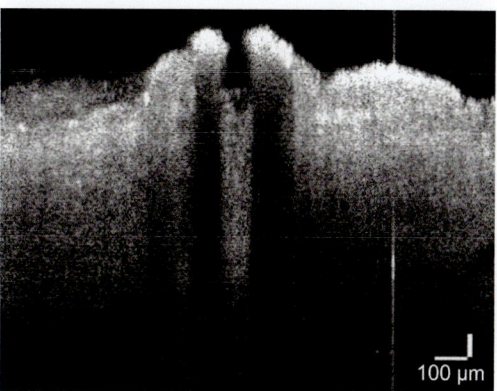

Fig. 2: Optical coherent tomography imaging demonstrating an ablative column caused by fractional carbon dioxide laser
(*Courtesy:* Weeranut Phothong, and Michael Evers)

Da), compared with larger peptide molecules (716, 2,190, and 2,354 Da)[16] through AFXL treatment. Incobotulinumtoxin A consisted of 150 KDa protein which contributes to therapeutic effect. On the other hand, onabotulinum toxin is manufactured including complexing protein which results in total molecular weight of 900 KDa.[17] Our previous unpublished data revealed no sweat reduction by Minors' iodine starch test after AFLX-assisted onabotulinum toxin delivery while our recent case series treatment highlighted an efficacy of incobotulinumtoxin A 50 units per palm (4 units/0.1 mL) in palmar hyperhidrosis treatment, compared to untreated palm (The manuscript is under reviewed by Lasers in Medical Science Journal).

One pass of $FXCO_2$ treatment was delivered using a pulse duration of 950 μs and an energy of 12.5 mJ. Microscopic ablative zones covered 5% skin surface of 10-mm by 10-mm spot size. According to our previous study, a fractional CO_2 laser set at this parameter created an average of 160 and 350 μm of vaporization and coagulation depth, respectively. Soon after laser treatment, toxin solution was gently applied over the treatment area and rubbed gently over the ablated columns for 3 minutes. The lag time between laser treatment and drug application is crucial since more than 90% length of the entire laser-ablated columns were shown to be filled rapidly by fibrin plug at 90 minutes after AFXL exposure.[18] Other than hyperhidrosis indication, AFXL-assisted BTX delivery for wrinkle treatment has also been studied. Mahmoud et al. compared AFXL-150 KDa BTX with AFXL-saline treatment and reported significant improvement on toxin side.[19] Rkein et al. applied poly-L-lactic acid in 19 patients without control group and reported scar improvement.[20] Further studies with randomized controlled trial designs are required for AFXL-assisted injectables since several indications can be improved by AFXL treatment alone.[21,22] In case of facial treatment, energy should be lowered to 10–12.5 mJ. In Asian or skin of color patients, treatment density should not exceed 5% to minimize the risk of postinflammatory hyperpigmentation.

POST-TREATMENT INSTRUCTION

Patients were instructed not to wash their hands until the next morning and apply petrolatum jelly four times a day for at least 7 days. Also, patient should avoid soaking or washing their hands with strong detergent. Although we found no patients experiencing hand muscle weakness, it is recommended to examine all possible adverse events at 2-week visit. After the second session with 2-week interval, authors found that the highest sweat reduction determined by starch test and visual analog scale (VAS) was noted at 2–4 weeks after the second treatment (52–89% reduction from baseline). Patient-based VAS noted 38% and 4% sweat reduction at 2 and 3 months after the second treatment, respectively. Hence, it is suggested to repeat the treatment every 1–2 months **(Figs. 3A and B)**.

USEFUL TIPS

- Ablative fractional laser can assist BTX delivery in palmar hyperhidrosis with an

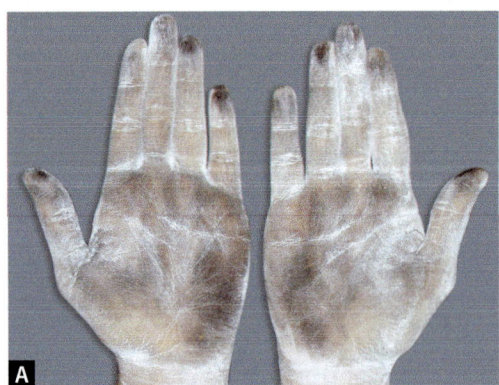
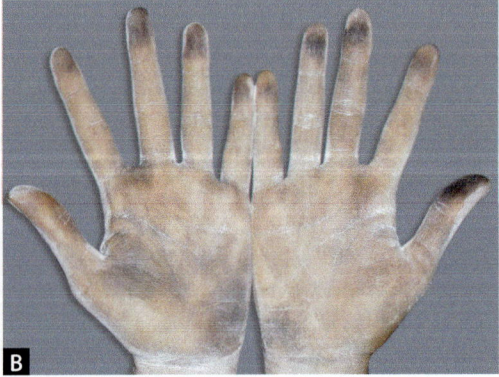

Figs. 3A and B: Iodine starch test photographs of the results in one patient at baseline, and on days 14 after injection the 1st treatment. (A) Severe bilateral palmar hyperhidrosis with uniform severe palmar sweating; (B) results of iodine starch test at 2 weeks after the first ablative fractional laser-assisted BTX-A delivery treatment on the right side, and untreated control on the left side.

(Courtesy: Woraphong Manuskiatti)

advantage of fast and tolerably painful procedure.
- Size of drug molecules affects penetration capability. The smallest size drug available is recommended.
- Fractional CO_2 laser is widely used due to deeper penetration and coagulative property.
- Ablative columns should reach the depth of superficial to mid dermis due to diffusion of toxin solution.
- Immediate application of toxin following laser treatment is emphasized.
- Although never reported in AFXL-assisted toxin delivery, hand muscle weakness is a possibility and should be checked for at the 14-day follow-up visit.
- Authors recommend treatment sessions every 1-2 months.

REFERENCES

1. Bernhard MK, Krause M, Syrbe S. Sweaty feet in adolescents-Early use of botulinum type A toxin in juvenile plantar hyperhidrosis. Pediatr Dermatol. 2018;35(6):784-6.
2. Campanati A, Giuliodori K, Martina E, et al. Onabotulinumtoxin type A (Botox®) versus Incobotulinumtoxin type A (Xeomin®) in the treatment of focal idiopathic palmar hyperhidrosis: results of a comparative double-blind clinical trial. J Neural Transm. 2014;121(1):21-6.
3. Weinberg T, Solish N, Murray C. Botulinum Neurotoxin Treatment of Palmar and Plantar Hyperhidrosis. Dermatol Clin. 2014;32(4):505-15.
4. Wanitphakdeedecha R, Ungaksornpairote C, Kaewkes A, et al. The comparison between intradermal injection of abobotulinumtoxinA and normal saline for face-lifting: a split-face randomized controlled trial. J Cosmet Dermatol. 2016;15(4):452-7.
5. Shah AR. Use of intradermal botulinum toxin to reduce sebum production and facial pore size. J Drugs Dermatol. 2008;7(9):847-50.
6. Phothong W, Wanitphakdeedecha R, Keskool P, et al. A case of dysphagia following botulinum toxin injection for neck rejuvenation. J Cosmet Dermatol. 2017;16(1):15-7.
7. Halachmi S, Ben Amitai D, Lapidoth M. Treatment of acne scars with hyaluronic acid: an improved approach. J Drugs Dermatol. 2013;12(7):e121-3.
8. Jacques SL, McAuliffe DJ, Blank IH, et al. Controlled removal of human stratum corneum by pulsed laser. J Invest Dermatol. 1987;88(1):88-93.
9. Manstein D, Herron GS, Sink RK, et al. Fractional photothermolysis: A New concept for cutaneous remodeling using microscopic patterns of thermal injury. Lasers Surg Med. 2004;34(5):426-38.
10. Bay C, Lerche CM, Ferrick B, et al. Comparison of Physical pretreatment regimens to enhance protoporphyrin ix uptake in photodynamic therapy. JAMA Dermatol. 2017;153(4):270.
11. Wenande E, Phothong W, Bay C, et al. Efficacy and safety of daylight photodynamic therapy after tailored pretreatment with ablative fractional laser or microdermabrasion: a randomized, side-by-side, single-blind trial in patients with actinic keratosis and large-area field cancerization. Br J Dermatol. 2019;180(4):756-64.
12. Haedersdal M, Erlendsson AM, Paasch U, et al. Translational medicine in the field of ablative fractional laser (AFXL)-assisted drug delivery: A critical review from basics to current clinical status. J Am Acad Dermatol. 2016;74(5):981-1004.
13. Nedelec B, Forget NJ, Hurtubise T, et al. Skin characteristics: normative data for elasticity, erythema, melanin, and thickness at 16 different anatomical locations. Ski Res Technol. 2016;22(3):263-75.
14. Ha RY, Nojima K, Adams WP, et al. Analysis of facial skin thickness: defining the relative thickness index. Plast Reconstr Surg. 2005;115(6):1769-73.
15. Alsantali A. A comparative trial of ice application versus EMLA cream in alleviation of pain during botulinum toxin injections for palmar hyperhidrosis. Clin Cosmet Investig Dermatol. 2018;11:137-40.
16. Lee WR, Shen SC, Al-Suwayeh SA, et al. Laser-assisted topical drug delivery by using a low-fluence fractional laser: imiquimod

and macromolecules. J Control Release. 2011;153(3):240-8.
17. Frevert J. Pharmaceutical, biological, and clinical properties of botulinum neurotoxin type A products. Drugs R D. 2015;15(1):1-9.
18. Kositratna G, Evers M, Sajjadi A, et al. Rapid fibrin plug formation within cutaneous ablative fractional CO_2 laser lesions. Lasers Surg Med. 2016;48(2):125-32.
19. Mahmoud BH, Burnett C, Ozog D. Prospective randomized controlled study to determine the effect of topical application of botulinum toxin A for crow's feet after treatment with ablative fractional CO2 laser. Dermatol Surg. 2015;41 (Suppl 1):S75-81.
20. Rkein A, Ozog D, Waibel JS. Treatment of atrophic scars with fractionated CO2 laser facilitating delivery of topically applied poly-L-lactic acid. Dermatol Surg. 2014;40(6):624-31.
21. Manuskiatti W, Iamphonrat T, Wanitphakdeedecha R, et al. Comparison of fractional erbium-doped yttrium aluminum garnet and carbon dioxide lasers in resurfacing of atrophic acne scars in Asians. Dermatol Surg. 2013;39 (1 Pt 1):111-20.
22. Manuskiatti W, Triwongwaranat D, Varothai S, et al. Efficacy and safety of a carbon-dioxide ablative fractional resurfacing device for treatment of atrophic acne scars in Asians. J Am Acad Dermatol. 2010;63(2):274-83.

SECTION 2

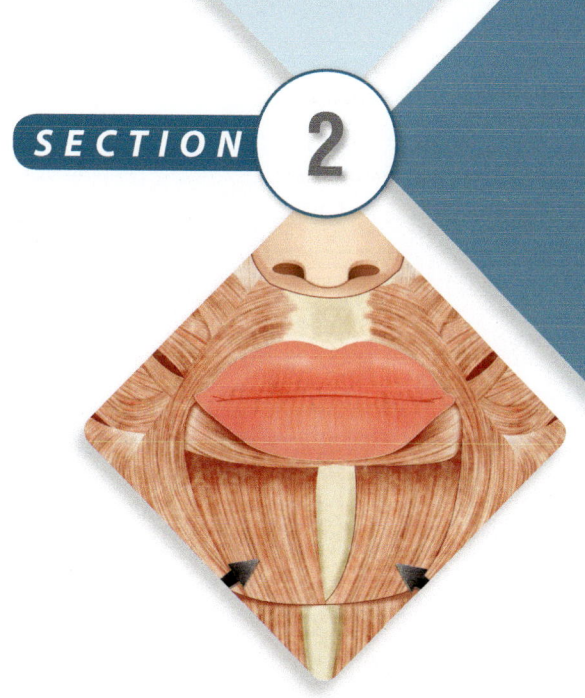

BOTULINUM TOXIN

SECTION OUTLINE

26. Neurotoxin Preparations
27. Frown Lines
28. Forehead Lines
29. Crow's Feet and Lower Eyelid
30. Brow Lift with Botulinum Toxin
31. Bunny Lines
32. Nose
33. Smoker's Lines (Lip Lines)
34. Gummy Smile-Botulinum Toxin
35. Botulinum Toxin for Marionette Lines
36. Dimpled Chin
37. Botulinum Toxin in Platysmal Bands
38. Nefertiti Lift
39. Botulinum Toxin in Masseteric Hypertrophy
40. Complications of Botulinum Toxin and their Management
41. Botulinum Toxin in Men
42. Microdosing in Botulinum Toxin
43. Neurotoxin Resistance

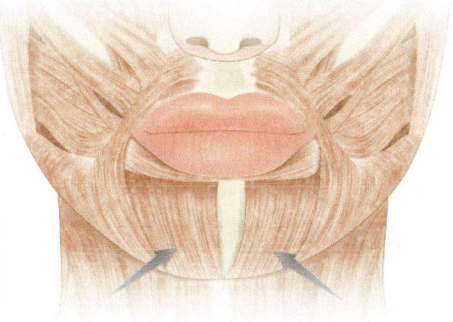

CHAPTER 26

Neurotoxin Preparations

Abhay Talathi

INTRODUCTION

Over the last three decades there has been a significant rise in patients receiving botulinum toxin injections for esthetic concerns.

Botulinum toxin type A is a very potent neurotoxin which inhibits the release of acetylcholine at the neuromuscular junction resulting in partial paralysis of the muscles.

The appropriate dose and precise placement of botulinum exotoxin A injections are the most important factors in optimizing the outcome. However, there are many preparatory steps which play a vital role in successful botulinum toxin results. This chapter focuses on such preparatory steps so as to improve the patient outcomes and increase patient satisfaction.

Over the past few years there has been an increase in the number of formulations of botulinum toxin type A available for cosmetic use. As an active biological protein no two toxin varieties shall be considered same. Every physician should be well-versed with correct scientific data about the product being used.

Correct patient alignment is the key to successful practice. Patients presenting for toxin treatment should be adequately informed and basic administrative formalities need to be completed.

DIFFERENT TOXINS[1]

Three varieties of US Food and Drug Administration (FDA)-approved botulinum toxin type A are available currently in India namely onabotulinum toxin type A (Botox), abobotulinum toxin type A (Dysport), and incobotulinum toxin type A (Xeomin).[1] Some other neurotoxins namely Neuronox and Siax (both from Korean manufacturers) and BTX-A from a Chinese manufacturer are also available.

Following **Table 1** illustrates differences in the three US FDA-approved toxins.[1-3]

DOSE EQUIVALENCE[1,4]

Each botulinum product is purified and manufactured using proprietary processes, resulting in unique, noninterchangeable agents that differ in molecular weight, uniformity of toxin complex size, protein content, and the presence of inactive ingredients. These differences can manifest as variations in performance characteristics including potency, duration of effect, adverse event profile, and diffusion.[4]

It is essential for a user to understand the efficacious dose of the toxin being used in clinic for a particular indication. Each manufacturer uses its own lethality tests so as to measure potency of the toxin.[3]

Based on their systematic review of the literature in 2009, Karsai and Raulin suggested that dose equivalences of 2.5 units abobotulinum toxin to 1 unit onabotulinum toxin should be used.[3]

Table 1: Comparisons of different US FDA-approved preparations of botulinum toxin type A.[1-3]

	Onabotulinum toxin (Botox)	Abobotulinum toxin (Dysport)	Incobotulinum toxin (Xeomin)
Strain of *Clostridium botulinum*	Hall strain	Hall strain	Hall strain
Purification method	Crystallization	Chromatography	Chromatography
Purification product	Botulinum neurotoxin (BoNT) A ~900 kDa complex protein	BoNT-A complex sizes <500 kDa	~150 kDa BoNT-A protein only
Available strengths	50 U and 100 U vials	300 U vials	50 U and 100 U vials
Excipients	*In 100 U vial:* • 900 μg sodium chloride • 500 μg human serum albumin	*In 500 U vial:* • 2.5 mg lactose • 125 μg human serum albumin	*In 100 U vial:* • 4.7 mg sucrose • 1 mg human serum albumin
Finishing	Vacuum dried	Freeze dried	Lyophilized
Storage recommendations before reconstitution	<8°	<8°	<25°
Dose equivalence	1 U	2.5 U	1 U

ONSET OF ACTION[5,6]

When given at their recommended doses, the times to onset of effect for abobotulinum toxin and incobotulinum toxin are similar, but abobotulinum toxin has a faster onset of effect than onabotulinum toxin.[5] In a study done by Brandt, 15% of subjects injected with abobotulinum toxin, onset of effect was seen as early as 24 hours, and in 35% of subjects, onset of effect was seen in 48 hours. The median time to onset of effect was 3 days for botulinum neurotoxin-A (BoNT-A).[6]

RECONSTITUTION AND INJECTION

Sterile 0.9% normal saline is used for reconstitution of all botulinum toxins. Precise reconstitution of the product is essential in order to ensure full potency when injected.[7]

Different dilutions are used by physicians worldwide; however in the Indian scenario considering the ease of injection the author recommends dilution with 2.5 mL normal saline for 100 units of onabotulinum toxin and incobotulinum toxin each and 3 mL normal saline dilution for 300 units of abobotulinum toxin.

Onabotulinum toxin is a vacuum dried powder so saline from the syringe need not be pushed into the vial whereas saline has to be pushed from syringe into abobotulinum toxin and incobotulinum toxin vials. Gently roll the vials to ensure uniform mixing of powder with saline.

As per the US FDA guidelines, reconstituted botulinum toxin has to be use in 24 hours, however as per some clinical data it is possible to refrigerate a partially used vial of botulinum toxin type A for 1 week without compromising its effectiveness.[8]

Different dose dilutions have been tried in a dose-dilution study in which a total dose of

Table 2: List of surgical materials used during neurotoxin treatment.

For injecting toxin	Surgical materials
Insulin 1 mL syringe/BD 1 mL syringe	Spirit/alcohol swabs
30 G 1/2 inch needles	Sterile gauze
	Marking pencils
	Head band
For toxin reconstitution	Ice compresses
Sterile normal saline	Topical antibiotic cream
5 cc disposable syringe	Topical anesthetic cream
24 G needle	Hand mirror for counseling

30 U was reconstituted in 1, 3, 5, or 10 mL, no differences in efficacy or safety were observed in treating glabellar rhytids in between groups.[9] The author recommends usage of multiple insulin syringes while injecting one patient so as to prevent blunting of needle tip and increase the comfort of injection. Here is an exhaustive list of surgical materials which can be used during neurotoxin treatment **(Table 2)**.

SUMMARY

It is clearly understood that the ultimate goal of neurotoxin treatment is patient satisfaction and best clinical outcome. Correct selection, dosing, and dilution of toxin in a perfectly prepared clinical setting is the key to achieve the ultimate goal.

REFERENCES

1. Ferrari A, Manca M, Tugnoli V, et al. Pharmacological differences and clinical implications of various botulinum toxin preparations: a critical appraisal. Funct Neurol. 2018;33(1):7-18.
2. Ramirez-Castaneda J, Jankovic J, Comella C, et al. Diffusion, spread, and migration of botulinum toxin. Mov Disord. 2013(13);28:1775-83.
3. Karsai S, Raulin C. Current evidence on the unit equivalence of different botulinum neurotoxin A formulations and recommendations for clinical practice in dermatology. Dermatol Surg. 2009;35(1):1-8.
4. de Almeida AT, De Boulle K. Diffusion characteristics of botulinum neurotoxin products and their clinical significance in cosmetic applications. J Cosmet Laser Ther. 2007;9(Suppl 1):17-22.
5. Nestor M, Ablon G, Pickett A. Key parameters for the use of abobotulinumtoxin A in aesthetics: onset and duration. Aesthet Surg J. 2017;37(Suppl 1): S20-31.
6. Brandt F, Swanson N, Baumann L, et al. Randomized, placebo-controlled study of a new botulinum toxin type A for treatment of glabellar lines: efficacy and safety. Dermatol Surg. 2009;35(12):1893-901.
7. Carruthers A, Cohen JL, Cox SE, et al. Facial aesthetics: achieving the natural, relaxed look. J Cosmet Laser Ther. 2007;9(Suppl 1):6-10.
8. Lizarralde M, Gutiérrez SH, Venegas A. Clinical efficacy of botulinum toxin type A reconstituted and refrigerated 1 week before its application in external canthus dynamic lines. Dermatol Surg. 2007;33(11):1328-33.
9. Carruthers A, Carruthers J, Cohen J, et al. Dose dilution and duration of effect of botulinum toxin type A (BTX-A) for the treatment of glabellar rhytids. Poster presented at the 2002 winter meeting of the American Academy of Dermatology. New Orleans, LA; February 2002.

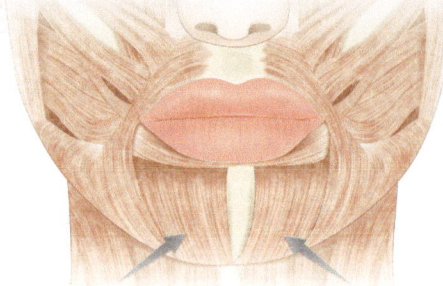

CHAPTER 27

Frown Lines

Varsha Vaidyanathan, Shilpa Garg, Rashmi Sarkar

INDICATIONS

Glabellar rhytides, also known as frown lines or eleven lines are the vertical lines appearing between the forehead and the eyebrows and are accentuated on frowning. They are a very common reason for cosmetic intervention in the form of botulinum toxin injection. These frown lines are graded on a four point clinical severity score as 0—no wrinkles, 1—mild wrinkles, 2—moderate wrinkles, and 3—severe wrinkles.[1]

ANATOMIC CONSIDERATIONS

The act of frowning is achieved by the combined action of the two corrugator supercilii muscles and the single procerus muscle. Upon contraction, they pull each individual brow downwards and medially. The procerus is responsible for the horizontal line at the glabellar area while the corrugators are responsible for the vertical lines.

Key vessels in the area are the supratrochlear and supraorbital arteries and veins which run vertically along the forehead very close to the frown area.

The supratrochlear nerve runs along the corrugator muscle and innervates the medial forehead. The supraorbital nerve runs underneath the frontalis fascia, leaves the orbital foramen, and ascends beneath the corrugator supercilii and the frontalis muscle while innervating the lateral forehead and scalp.

DESIRED OUTCOMES[2]

- Smooth glabellar area with very few lines and wrinkles
- Female eyebrow:
  – Lies over the supraorbital margin
  – Slightly arched as compared to a male brow
  – Medial part (head) a little lower than the lateral part (tail).
- Male eyebrow:
  – Obscures the supraorbital margin
  – Lower and flatter than the female eyebrow
  – No arch
  – Medial and lateral ends lie at the same horizontal level or the medial end may be slightly lower.

INJECTION TECHNIQUES[2]

Typically, insulin syringes or 1 mL syringes with 30G needles are used for injecting.

There are five injection sites for the glabellar complex **(Fig. 1)**. One single injection centrally within the procerus muscle (1), one injection for each lateral corrugator—1 cm above the

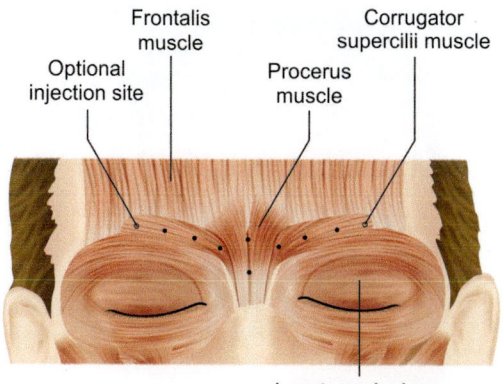

Fig. 1: Suggested injection sites for frown lines.

orbital rim at the mid-pupillary line (2,3), one injection for each medial corrugator—midway between the sites for procerus and lateral corrugators (4,5).

Some patients may require an additional injection midway between the medial and lateral corrugators (6,7).

After explaining the procedure to the patient, written consent is obtained. Preprocedure photographs must be taken in good lighting with the patient frowning. Apprehensive patients can be given prior ice packs or topical anesthesia to numb the area. The skin is cleaned with alcohol swabs. The patient is then asked to stare straight ahead while frowning maximally to better delineate the procerus and the corrugators, as well as to fix the mid-pupillary line. As explained above, the sites of injection are chosen and marked with a skin marking pencil. To avoid complications, a good grasp of the regional anatomy is essential. It is recommended that aspiration is done at each site to ensure the needle is not placed intravascularly.

For the procerus, the skin between the eyebrows is pinched with the noninjecting hand and the injection is given in the middle of the muscle with the needle angled upwards and inserted till one-half of the needle length. As the muscle is not very deep, the needle need not be inserted fully.

For the medial corrugators, the skin is pinched using the thumb and forefinger to isolate the muscle. The thumb rests on the superior orbital rim to prevent accidental injection below the rim which can lead to the complication of lid ptosis. As the muscle is deep, the full length of the needle is inserted while being angled upwards and laterally.

For the lateral corrugators, the skin is pinched and owing to the superficial nature of the muscle here, only one-third of the needle length is inserted while angled laterally upwards.

At each of the injection sites, the injecting hand can be steadied by placing it on the patient's face.

Injection into the glabellar complex allows diffusion of botulinum toxin into the lower part of the frontalis muscle and lessens the lines on the lower part of the forehead. This also acts to achieve a brow lift due to the relaxation of the procerus, corrugators, medial belly of frontalis and consequent strengthening of the lateral belly of frontalis which acts to lift up the lateral ends of the eyebrows (**Figs. 2A and 2B**).

To achieve a further brow lift especially in female patients, 3 U can be injected at the tail end of the eyebrow to target the superior fibers of the orbicularis oculi which act to depressor the end of the eyebrow while tightly contracted. Relaxation of these fibers will tend to lift up the lateral part of the eyebrow.

In men, a brow lift can give rise to a feminine appearance. To achieve a straighter brow, 3 U can be injected 1–1.5 cm above the

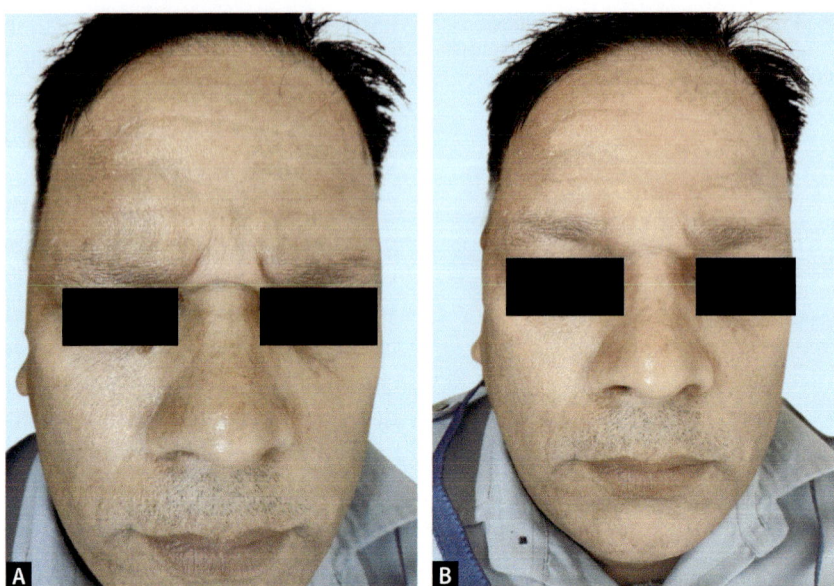

Figs. 2A and B: (A) Frown lines before botulinum toxin injections; (B) Smoothness after botulinum toxin injections.
(*Courtesy*: Rashmi Sarkar)

lateral eyebrow at the junction of the frontalis, temporalis, and orbicularis oculi muscles.

Botulinum toxin can be used along with fillers for an overall cosmetic improvement. Botox is generally given first to deal with the dynamic component and then at a later date, injectable fillers are used. If used in the same session, the filler is injected first, massaged well into the face and after a few minutes, Botox is injected.

In women, approximately 4 U of Botox is injected at each of the five sites to a total of 20 U which can increase to 24 U. Males generally require higher doses from 20 U to 40 U depending upon strength of muscle contraction. There are studies where men have received up to 80U in the glabellar complex with no complications.

The response is seen within 1–14 days and lasts for 3–4 months at which time the botulinum toxin can be reinjected.[3-5]

PRECAUTIONS

Ptosis can result due to diffusion of botulinum toxin into the levator palpebrae muscle during injection of the corrugators. To prevent this diffusion, a thumb must be placed below the orbital rim during injection. Ptosis presents within 2–7 days of injection and can last up to 6 weeks. Eye drops containing alpha adrenergic agents like 0.5% apraclonidine or 2.5% phenylephrine are used 2–3 times a day till the ptosis resolves. The mechanism of action is the stimulation of Muller's muscles to help elevate the ptotic eyelids.

It is better to initially undercorrect rather than overcorrect as the undertreatment can be dealt with in a later session whereas the overtreatment leads to unpleasant cosmesis and runs the risk of complications. Overcorrection at the glabella can lead to lifting of the eyebrows laterally as explained earlier, giving rise to a Mephisto or Spock appearance. This is particularly undesirable in males. To combat this, 3U are given above the lateral eyebrow.

POSTINJECTION INSTRUCTIONS

Patient should be instructed to avoid massaging the area after the injections as this can lead to diffusion of the botulinum toxin to unwanted areas. Antibiotic cream can be applied to the injected areas. Patients can resume all daily activities.

General nonspecific early complications include headache, bruising, swelling, pain, and redness at the injection sites. These are self-resolving and not a matter of great concern. Late complications include chronic inflammation, infection at the injection site, hypertrophic scarring, and granuloma formation as a rare complication.

USEFUL TIPS

- Glabellar lines are amongst the most common indications of Botox.
- Lateral corrugators lie very superficially so only one-third of the needle length is inserted; procerus is less superficial so one-half of the needle length is inserted while the medial corrugators are deep therefore, the full needle length is inserted.
- Due care needs to be taken regarding the appearance of the eyebrows while injecting the glabellar lines to avoid unpleasant cosmesis.
- A thumb needs to be pressed below the orbital rim while injecting to avoid diffusion into levator palpebrae and hence ptosis.
- Better to undercorrect than overcorrect.

REFERENCES

1. Honeck P, Weiss C, Sterry W, et al; Gladys Study Group. Reproducibility of a four-point clinical severity score for glabellar frown lines. Br J Dermatol. 2003;149(2):306-10.
2. de Maio M, DeBoulle K, Braz A, et al; Alliance for the Future of Aesthetics Consensus Committee. Facial Assessment and Injection Guide for Botulinum Toxin and Injectable Hyaluronic Acid Fillers: Focus on the Midface. Plast Reconstr Surg. 2017;140(4):540e-550e.
3. Monheit G, Carruthers A, Brandt F, et al. A randomized, double-blind, placebo-controlled study of botulinum toxin type A for the treatment of glabellar lines: determination of optimal dose. Dermatol Surg. 2007;33(1 Spec No.):S51-9.
4. Carruthers A, Carruthers J. Prospective, double-blind, randomized, parallel-group, dose-ranging study of botulinum toxin type A in men with glabellar rhytids. Dermatol Surg. 2005;31(10):1297-303.
5. Carruthers A, Carruthers J, Said S. Dose-ranging study of botulinum toxin type A in the treatment of glabellar rhytids in females. Dermatol Surg. 2005;31(4):414-22.

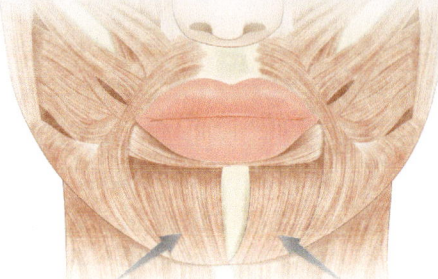

Forehead Lines

Richa Ojha Sharma, Rashmi Sarkar

INDICATIONS

The first report of the esthetic utility of botulinum toxin was published in 1992.[1] Among the several esthetic uses of botulinum toxin, its utility for treating forehead lines remains foremost. The aim of injecting the forehead with botulinum toxin is primarily to relax the frontalis muscle and reduce horizontal forehead creases. The technique of treatment of forehead with botulinum toxin has evolved considerably in the past 2 decades. No longer is the frozen and plastic look appreciated by the patient or the esthetic physician. A conservative approach to preserve some mobility of the frontalis, while maintaining a delicate balance between the elevator and the depressors of the forehead has led to finer esthetic outcomes such as increasing forehead height, sculpting and reshaping of eyebrows, and managing eye aperture. Improvement in skin texture and a certain "shine" are additional benefits with botulinum toxin treatment.[2]

ANATOMIC CONSIDERATIONS

Understanding the anatomy of the forehead muscles and the effect of the synergy of the upper face musculature on brow position and shape can help deliver finer results upon injecting and can prevent complications.

Frontalis

The frontalis muscle is the only elevator of the brows. It is a broad, symmetrical, roughly rectangular muscle with vertically oriented muscle fibers in the forehead. It originates in the galea aponeurotica at the coronal suture superiorly and inserts into the superficial fascia of the skin where it meets the muscles at the glabella. The medial fibers intermingle with the procerus while the intermediate fibers mingle with the corrugator supercilii and orbicularis oculi.[3] The glabellar complex muscles are the depressors of the brow.

The Role of Levator Palpebra Superioris

The levator palpebra superioris (LPS) causes eyelid lifting, while the frontalis causes eyebrow lifting. The tone of the LPS determines the baseline activity of the frontalis. If the LPS is weak, there is ptosis of the eyelid and the frontalis compensates by contracting to raise the eyelid. This causes higher and more arched eyebrows and deeper wrinkles in that area of the forehead.[4]

INJECTION TECHNIQUE

Assessment

- Assess the facial expression at rest and during animation.

- *Perform the stretch test:* If stretching the area with the hand improves the wrinkles, then the chances of improvement with botulinum toxin are better.
- Palpate the muscles to assess their thickness and tonicity.
- Check the position of the brow.
- *Check the position of the eyelid:* In static position, the upper eyelid must cover about 2 mm of the corneoscleral limbus. If it covers more than 2 mm, it denotes that the LPS is weak. In such cases botulinum toxin injections should be placed further from the area of the upper eyelid than usual, should contain a lower dose, or should be omitted altogether.[4]
- Look for any asymmetries in the face and make the patient aware of these before injecting.
- Click clear photographs of the patient at rest and during animation.

Discussion

- Always ask the patient what his/her desires pertaining to esthetic outcome are.
- Patients with thick and heavy foreheads, those with low brows, or with ptotic eyelids must be told of the possibility of eyelid heaviness and of difficulty to spontaneously raise the brows following treatment.

Technique

Botulinum toxin on the forehead is a more tailored approach than elsewhere over the face. Dose and injection technique must be individualized based on the variable anatomy and function of the musculature, while respecting patient aspirations.[5] The key points of injection technique are listed in **Table 1**. It is now recommended to treat the glabellar lines too in order to manage the

Table 1: Injection techniques for forehead.

		Key points
Dose	• 8–10 units in females • 10–20 units in males	Avoid over injecting as it may lead to frozen look and brow heaviness
Pattern	*Females:* V-shaped distribution—5–8 points—1–2 units per point, along with an extra point laterally[6] **(Figs. 1A and B)** *Males:* Span the forehead in zigzag pattern along alternate lines at 6–10 points, 1–1.5 cm apart—0.5–1 unit per point **(Fig. 2)** Avoid injecting 1–2 cm above the brow (3–4 cm above bony orbital ridge)	• Going too far lateral in females leads to a flat eyebrow but staying too medial will leave the lateral lines uncorrected and cause quizzical look.[8] • In men, a flatter eyebrow is more desirable. It is inadvisable to leave the external part of the frontalis untreated in men.
Point of deposit	• In older individuals or those with brow ptosis, inject intradermal (ID)—raise a wheal or bleb • In younger individuals—intramuscular (IM)	• IM injection causes more robust paralyzing of frontalis but leads to heavier feeling in forehead • ID injections prevent heaviness of brows, but at the cost of lesser longevity of effect
Botulinum toxin brow lift	A slight amount of lateral eyebrow elevation can be induced by sparing the lateral fibers of the frontalis. Ideally, the lateral fibers of orbicularis oculi must also be simultaneously injected for a full effect	This subtle lateral flare causes an appealing change in the appearance of the face although this might be at the expense of an incomplete reduction in the lateral forehead creases

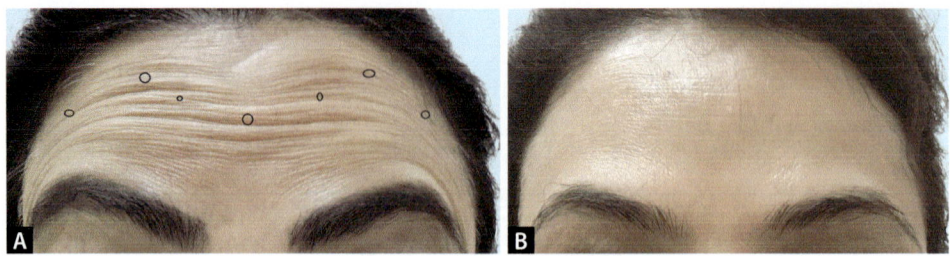

Figs. 1A and B: (A) V-shaped distribution of injection points, and two points placed laterally to avoid quizzical look; (B) Correction of forehead lines with maintenance of correct brow arch after Botox injection.

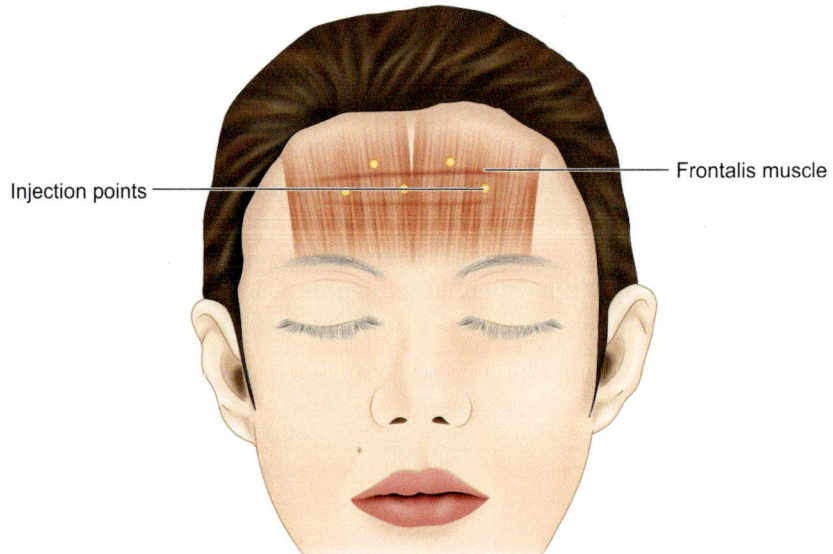

Fig. 2: Zig-zag injection pattern for males.

brow shape and eyebrow position better.[6] Theoretically, maximum effect of botulinum toxin would occur when the toxin is deposited deep intramuscularly. However, lately it has been observed that intradermal injections lead to two important differences:
- Reduced chances of eyebrow ptosis and eyelid heaviness, and
- Improvement in skin texture, pore size, and greasiness of skin.[7]

Precautions

Injecting the frontalis has a direct impact on the brow position **(Table 2)**.

A few basic precautions such as those listed in **Box 1** help to minimize complications and refine the results.

FOLLOW-UP

Assess after 10 days. If needed, one may inject 4–6 units into unresponsive parts of the frontalis

Table 2: Effect of forehead botulinum toxin on brow position.

Brow position/shape	Reason
Brow ptosis	Excessive weakening of the frontalis without a corresponding weakening of the depressors. High doses or too low placement of toxin in forehead. Avoid injections in the 1 cm area above the brow (2 cm for beginner injectors).
Flattened brow	Too much botulinum toxin over the lateral brow
"Mephisto" or "Spock" effect	Too much botulinum toxin in the medial forehead, and none in the lateral, causing the lateral fibers to compensate and lift up the lateral brow causing an abnormally quizzical look

Box 1 Precautions to be taken while injecting forehead lines with botulinum toxin.

Precautions
- Stay superior to the most inferior forehead line or 3–4 cm above the orbital margin (2 cm above the brow)
- Do not use over-diluted toxin
- Inject the lateral fibers lateral only in the upper part of the forehead, and not in the lower
- Inject a small amount in the procerus
- Staying too central in the forehead will lead to quizzical expression
- Use low doses in forehead. You can always touch up later

and 2–4 units of botulinum toxin may have to be injected laterally, if quizzical brow shape occurs. A check for eyebrow ptosis must be done. Brow ptosis may persist for up to 3 months. The patient may not recognize the brow drop but may report an angrier or more depressed look after the procedure.

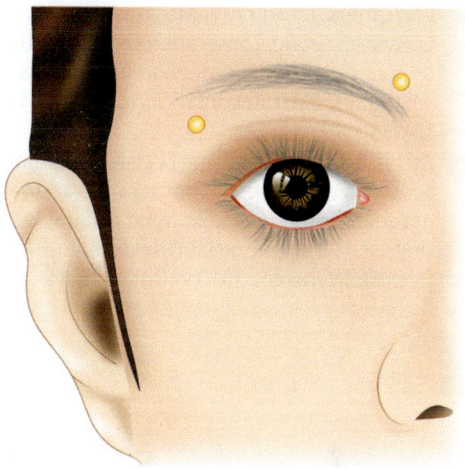

Fig. 3: Points of injection to correct brow ptosis.

Brow ptosis can be corrected by injecting 1–2 units botulinum toxin 2–3 mm intradermally laterally below the brow; and 1–2 units deep into the medial end of the brow as shown in **Figure 3**.[9]

REFERENCES

1. Carruthers A, Carruthers J, Cohen J. A prospective, double-blind, randomized, parallel-group, dose-ranging study of botulinum toxin type a in female subjects with horizontal forehead rhytides. Dermatol Surg. 2003;29(5):461-7.
2. Raspaldo H, Baspeyras M, Bellity P, et al; Consensus Group. Upper- and mid-face anti-aging treatment and prevention using onabotulinumtoxin A: the 2010 multidisciplinary French consensus – part 1. J Cosmet Dermatol. 2011;10(1):36-50.
3. Lorenc ZP, Smith S, Nestor M, et al. Understanding the functional anatomy of the frontalis and glabellar complex for optimal aesthetic botulinum toxin type A therapy. Aesthetic Plast Surg. 2013;37(5):975-83.
4. Ezure T, Amano S. The severity of wrinkling at the forehead is related to the degree of ptosis of the upper eyelid. Skin Research and Technology. 2010;16(2):202-9.

5. Carruthers J, Fagien S, Matarasso SL; Botox Consensus Group. Consensus recommendations on the use of botulinum toxin type A in facial aesthetics. Plast Reconstr Surg. 2004:114(6):1S-22S.
6. Ascher B, Talarico S, Cassuto D, et al. International consensus recommendations on the aesthetic usage of botulinum toxin type A (Speywood Unit): Part I. Upper facial wrinkles. J Eur Acad Dermatol Venereol. 2010;24(11):1278-84.
7. Jun JY, Park JH, Youn CS, et al. Intradermal injection of botulinum toxin: a safer treatment modality for forehead wrinkles. Ann Dermatol. 2018;30(4):458-61.
8. Vartanian AJ, Dayan SH. Complications of botulinum toxin A use in facial rejuvenation. Facial Plast Surg Clin North Am. 2005;13(1):1-10.
9. Redaelli A, Forte R. How to avoid brow ptosis after forehead treatment with botulinum toxin. J Cosmet Laser Ther. 2003;5(3-4):220-2.

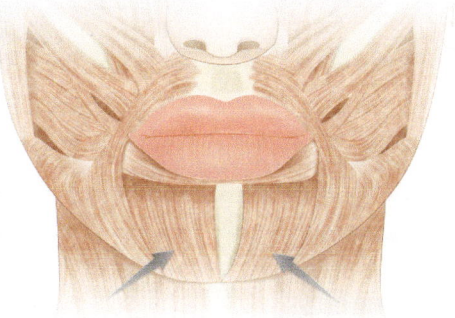

CHAPTER 29

Crow's Feet and Lower Eyelid

Nidhi Sharma

INDICATIONS

Crow's feet is one of the simplest and most satisfying applications of botulinum toxin (BTX). These are wrinkles that form around the eyes and are also known as crow's feet lines (CFL) or lateral canthal lines (LCL). Crow's feet develop due to the repeated contraction of orbicularis oculi, the facial muscle predominantly involved in smiling.[1]

ANATOMIC CONSIDERATIONS

Classification of Crow's Feet Patterns (Figs. 1A to D)

Four pattern types are identified for CFL:[2]
1. Full fan
2. Lower fan
3. Central fan
4. Upper fan.

The first three patterns namely the full fan, lower fan, and central fan constitute 90% of the CFL. In a full fan **(Fig. 3)**, lines project from the lateral canthus and extend into both superior malar area and tail of the brow. In the lower fan, lines are restricted to the lateral canthus and superior malar area. In the central fan, lines are confined to the lateral canthal area but do not extend into the superior malar area or lateral third of the brow. In the upper fan **(Fig. 4A and B)**, lines are confined to the lateral canthus and extend toward or into the lateral third of the brow.

The orbicularis oculi is a broad muscle composed of concentric striated fibers having three subparts.[3]
1. *Lacrimal portion:* Smallest innermost portion that runs deep into the lacrimal sac and inserts on the upper and lower eyelids at the tarsal plates.
2. *Palpebral portion:* Raises the eyelid and controls the involuntary action of blinking.
3. *Orbital portion:* Surrounds the orbit with concentric fibers and blends into the frontalis and extends to the masseter.

INJECTION TECHNIQUE[4,5]

Treatment of crow's feet for BTX has been US Food and Drug Administration (US FDA) approved for onabotulinum toxin and A. The presence of different CFL patterns enable that it is possible to customize treatment with a total of 20–30 U dose based on type of line pattern **(Figs. 5A and B)**. Two types of injection techniques can be used—CFL injection pattern and the modified CFL injection pattern **(Figs. 2A and B)**.

Crow's Feet Lines Injection Pattern[4,5]

The first injection is given in the orbicularis oculi at the level of the lateral canthus,

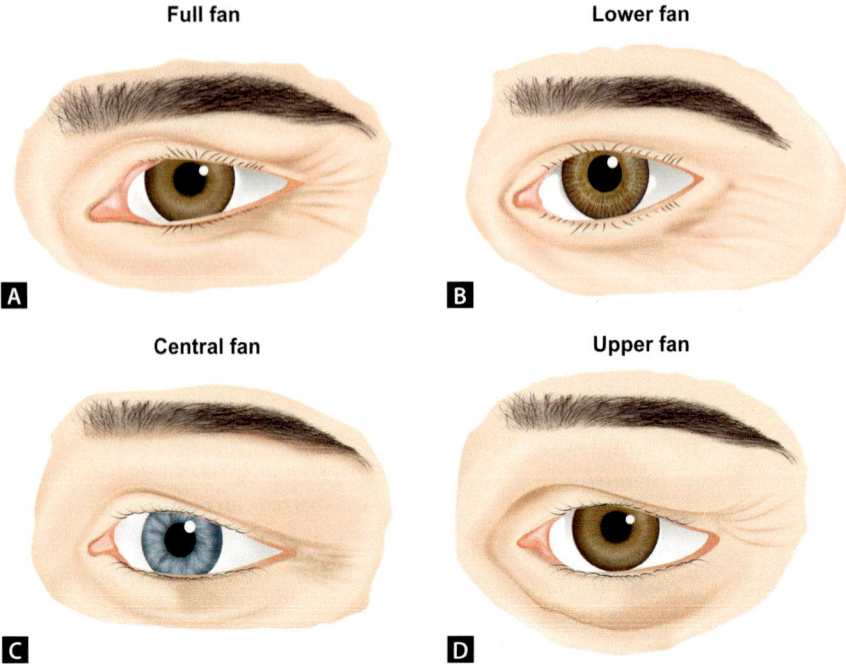

Figs. 1A to D: Classification of crow's feet lines patterns in untreated patients. (A) In a full-fan pattern; (B) Lines project from the lateral canthal area and extend into both the superior malar area and the tail of the brow. In a lower-fan pattern; (C) Lines are predominantly confined to the lateral canthal area and the superior malar area. In a central-fan pattern, lines are predominantly confined to the lateral canthal area and do not extend into the superior malar area or lateral third of the brow; (D) An upper-fan pattern has lines predominantly confined to the lateral canthal area and extends toward or into the lateral third of the brow.

1.5–2 cm temporal to the lateral canthus and just temporal to the lateral orbital rim. The second injection is 1–1.5 cm above the first injection and marked at 30° angle medially. The third injection is 1–1.5 cm below the first injection site at an approximately 30° angle medially.

Modified Crow's Feet Lines Injection Pattern[4,5]

When CFLs are below the lateral canthus, three injections may be given in a line angling from superoposterior to anteroinferior. The injections are given with the needle bevel tip pointed up and oriented away from the eye. Each injection is .1 mL in volume and contains 4 U of onabotulinumtoxin A. Injections should be placed as a wheal superficially into the dermis **(Fig. 2)**.

PRECAUTIONS[6]

Before administering BTX injections, it is necessary to make an assessment of the CFL at rest and while the patient is making deliberate muscle contraction such as during smiling. Cleansing with alcohol prior to treatment in addition to good lighting, magnification and stretching the skin may help to identify any superficial vessels along the treatment area. Needles should be changed frequently to prevent them from getting blunt. Injections should be kept superficial to minimize

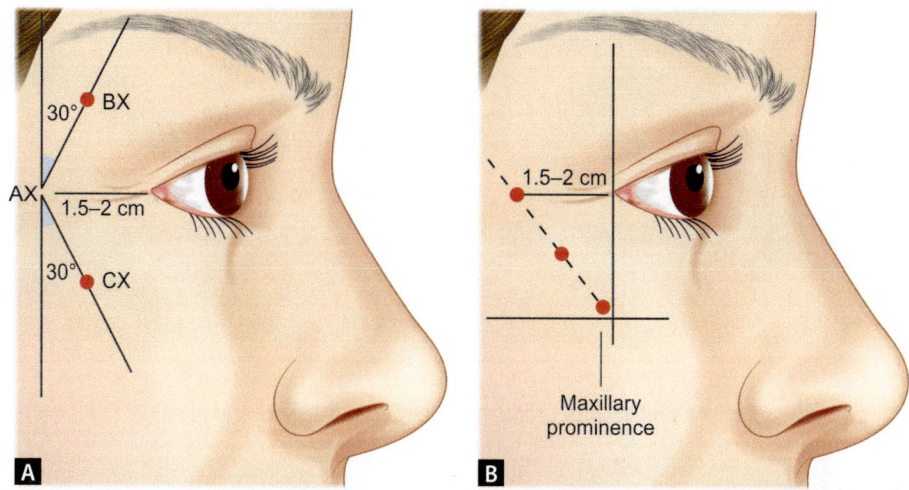

Figs. 2A and B: Injection pattern and allowed modification for the treatment of crow's feet lines (CFL). (A) CFL injection pattern. The first injection was in the orbicularis oculi at the level of the lateral canthus, at least 1.5–2.0 cm temporal to the lateral canthus and just temporal to the lateral orbital rim (marked as AX). The second injection was 1.0–1.5 cm above this first injection site and at an approximately 30° angle medially (marked as BX). The third injection was 1.0–1.5 cm below the first injection site at an approximately 30° angle medially (marked as CX); (B) Modified CFL injection pattern. When CFL are below the lateral canthus, 3 injections may be given in a line angling from superoposterior to anteroinferior. The first injection is made in the same manner as described above for site AX. The anteroinferior injection point should be lateral to a line drawn vertically from the lateral canthus and superior to the maxillary prominence. A third injection point should be positioned at the midpoint along a line connecting the superoposterior and anteroinferior injection points.

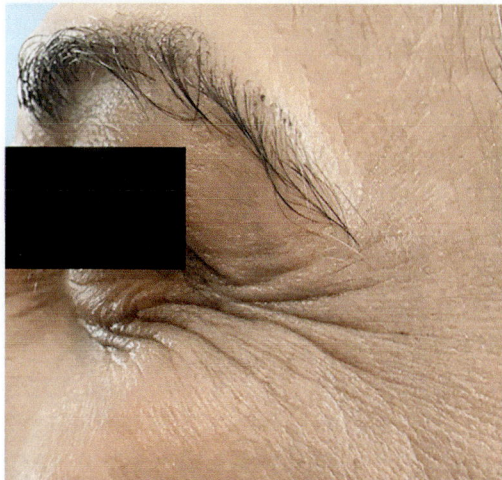

Fig. 3: Full-fan pattern of crow's feet lines (CFL) in a 63-year-old female. This pattern is commonly seen in older patients with greater CFL severity.

the risk of direct injection into nearby lip elevators including the zygomaticus major and minor muscles. Injecting below the level of superior zygomatic arch should be avoided to prevent complications such as ipsilateral facial paralysis and lip ptosis. To prevent inadvertent injections into the frontalis, injections should be performed at least 1 cm above the eyebrow. Ecchymosis can be minimized by avoiding aspirin and drugs that inhibit platelet function for ~10 days before injection. Limiting the number of injections, and applying postinjection digital pressure (without manipulation) will assist in reducing the severity of bruising. When treating CFL, candidate selection is crucial and the injector should avoid patients with

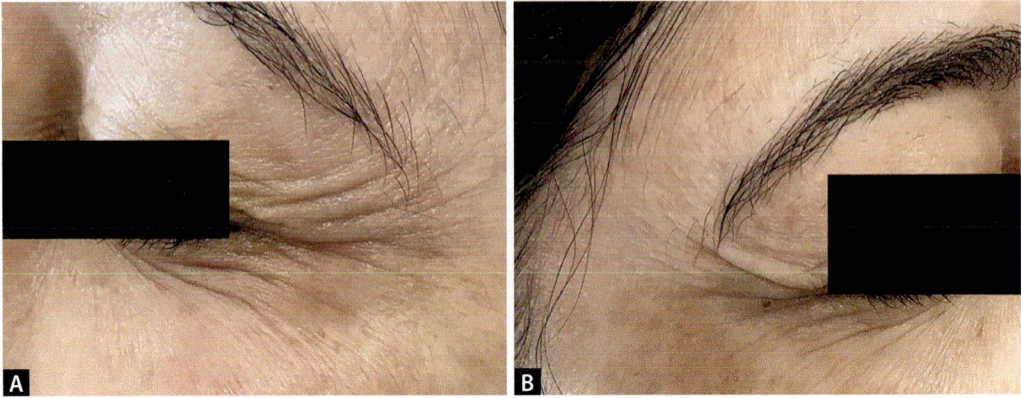

Figs. 4A and B: Upper-fan pattern of CFL in a 56-year-old female.

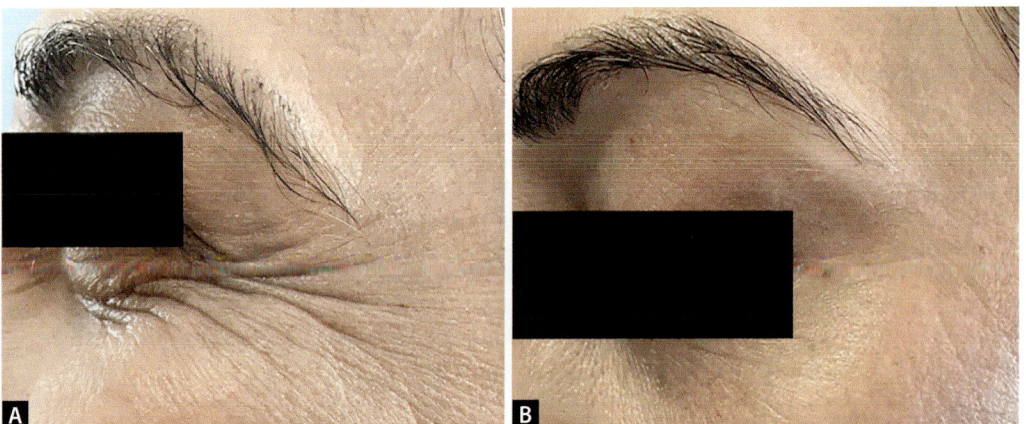

Figs. 5A and B: Pre- and post-treatment photograph of a 63-year-old female with CFL treated with 12 U of BTX each side.

(BTX: botulinum toxin)

dry eyes, prominent eye bags, scleral show, or morning eyelid edema. In addition, patients need to have a positive snap test and preferably good skin elasticity.

COMPLICATIONS

Eyelid ptosis can occur rarely as a result of migration of the toxin into the levator palpebrae superioris muscle. Both eyelid and eyebrow ptosis may also occur as a result of inadvertent weakening of the frontalis muscle secondary to the diffusion of toxin. Upper lip ptosis can occur due to direct injection or diffusion of the toxin into zygomaticus major and minor or levator labii superioris muscles. These complications are temporary and usually improve within 4–8 weeks.

USEFUL TIPS

- Evaluate lid laxity with a snap text. Laxity indicates the potential for developing an ectropion, and lower eyelid injections may be avoided.
- Ask the patient to animate during injections in order to carefully assess the line patterns.

- Exercise caution in patients who have dry eyes or have undergone surgery.
- Avoid the area below the zygomatic arch. Injection into this area has the potential to cause lip and cheek ptosis.
- Start with low doses. Apply pressure after each injection and use ice to help avoid ecchymoses.

BOTULINUM TOXIN INJECTIONS IN THE LOWER EYELID[7]

Botulinum toxin injections in the lower eyelid area when properly administered can provide a dramatic improvement **(Fig. 6)**. For periocular wrinkles, it is advised to start with 2 U in the lower lid along with 12 U in the crow's feet area. 2 U of BTX in the lower eyelid can reduce the periorbital wrinkles and widen the eye. Increasing doses of BTX in the lower eyelid can increase palpebral aperture and decrease lower lid folds. However, increasing the dose beyond 4 U may be associated with side effects such as scleral show or lower lid edema giving a sad look to the patient. Patients who desire improvement of the lower eyelid wrinkles or eye widening are therefore initially treated with 2 U placed in the midpupillary line. A follow-up can be done approximately 2–4 weeks later and if the patient desires further eyelid widening or improvement in their lower eyelid rhytids, an additional 2 U may be placed into the lower lid. Symptoms such as dryness of the eyes or problems with sphincter function of the orbicularis must be assessed before supplementing the patient with an additional 2 U in the lower eyelid. All patients should have an acceptable snap test before treatment.

Injection Technique for Lower Eyelid

Following a lateral approach, the tip of the needle is advanced to the midpupillary point and 2 U of BTX is injected subdermally just lateral to the midpupillary point 3 mm inferior to the lash margin.

Precautions

- The "snap test" entails gently tugging down on the lower eyelid and then releasing the eyelid.[8] If the lid only slowly or partially returns to its rest position, this is indicative of decreased elasticity, which should preclude treatment.
- If faced with incipient bruising, the injector should immediately apply firm pressure with a gauze and fingertip for several seconds.
- Injections under the eye should be very superficial because the relevant muscles (orbicularis) are thin and right under the dermis.
- Injections of more than 2 U per eye should be avoided in patients with pre-existing dry eye symptoms or Sjogren's syndrome. Dry

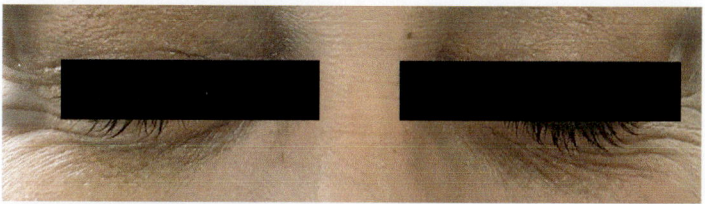

Fig. 6: Lower eyelid wrinkles along with CFL in an elderly female patient.

eye is the most common complication in middle-aged to older women[9] and before administering infraorbital injection in such patients, it may be reasonable to elicit this relevant history.

REFERENCES

1. Charles Finn J, Cox SE, Earl ML. Social implications of hyperfunctional facial lines. Dermatol Surg. 2003;29(5):450-5.
2. Kane MA. Classification of crow's feet patterns among Caucasian women: the key to individualizing treatment. Plast Reconstr Surg. 2003;112(Suppl 5):33S-9S.
3. Ascher B, Talarico S, Cassuto D, et al. International consensus recommendations on the aesthetic usage of botulinum toxin type A (Speywood Unit)–Part II: Wrinkles on the middle and lower face, neck and chest. J Eur Acad Dermatol Venereol. 2010;24(11):1285-95.
4. Carruthers A, Bruce S, de Coninck A, et al. Efficacy and safety of onabotulinumtoxinA for the treatment of crow's feet lines: a multicenter, randomized, controlled trial. Dermatol Surg. 2014;40(11):1181-90.
5. Moers-Carpi M, Carruthers J, Fagien S, et al. Efficacy and safety of onabotulinumtoxinA for treating crow's feet lines alone or in combination with glabellar lines: a multicenter, randomized controlled trial. Dermatol Surg. 2015;41(1):102-12.
6. Lowe NJ, Ascher B, Heckmann M, et al. Double-blind, randomized, placebo-controlled, dose-response study of the safety and efficacy of botulinum toxin type A in subjects with crow's feet. Dermatol Surg. 2005;31(3):257-62.
7. Timothy F, Jean C, Alastair C, et al. Botulinum A toxin (BOTOX) in the lower eyelid. Dermatol Surg. 2003;29:943-50.
8. Klein AW. Treatment of wrinkles with Botox. In: Kreyden OP, Boni R, Burg G (Eds). Hyperhidrosis and Botulinum Toxin in Dermatology. Basel: S. Karger; 2002. pp. 189-217.
9. Nelson JD. Diagnosis and treatment of the dry eye: a clinical perspective. Adv Exp Med Biol. 2002;506:1067-78.

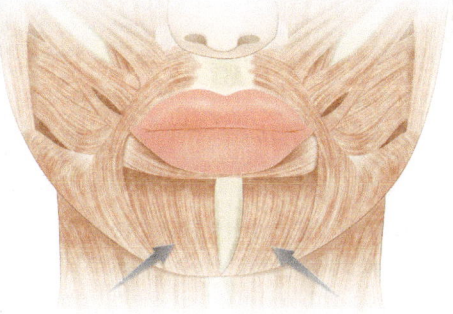

CHAPTER 30

Brow Lift with Botulinum Toxin

Jaishree Sharad

INTRODUCTION

Eyebrows positioned properly mark an important aspect of beauty and youthfulness.

Well-demarcated eyebrows usually arch slightly at the junction of the medial two-thirds and lateral one-third of the face. However, males usually prefer to have horizontal eyebrows. Eyebrow dimensions also vary with ethnicity. Shape of the eyebrows is also a mark of fashion and may change from time to time.

The overall esthetic balance of the face can change with eyebrow asymmetry, change in brow position and fullness. The eyebrows may be asymmetrical from the beginning and this asymmetry becomes more evident as one ages.

Brow ptosis is common with aging due to loss of soft tissue support, bone resorption, and gravity. Sometimes, brow ptosis may be genetic too. Brow ptosis can also be a result of diffusion of botulinum toxin (BTX) into lower fibers of the frontalis muscle close to its insertion when the neurotoxin is injected within 1 cm of the bony superior orbital rim.

Brow ptosis gives a sad and tired look. Lateral hooding of eyelids due to eyebrow ptosis results in prominent skin folds and crow's feet.

Injecting BTX is the simplest and quickest technique for a brow lift.

RELEVANT ANATOMY[1]

Brow position is dependent on the interplay between the muscles that elevate the brow and those muscles that depress the brow.

The frontalis muscle is the only muscle on the forehead responsible for brow elevation.

Corrugator supercilii, procerus, and depressor supercilii are medial brow depressors. Lateral fibers of orbicularis oculi are lateral brow depressors. It is important to understand the anatomy of these muscles in detail to be able to create the desired brow lift.

By treating the brow depressors, an unopposed action of the frontalis on the brows is seen elevating their position. The frontalis muscle elevates the eyebrows and the skin of the forehead. It originates on the galea aponeurotica along the coronal suture and inserts in the dermis at the level of the supraorbital ridge of the frontal bone where it interdigitates with fibers of procerus, corrugator supercilii, and orbicularis oculi muscles.

The corrugator supercilii muscle adducts and slightly depresses the eyebrow thus moving it medially and inferiorly. It originates at medial supraorbital ridge of the frontal bone, runs obliquely in a superior lateral direction and inserts in the skin, interdigitating with fibers of frontalis. It is deep centrally and gets more superficial at the point of insertion.

The procerus is a thin depressor muscle that pulls the medial part of the brow down causing horizontal wrinkles on the bridge of the nose. It originates over the periosteum of the nasal bone and inserts into the dermis of the glabella. Finally the depressor supercilii originates from the nasal process of the frontal bone and inserts into the skin beneath the medial head of the brow.[2]

Orbicularis oculi: The orbicularis oculi muscle arises from three sites—(1) from the nasal part of the frontal bone, (2) from the frontal process of the maxilla, and (3) between these two sites, from the medial palpebral ligament. The fibers then pass around the orbit in concentric loops and insert at the origin itself.

The forehead and eyebrow positions are dependent on the frontal bone, the supraorbital rims, and the zygoma. The frontalis, corrugator, procerus, and lateral fibers of orbicularis oculi muscles also influence the position of the eyebrows. It is important to understand the eyebrow shape and its position with respect to the supraorbital rim to be able to create a brow lift. The eyebrows should be 5-6 cm below the hairline. The medial and lateral ends of the eyebrow should lie at the same horizontal level. In women, the eyebrow should lie above the supraorbital rim and in an arch shape with its highest point at the level of the lateral limbus of the eye at approximately the junction of the medial two-thirds and the lateral third of the eyebrow **(Fig. 1)**. In men, the arch must be smaller and lie slightly lower at the level of the supraorbital rim. Eyebrows also tend to be heavier in men than in women **(Fig. 2)**.[3]

INJECTION TECHNIQUES
Medial Brow Lift

The medial brow depressors namely procerus, depressor supercilii, and medial fibers of corrugator supercilii can be injected to cause a medical brow elevation **(Fig. 3)**.[4] Dose depends on the amount of elevation required and also on the existence of frown lines. Usually 4 U of BTX perpendicular into the procerus and 2 U each into the depressor

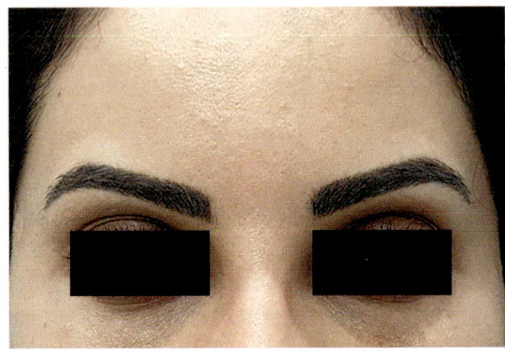

Fig. 1: Female brow.

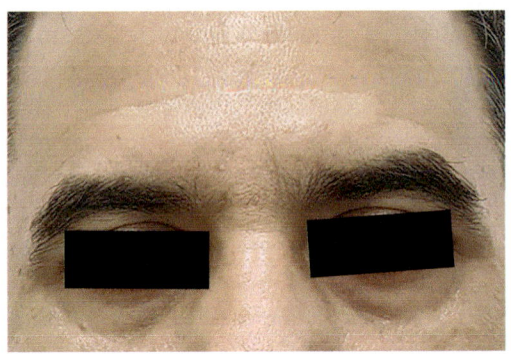

Fig. 2: Male brow.

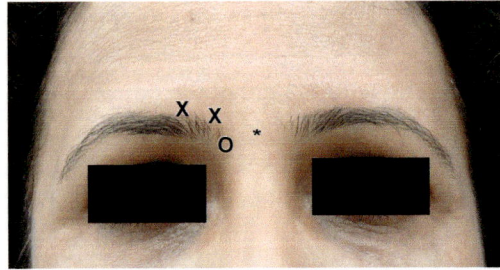

Fig. 3: Injection points for medial brow lift. (X: corrugator supercilii muscle, *: procerus muscle, O: depressor supercilii muscle)

supercilii and medial fibers of corrugator supercilii cause good medial brow elevation. To ensure brow elevation, it is necessary to inject those fibers of corrugators that are at, or below, the level of the brow. It is equally important to avoid injecting frontalis fibers which may otherwise lift the brow. The procerus muscle bulges between the medial brows. The injection technique is similar to that of the corrugator supercilii. The area between the medial heads of the brow, just above the radix and the area 2–3 cm superior are the typical injection sites. The depressor supercilii muscle stretches between the nasal process of the frontal bone and the medial head of the brow. This muscle is treated by a single injection of BTX just inferior and lateral to the medial head of the brow.[5]

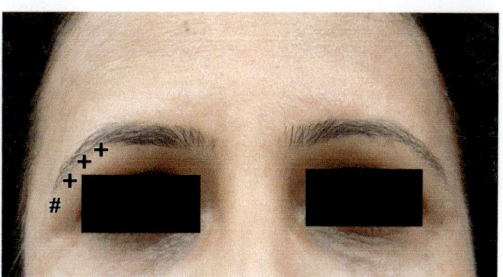

Fig. 4: Injection points for lateral brow lift.
[+: lateral fibers of orbicularis muscle, #: lateral fibers of orbicularis muscle (causing crow's feet)]

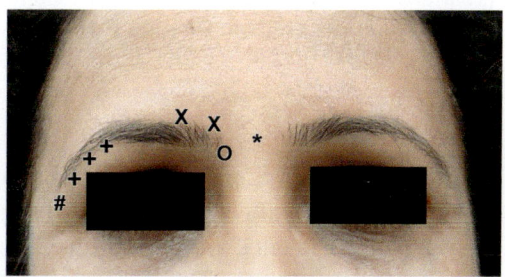

Fig. 5: Injection points for entire brow lift.
[X: corrugator supercilii muscle, *: procerus muscle; 0: depressor supercilii muscle, +: lateral fibers of orbicularis muscle, #: lateral fibers of orbicularis muscle (causing crow's feet)]

Lateral Brow Lift

Elevation of only the lateral brow can be accomplished by selectively treating the lateral brow depressors.[6] 2–3 U of BTX injected subdermally into lateral fibers of orbicularis oculi will elevate the lateral brow. Accentuation of the desired lateral brow elevation can be achieved by the additional weakening of the medial brow elevators to lower the medial brow, creating the illusion of higher lateral brows. Limit the total injection to each lateral brow area to less than 10 U of BTX **(Fig. 4)**.

Entire Brow Lift

Elevation of the entire brow complex can be achieved by injection of BTX into the medial and lateral brow depressors. In general, there is 1–3 mm of brow elevation with BTX **(Fig. 5)**.[7,8]

Arched Brow Lift

The orbicularis is injected in two to three sites just inferior to the eyebrow starting at the highest point of the brow and moving laterally half a centimeter apart.

Additionally, crow's feet if present should also be injected for a better lift.[9] The arch may be further accentuated by selective weakening of the medial frontalis muscle. This is done by injecting about 3 U of BTX in only the middle part of the frontalis muscle in order to lower the medial brow **(Fig. 6)**. 1–2 U are injected at each injection site.

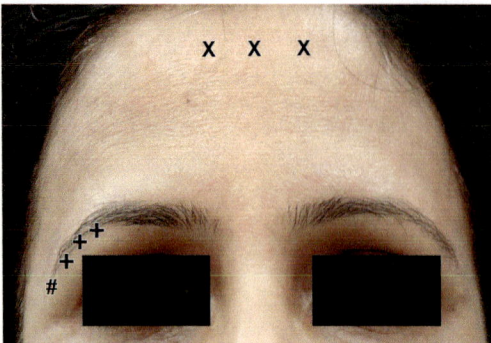

Fig. 6: Injection points for arched brow lift.
[+: lateral fibers of orbicularis muscle, #: lateral fibers of orbicularis muscle (causing crow's feet), X: middle fibers of frontalis muscle]

PRECAUTIONS

It is important to remember that treatment of the frontalis can affect brow position. The brow position can fall if the lower 2 cm of the frontalis muscle is treated with BTX. Do not be tempted to inject the frontalis in order to treat the most inferior horizontal forehead wrinkle. Diffusion of the toxin across the orbital septum can weaken the levator palpebrae muscle resulting in lid ptosis. Hence, stay above the orbital rim and do not point your needle downward toward the rim.

SIDE EFFECTS[10]

- Lid ptosis
- Asymmetrical eyebrow.

USEFUL TIPS

- Not all patients obtain the same degree of brow elevation with BTX.
- Patients with severe brow ptosis may not improve significantly.
- Patients with thick skin folds over upper lid may not respond to neurotoxin.
- Overtreatment of frontalis will negate the results obtained by injecting depressors.
- Individuals who use the frontalis muscle to compensate for underlying brow ptosis will not show much improvement in chemical brow lift with BTX. It is better not to attempt a chemical brow lift in such individuals.
- The orbicularis oculi muscle is closely adherent to the overlying skin, hence subdermal injections should be given to create a wheal.
- Load only as many units you want to inject per insulin syringe and inject slowly so that you do not overdose by mistake.
- Avoid injecting if there are excessive skin folds.
- Avoid injecting if there is lid ptosis.
- Avoid in patients with unrealistic expectations.
- Examination at rest and in motion is very important to see the brow and muscle position.
- Photographs must be taken before planning the injection not only for documentation but also for a final assessment.

CONCLUSION

Botulinum toxin can be used to create a chemical brow lift. There is a dynamic interaction between depressor and elevator muscles which should be understood. One must have thorough knowledge of the anatomy of these muscles. Patients must be carefully evaluated and selected for a brow lift with BTX as all patients may not respond well. Excessive brow droop, hooding, or lid ptosis may need surgical intervention.

REFERENCES

1. França K, Lotti T. Botulinum toxin. Advances in Integrative Dermatology, 1st edition. Chichester: John Wiley & Sons Ltd; 2019.

2. Daniel RK, Landon B. Endoscopic forehead lift: anatomic basis. Aesthet Surg J. 1997;17(2):97-104.
3. de Maio M, Berthold R. Eyebrow. Injectable Fillers in Aesthetic Medicine. Berlin: Springer-Verlag; 2006. pp. 34-6.
4. Sharad J. Botulinum toxin: Upper face indications. Aesthetic Dermatology: Current Perspectives, 1st edition. New Delhi: Jaypee Brothers Medical Publishers (P) Ltd; 2018.
5. Chen AH, Frankel AS. Altering brow contour with botulinum toxin. Facial Plast Surg Clin North Am. 2003;11(4):457-64.
6. Savant S. Botulinum toxin. Textbook of Dermatosurgery and Cosmetology: Principles and Practice, 3rd edition. Mumbai: Bhalani Publication; 2018.
7. Huilgol SC, Carruthers A, Carruthers JD. Raising eyebrows with botulinum toxin. Dermatol Surg. 1999;25(5):373-5.
8. Huang W, Rogachefsky AS, Foster JA, et al. Browlift with botulinum toxin. Dermatol Surg. 2000;26(1):55-60.
9. Frankel AS, Kamer FM. Chemical browlift. Arch Otolaryngol Head Neck Surg. 1998;124(3):321-3.
10. Viswanath V. Botulinum toxin. Cosmetic Dermatology: A Practical and Evidence-Based Approach. New Delhi, CBS Publishers and Distributors (P) Ltd; 2012.

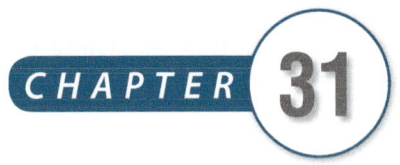
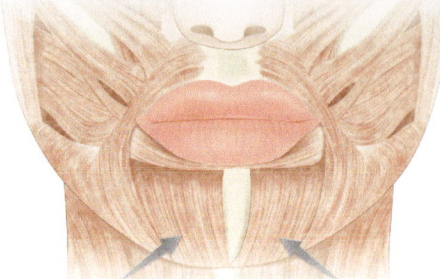

Bunny Lines

Sonali Langar

INDICATIONS

Nasoglabellar lines **(Fig. 1)** are oblique rhytides running inferomedially over the upper lateral walls of the nasal bridge when a person squints, smiles, laughs, or frowns. These wrinkles may be present naturally in an individual due to aging or may appear or accentuate after botulinum toxin (BTX) treatment of the glabellar frown region. When occurring naturally as a part of chronological aging, these rhytides are termed as "bunny lines" or "scrunch lines". However, when these occur as a part of compensatory phenomena following treatment of the glabellar frown region with BTX, these are referred to as the "Botox sign" **(Fig. 2)**.

Paresis in the glabellar frown region leads to unopposed overaction of transverse nasalis muscle causing nasoglabellar lines to appear.[1,2] Interestingly glamour industry watchers keep a keen eye on scrutinizing the presence of bunny lines with smoothened out glabellar region in celebrities indicating the tell-tale sign of BTX treatment done.

Bunny lines should not be confused with transverse lines that occur across the nasal root in some people **(Fig. 3)**. These horizontal lines do not originate from the nasalis muscle but arise due to contraction and downward pull of the procerus muscle when an individual frowns.[3]

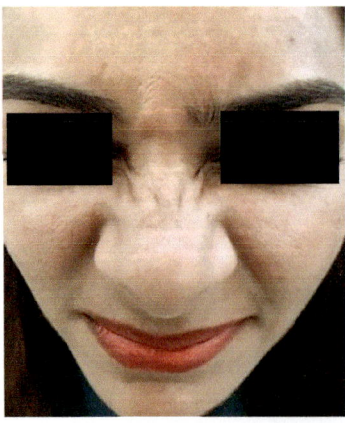

Fig. 1: Bunny lines in a 38-year-old female patient. These rhytides run obliquely and inferomedially over the upper lateral wall of the nasal bridge.

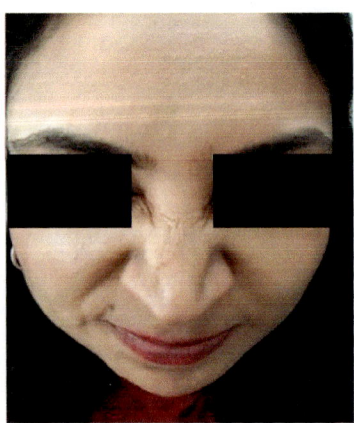

Fig. 2: "Botox sign" in a 40-year-old female. Isolated presence of bunny lines with smoothened glabellar frown and forehead region 3 weeks after BTX treatment of upper face.

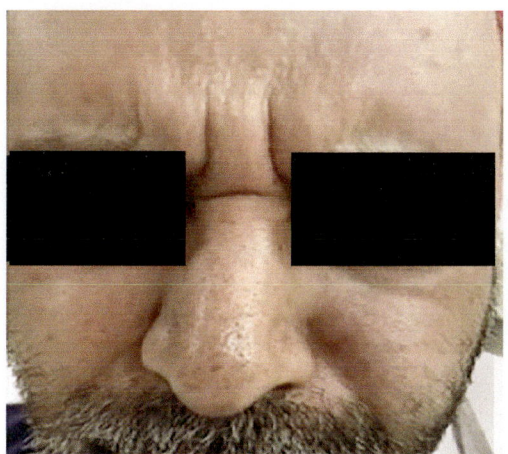

Fig. 3: Transverse line across the nasal root in a 45-year-old patient. These rhytides originate from contraction and downward pull of procerus muscle.

ANATOMIC CONSIDERATIONS

The nose contains three main muscles **(Fig. 4)**.
1. Procerus
2. Nasalis
3. Depressor septi.

The procerus arises in the midline from the upper aspect of the nasal bone and cartilage and inserts into the skin of the lower part of the forehead between the corrugators and into the frontal belly of occipitofrontalis. It helps to pull the medial eyebrow down.

The nasalis is a paramedian muscle which originates from the maxilla and runs across the nasal bridge expanding into a thin aponeurosis where it becomes continuous with the contralateral muscle of the opposite side. This muscle is somewhat horseshoe shaped, with the upper transverse portion also known compressor naris fanning diagonally across the nasal dorsum and two lower lateral parts also known as the dilator naris traversing vertically down the sides of the ala of the nose.

The depressor septi nasi originates in the incisive fossa of the maxilla and inserts into the nasal septum and posterior aspect of dilator naris. Contraction of this muscle pulls the nasal tip down and constricts the nostril aperture.[4,5]

Though not a part of nose, levator labii superioris alaeque nasi (LLSAN) and levator labii superioris (LLS) need to be mentioned here as they run closely along the side of the nasal bridge **(Fig. 4)**. LLSAN originates from the frontal process of the maxilla near the inner canthus of the eye and inserts into the skin of lateral part of the ala of nose and upper lip. It is responsible for dilating the nostrils and elevation of upper lip. LLS originates from the infraorbital margin of the maxilla and inserts into the skin of the upper lip. It is responsible for elevation of the upper lip and portrayal of facial expression of worry and anxiety.[6]

CAUSE OF NASOGLABELLAR LINES

The nasoglabellar lines arise from the nasalis muscle. Nasalis muscle can be distinguishably categorized into two parts, the upper transverse part known as compressor naris fanning diagonally across the nasal dorsum and two lower parts known as the dilator naris traversing vertically down the sides of ala of the nose. Nasalis fibers originate from either side of the maxilla, course medially and superiorly expanding into an aponeurosis over the bridge of the nose interdigitating with the contralateral muscles of the opposite side. Inferiorly they descend into the nasolabial groove, where they intervene with the muscular elevators of the upper lip LLSAN and LLS. The transverse fibers (compressor naris) depress the cartilaginous part of the nose, drawing the ala toward the nasal septum.[7]

The action of compressor naris can be elicited by asking the patient to frown, laugh, smile, or squint forcibly mimicking intense

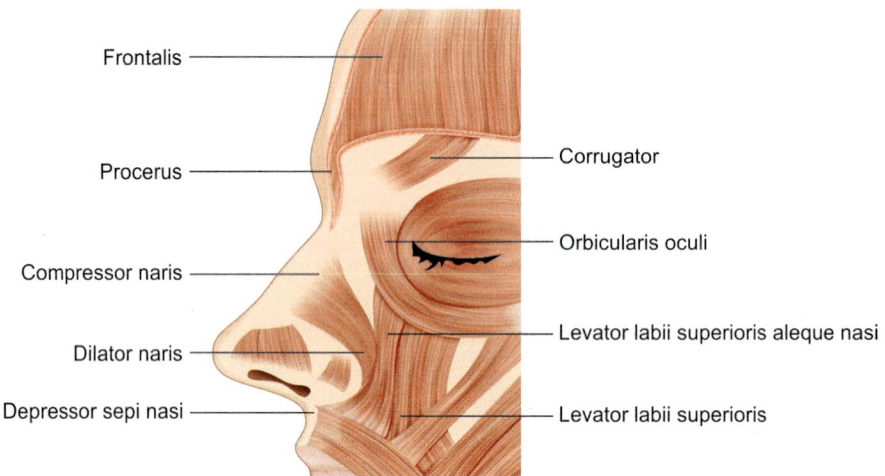

Fig. 4: Diagrammatic lateral view of muscular anatomy of face in relation to bunny lines.

bright light falling on the eyes. In doing so if bunny lines become prominent, it is most likely that the patients will produce them more avidly after their glabellar lines are treated with BTX due to unopposed action of the nasalis ("Botox sign"—**Fig. 2**). Hence, such naturally occurring nasoglabellar lines should be treated simultaneously at the same session of treatment of glabellar frown lines. If not treated so, the patient more than likely may put the discredit on the physician for their presence later.[8]

INJECTION TECHNIQUES

The patient sits upright or in a semirecumbent position. Prior topical anesthesia or ice can be applied to allay pain during the procedure. The patient is asked to wrinkle up the nose by squinting or frowning. Assess the location and strength of the nasalis muscle. A single point injection of BTX is placed superficially on either side of the nasal wall **(Fig. 5)**. Assessing the proper location and activity of muscle contractions during frowning or squinting is essential in determining the total dose of

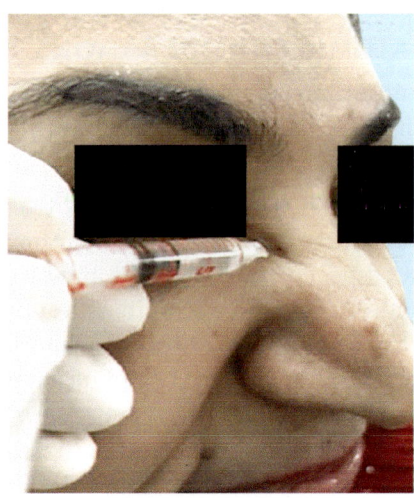

Fig. 5: Technique of botulinum toxin (BTX) injection. 3–5 U of BTX are placed anteriorly and medially on the dorsum of the nose away from the nasofacial groove.

BTX to be administered. Usually 2–5 U of onabotulinumtoxinA and incobotulinumtoxin A injected superficially in the subcutaneous plane are sufficient to relax the lines **(Figs. 6A and B)**. Patients who spend most of their time in sun, constantly squinting their eyes require a higher dose of BTX due to more extensive

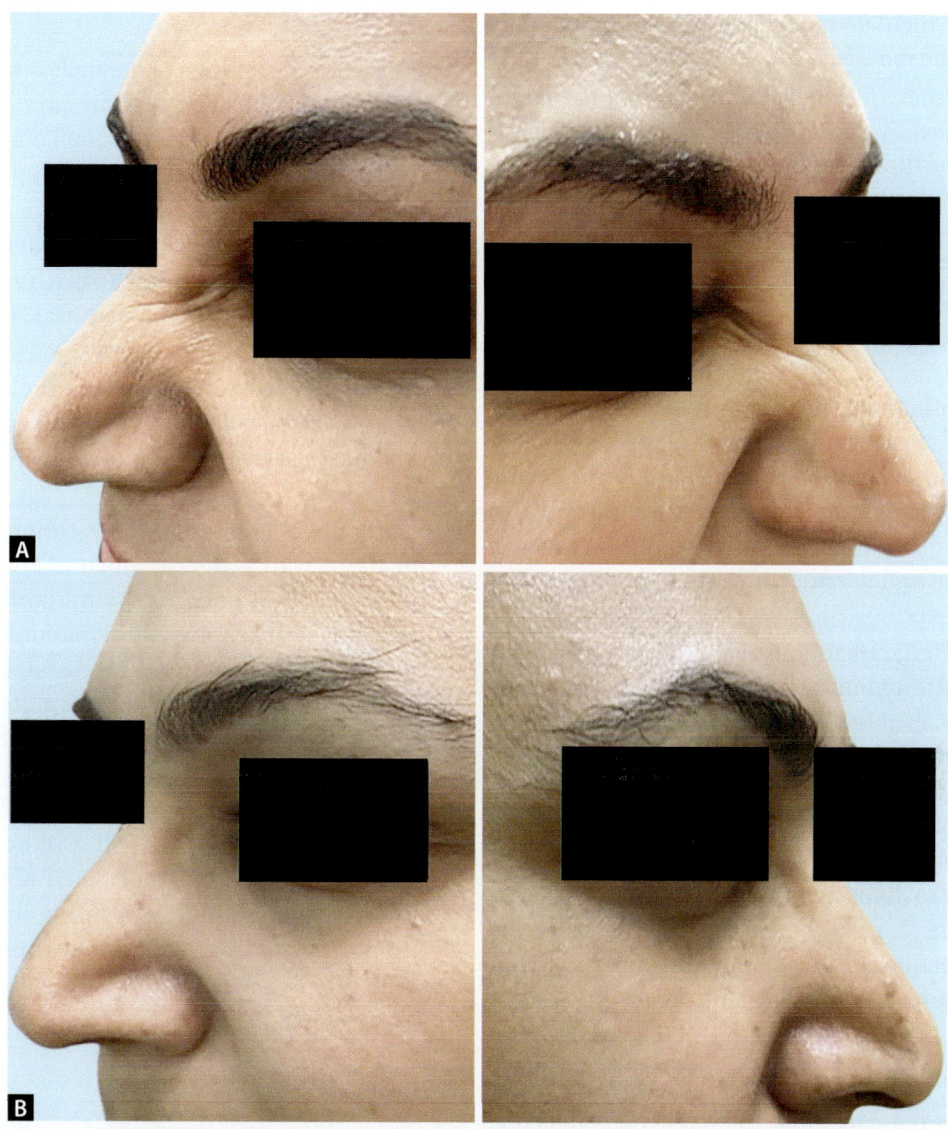

Figs. 6A and B: Pre- and post-treatment photographs of treated "bunny" lines. Significant improvement in rhytides 2 weeks following 3 U of botulinum toxin injection.

lines formed by hypertrophic nasalis. In such cases more injections can be placed taking care that the injection points remain medial to LLSAN at or near the level of the nasal bones and upper lateral cartilages of the nose.[9]

PRECAUTIONS

Injections should be placed in the subcutaneous plane, anteriorly and medially on the bony dorsum of the nose. The injections should also be well anterior and medial to the angular vein which runs superolaterally to the nasalis.

Injecting toxin too low along the nasal sidewalls carries a risk of toxin diffusion into upper lip elevators. Extension of BTX to these muscles can cause flattening of nasolabial fold, upper lip ptosis and lip asymmetry leading to difficulties in eating and speaking. Injecting toxin too near the inner canthus of eye may involve the medial palpebral portion of the orbicularis oculi subsequently leading to a diminution in the action of the lacrimal pump causing epiphora. Spread of toxin to medial rectus can lead to diplopia. Enthusiastic massage to the area after injecting can also produce the same adverse results, even if dose and the injection technique have been correct.[10,11]

Under treatment of one side of nasalis can lead to asymmetrical sniffing which may not be perceivable by the patient. It can be rectified by placement of a small correction unit of BTX in the undertreated side. Overenthusiastic treatment of one side can lead to ipsilateral flattening of nasolabial fold and upper lip ptosis due to diffusion in surrounding musculature. Therefore, playing safe is advisable to start the injections in conservative dosing, and to not wander off laterally along the nasal wall.

POSTINJECTION INSTRUCTIONS

Firm pressure should be applied after injecting to prevent bruising. Vigorous message of the area should be avoided to prevent diffusion of the toxin to surrounding musculature. Utmost care should be taken to avoid diffusion or unintentional injection into LLSAN and LLS, which are lip elevators running parallel along the side of the nose in the nasolabial groove **(Fig. 4)**.[10]

USEFUL TIPS

- Nasoglabellar lines occur naturally in some patients and in some they are produced or accentuated by treating glabellar frown lines with BTX injections due to unopposed action of nasalis.
- It is imperative to treat nasoglabellar lines along with the glabellar frown region in suitable patients or else risk their accentuation post-treatment.
- Injections have to be kept superficial as this area is vascular to avoid bruising. Do not massage vigorously or in a downward direction.
- Normally 2–5 units of BTX on either side of nasal wall gives the desired results in majority of patients. Some patients may however require additional units of BTX along the proximal and distal nasal bridge to attenuate different patterns of nasoglabellar lines arising from hypertrophic nasalis.
- Injections should be placed medially and anteriorly on the nasal wall as too low and lateral placements, near or into the nasofacial fold may result in upper lip ptosis and lip asymmetry leading to difficulty in speaking and eating due to involvement of LLSAN and LLS.

REFERENCES

1. Fagien S. Botox for the treatment of dynamic and hyperkinetic facial lines and furrows: adjunctive use in facial aesthetic surgery. Plast Reconstr Surg. 1999;103(2):701-13.
2. Manaloto RM, Alster TS. Periorbital rejuvenation: a review of dermatologic treatments. Dermatol Surg. 1999;25(1):1-9.
3. Small R, Hoang D (Eds). A Practical Guide to Botulinum Toxin Procedures, 1st edition. Philadelphia: Wolters Kluwer; 2012.

4. Carruthers J, Fagien S, Matarasso SL. Consensus recommendations on the use of botulinum toxin type A in facial aesthetics. Plast Reconstr Surg. 2004;114:(Suppl 6)1S-22S.
5. Wieder JM, Moy RL. Understanding botulinum toxin. Surgical anatomy of the frown, forehead, and periocular region. Dermatol Surg. 1998; 24(11):1172-4.
6. Le Louarn C. Botulinum toxin A and facial lines: the variable concentration. Aesthetic Plast Surg. 2001;25(2):73-84.
7. Janfaza P, Cheney ML. Superficial structures of the face, head, and parotid region. In: Janfaza P, Nadol JB, Galla RJ (Eds). Surgical Anatomy of the Head and Neck. Philadelphia: Lippincott Williams and Wilkins; 2000. pp. 1-48.
8. Carruthers A, Carruthers J. Clinical indications and injection technique for the cosmetic use of botulinum A exotoxin. Dermatol Surg. 1998;24(11):1189-94.
9. Blitzer A, Binder WJ. Current practices in the use of botulinum toxin in the management of facial lines and wrinkles. Facial Plast Surg Clin North Am. 2001;9:395-404.
10. Carruthers J, Fagien S, Matarasso SL; Botox Consensus Group. Consensus recommendations on the use of botulinum toxin type A in facial aesthetics. Plast Reconstr Surg. 2004;114:1S-22S.
11. Tamura BM, Odo MY, Chang B, et al. Treatment of nasal wrinkles with botulinum toxin. Dermatol Surg. 2005;31(3):271-5.

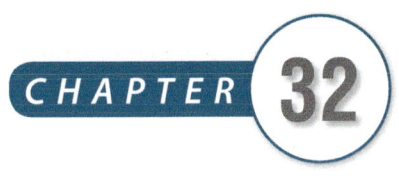
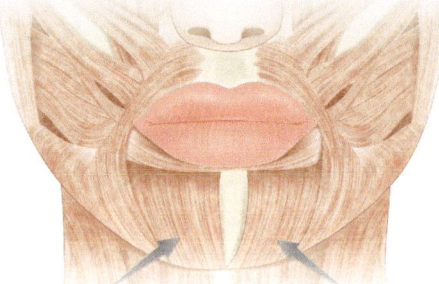

Nose

Indu Ballani

INTRODUCTION

Nose is an important esthetic unit of the face. With greater awareness of facial esthetics more people are opting for nonsurgical procedures for nose beautification. These procedures can be done to enhance nasal esthetics thereby reducing need for rhinoplasty in some cases. Nose being an important landmark of face, even small changes may result in change of appearance. With the increase in nonsurgical procedures it is now possible to enhance its esthetics by combining various modalities like fillers, threads, and neuromodulators.

Botulinum toxin (BTX) type A has been commonly used to treat expression lines on the face for more than 25 years leading to rejuvenated and youthful appearance. Upper face lines are the most common indications for injecting BTX. Now it is also being used on lower face, neck, and the nose. In this chapter we will be discussing use of BTX in nasal esthetics.

The dosages advised in this chapter are mainly for onabotulinum toxin.

MAIN INDICATIONS FOR USE OF BOTULINUM TOXIN ON NOSE

Bunny lines on sides of nose are the most common indications for which patients seek

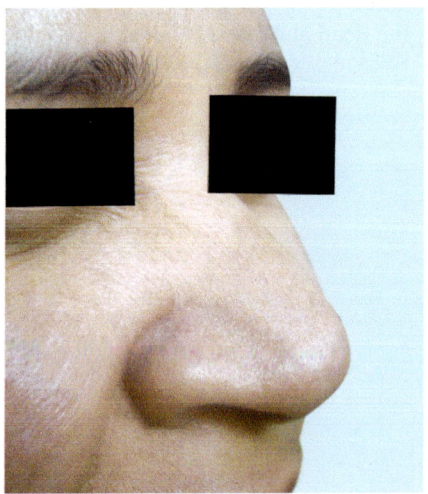

Fig. 1: Bunny/Nasoglabellar lines.

treatment (**Fig. 1**). Slight nasal tip elevation is also possible with the toxin. Nasal flutter or dilatation of nostrils which occurs in some people during emotional outbursts can also be controlled by injecting BTX. Another indication is nasal dorsum hyperhidrosis or excessive sweating on nose.

ANATOMY

A good knowledge of the anatomy of nose and muscle attachments is an essential prerequisite for anyone who wishes to inject BTX on targeted areas.

Table 1: Anatomy and functions of muscles on and around the nose.

Muscles	Origin	Insertion	Action
Procerus	Nasal bone	Dermis of glabella between brows	Pulls medial end of eyebrow downward
Levator labii superioris alaeque nasi	Frontal process of maxilla	Nasal cartilage and upper lip	Lifting upper lip and wing of nose
Nasalis = Two parts • Transverse nasalis/compressor naris • Alar part/dilator naris	• Maxilla over canine tooth • Maxilla below and medial to compressor naris	• Dorsum of nose interlace with fibers from contralateral side • Alar cartilage of nose	• Draws the nasal sidewalls upward and medially, compresses nostrils • Moves the nasal ala outward and downward opening the nostrils during inspiration
Depressor septi	Maxilla above the central incisor	Cartilaginous nasal septum	Pulls the nasal tip down

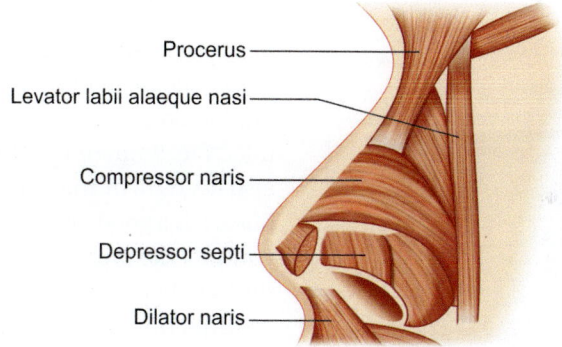

Fig. 2: Muscles of the nose.

Table 1 summarizes the anatomy and functions of muscles on and around the nose (Fig. 2).

INJECTION TECHNIQUES (FIG. 3)
Bunny Lines or Nasoglabellar Lines

The muscles creating these bunny lines are the transverse or compressor nasalis and part of levator palpebrae superioris alaeque nasi. Sometimes a prominent horizontal line on the nose may be formed due to contraction of procerus muscle. This is different from bunny lines and gets corrected when the procerus muscle is injected for relaxing frown lines on the forehead.

It is very important to have a proper assessment before injecting as dynamic lines (lines formed during expression) benefit more than static lines. Simultaneous contraction of glabella and orbicularis oculi muscle should also be noted as injecting microbotox around the eyes in the lower eyelid area enhances results. Injections of bunny lines also help to alleviate medial lines under the eye.

One hundred units of Botox vial are generally reconstituted in 2.5 mL of sterile saline without preservative, for upper face use. For the nose

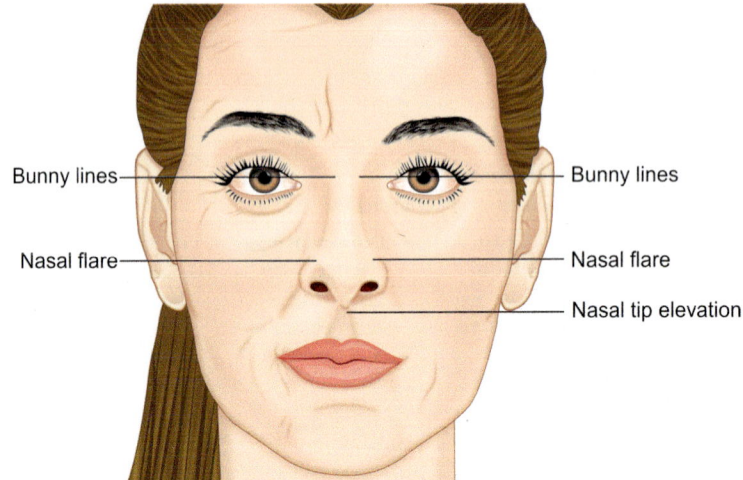

Fig. 3: Injection points on nose.

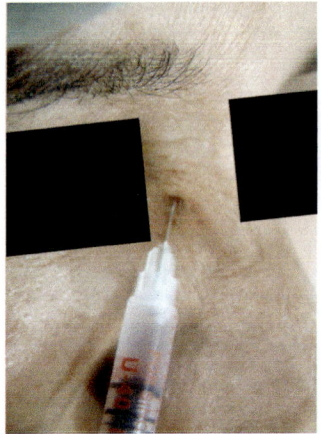

Fig. 4: Injection point for Bunny lines.

it is recommended to formulate in 1 mL saline to avoid diffusion into the surrounding areas. Practically this is often not possible as we are using the same reconstituted vial for other areas at the same time. Hence, we can use the 2.5 mL formulation but inject low doses as a precaution. 31-gauge insulin syringes having needle length 6 mm are used for injection.

Two lateral injection sites one on each side of the nose **(Fig. 4)**. Upper limit for these points is the nasion (do not go above medial canthi of eye) lower limit is halfway between nasion and tip. Only one-third part of the needle depth is inserted and 1–2 units are injected in muscle. Blebs are visible on injection. Sometimes a third point on dorsum also needs to be injected if there are too many lines. It is a good practice to ask the patients to contract the muscles and mark the points on the lines before injecting. Immediate massage on injection points should be avoided to prevent diffusion.

Elevation of Nasal Tip

Preprocedure assessment is very important. In some persons the nasal tip may show a dip on certain expressions along with pulling up of upper lip. This is due to contraction of depressor septi muscle therefore injecting this muscle gives good results. At times, the dip in nasal tip might be accompanied with flaring of nostrils due to action of dilator naris in conjunction with depressor septi. The action of muscles should be observed carefully to see if relaxation of these muscles would help in elevating the tip as an anatomical dip without increased activity of muscles would not be benefitted by Botox injection.

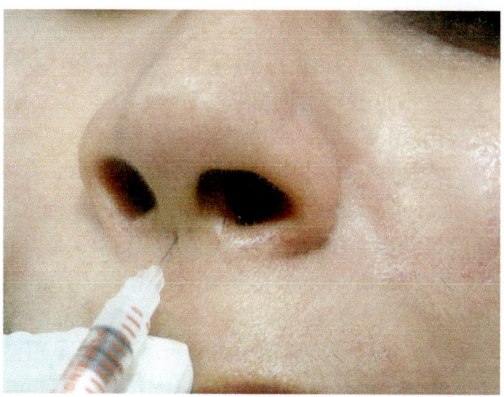

Fig. 5: Injection point for nasal tip elevation.

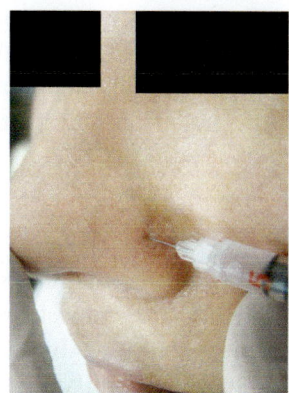

Fig. 6: Injecting dilator naris muscle for reducing flare.

Four-to-five units of Botox are injected on nasal tip where it inserts into the cartilage at the base of the columella **(Fig. 5)**. It is important to observe that only half depth of the needle of the insulin syringe of 6 mm length goes in, so that it is inserted into the muscle. The muscle may be stretched by pulling down the upper lip while injecting. Topical anesthesia may be applied. This injection should be avoided in patients having a long upper lip as it might make it longer by raising the nasal tip.

Nasal Flutter

The muscle causing this dilatation or flutter is the dilator naris which covers the nasal ala inserting into alar cartilage and skin of nostrils.

Two-to-four units on each side over the nasal ala are injected into the muscle subcutaneously **(Fig. 6)**.

Nasal Dorsum Hyperhidrosis

Excessive sweating when seen on face usually affects the forehead, cheeks, lips, scalp, and nose. This may sometimes be very embarrassing or humiliating. BTX blocks the release of acetylcholine in synapses which regulates the production of sweat by eccrine glands. Starch iodine test is done to identify and mark the area of excessive sweating. Injections for this indication are given intradermal as no muscles are responsible.

Topical anesthesia is essential as pricks are painful. In this procedure we use mesobotox. For this the normally formulated botox in 2.5 mL saline is withdrawn in insulin syringe and further diluted with saline in the syringe in ratio of 1:3. The pricks should be intradermal so that raised blebs with surrounding wheals lasting for 2–3 hours. Patient should be counseled about this.

PRECAUTIONS AND COMPLICATIONS
Bunny Line Injections

If the lateral injection points sometimes become too lateral then the levator labii superior alaeque nasi (LLSAN) may get affected leading to lip ptosis which causes asymmetry while smiling. Rarely the zygomatic muscle or levator labii superioris may be affected leading to oral incompetence creating problems in eating and talking. If more than 5 units are injected there is a risk of diffusion into the fibers of orbicularis oculi, diminishing the pump effect of lac-sac causing excessive tear secretion. Blurred vision may result if there is diffusion to medial rectus muscle of the eye. No corrective treatments are available for these complications. They usually resolve spontaneously with time. An ophthalmologist consultation may be required to prevent corneal injury.

Nasal Tip Injection

Avoid injecting more than 4 units as diffusion into the orbicularis oris muscle may occur. Diffusion into levator labii superioris may cause some difficulty in talking or eating. Sometimes upper lip may become too elongated or flat leading to patient dissatisfaction from esthetic point of view. Raising the tip may sometimes lead to flared nostrils due to overaction of dilator naris giving appearance of "piggy nose". In such cases dilator naris can be injected on follow-up for better results.

Nasal Flutter

Complications usually not seen if correct technique is used.

Nasal Hyperhidrosis

There may be chances of bruising at some points. If by accident a prick gets deeper and muscle gets injected there might be asymmetry due to muscle action at that point being affected.

Postinjection Instructions

Bruising is a possibility after any injection. Patient should be counseled that the results would be evident after 4–7 days, maximum effect being observed at 2 weeks. The patient should be asked to avoid facial massage and steam, sauna for 7 days. Heavy exercise is avoided for 48 hours. Sudden bending forward is avoided for 4 hours.

USEFUL TIPS

- Nose injection of BTX is not a very common indication asked by the patient but injectors should assess properly and counsel accordingly for best results.
- Careful assessment and preprocedure photographs are essential as results are subtle especially in case of nasal tip elevation.
- *Injecting bunny lines,* when doing glabella and forehead injections, enhances overall results of upper face botulinum treatment.
- Mesobotox for nasal hyperhidrosis gives added advantage of tightening pores and giving a brighter rejuvenated appearance to the injected person.

SUGGESTED READINGS

1. Benedetto AV. Botulinum toxin in clinical medicine. Clin Dermatol. 2003;21(6):465-8.
2. Blugerman G, Schavelzon D, D'Angelo S. Multiple eccrine hidrocystomas: a new therapeutic option with botulinum toxin. Dermatol Surg. 2003;29(5):557-9.
3. Carruthers J, Carruthers A. Practical cosmetic Botox techniques. J Cutan Med Surg. 1999;3 (Suppl 4):S49-52.
4. de Maio M, DeBoulle K, Braz A, et al. Facial assessment and injection guide for botulinum toxin and injectable hyaluronic acid fillers: focus on the midface. Plast Reconstr Surg. 2017;140(4):540e-50e.
5. Letourneau A, Daniel RK. The superficial musculoaponeurotic system of the nose. Plast Reconstr Surg. 1988;82(1):48-57.
6. Schavelzon D, Blugerman G, Wexler G, et al. Botulinum toxin in the nasal area. Rhinoplasty. UK: IntecOpen; 2016.
7. Small R, Hoang D. Treatment areas: bunny lines. A Practical Guide to Botulinum Toxin Procedures, 1st edition. Philadelphia: Lippincott Williams and Wilkins; 2012.
8. Tamura BM, Odo MY, Chang B, et al. Treatment of nasal wrinkles with botulinum toxin. Dermatol Surg. 2005;31(3):271-5.
9. Zide BM. Nasal anatomy: the muscles and tip sensation. Aesthetic Plast Surg. 1985;9(3):193-6.

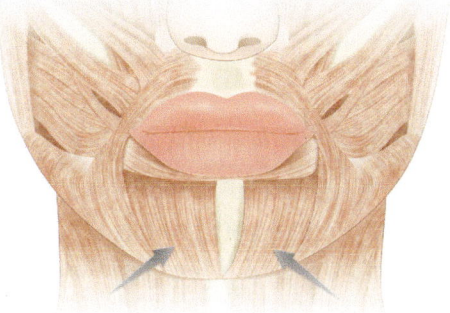

CHAPTER 33

Smoker's Lines (Lip Lines)

Gulhima Arora, Sandeep Arora

INTRODUCTION

Lips, along with the perioral area, are considered to be an important part of facial esthetics. Smoker's lines (lip lines) which are also called "lipstick lines" or "perioral rhytides" are wrinkles that appear around the mouth due to aging **(Fig. 1)**. Chronological as well as chronic photoaging are responsible for the attenuation of the youthful appearance of the perioral area. Skeletal resorption of the maxilla, loss of muscle tone of the orbicularis oris muscle, loss of fat pads and skin aging due to loss of elastic and collagen fibers, all contribute to the aging of this region.[1]

Smoking, exposure to environmental factors like sunlight and pollution, and hereditary factors[2] also contribute to the formation of smoker's lines. People of certain occupations like those who play wind instruments are more prone to develop these lines.[1,3] The normal physiology of the orbicularis oris muscle due to its repetitive action during eating and talking itself leads to exaggerated wrinkling of this area. This muscles' hyperactivity, thus is an important determinant in development of the signs of aging in this area.[2]

Aging of this area results in the development of fine perioral lines and wrinkling, with changes in the lip causing flattening of the cupid's bow, elongation and flattening of

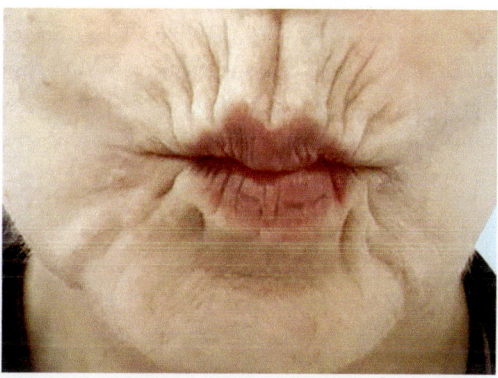

Fig. 1: Smoker's lines.

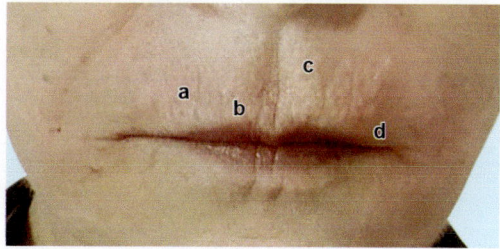

Fig. 2: Age-related changes of the perioral region. (a) Perioral fine lines and wrinkling, (b) Flattening of the cupid's bow, (c) Elongation and flattening of the philtral column, and (d) Inversion of the lips.

the philtral column, and inversion of the lips along with the formation of marionette lines **(Fig. 2)**.[1]

Improvement of the skin around the mouth and addressing dental esthetics, in part, can restore the youthful appearance. Botulinum toxin, for hyperdynamic wrinkles around the mouth, has proved to be a rapid and gratifying minimally invasive technique for this indication.

ANATOMIC CONSIDERATIONS

The bony structure of the perioral region is formed by the maxilla and mandible. Teeth as hard structures affect the esthetics of this area.[1,4] There are 12 muscles that directly affect the perioral area **(Fig. 3)**. They are divided into three groups depending on whether they insert into the modiolus, upper lip or lower lip. The muscles which insert into the upper lip also insert into the fibers of the orbicularis oris, and are responsible for the elevation of the upper lip. The muscles which insert into the lower lip are responsible for depressing the lower lip.[5]

The main muscle that is responsible for the development of the smoker's lines is the orbicularis oris muscle. Since injections of botulinum toxin are injected into this muscle and target this muscle primarily, it is important to be well-versed with the anatomical aspects of the muscle **(Table 1)**[1,5,6] as well as the related fat compartments.[7]

The blood supply to the perioral area is through the superior and inferior labial

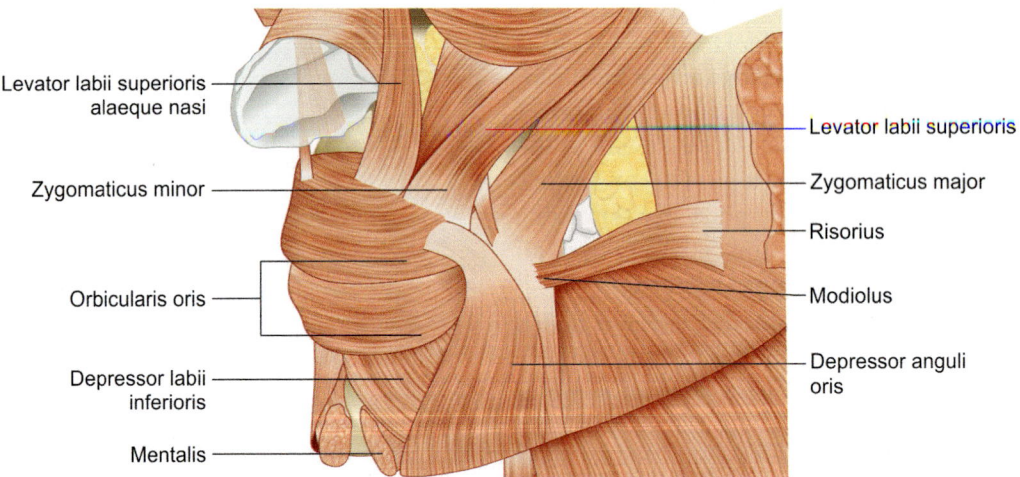

Fig. 3: Muscles of the perioral area.

Table 1: Orbicularis oris.				
Origin	Insertion	Innervation	Action	Features
Maxilla and mandible, anterior portion of modiolus	Have dermal insertions 4–5 mm away from the midline. On contraction this pulls the skin medially to accentuate the philtral columns. It forms the lip muscle	Buccal and mandibular branches of facial nerve	Purses the lips and presses them against the teeth. Deeper fibers act as oral sphincter. Influences speech, blowing, smiling	It is a sphincteric muscle

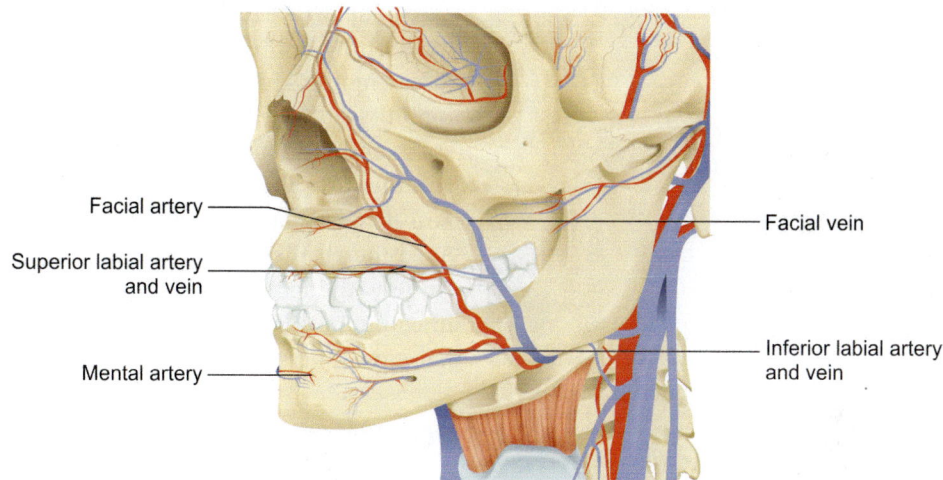

Fig. 4: Blood supply of the perioral area.

arteries (branches of the facial artery) and their branches, the mental arteries **(Fig. 4)**. The maxillary and mandibular branches of the trigeminal nerve are the main sensory nerves of perioral area. The facial nerve is the main motor nerve.

INJECTION TECHNIQUES

Assessment of the patient at rest as well as in animation is crucial. Marking is done with the patient asked to purse his/her lips, as this accentuates the wrinkles, showing the ridges **(Fig. 1)**. It is best to assess and treat in the sitting or semi-reclined position. A history about their occupation and hobbies is essential.

Marking should include four points on the upper lip and two on the lower **(Fig. 5)**. The points marked should be within 5 mm of the vermilion border, or in the "white roll."[8] Additional points can be marked if the periphery of the orbicularis oris muscle is to be targeted. These are around 7–10 mm from the vermillion border, in the "outer orbicularis oris."[8] The number of injection points is tailor-

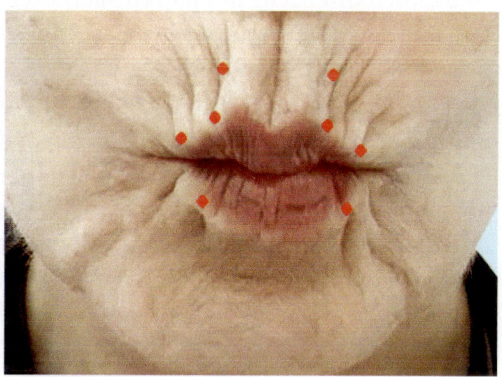

Fig. 5: Injection points recommendation 1.

made according to each patient's needs. Trevedic et al. recommend an initial four point injection treatment, with each point lying the middle third of the lip on each side **(Fig. 6)**.[9] The points marked should be away from the center as well as at least 1 cm medial to the oral commissures.

Anesthesia can be in the form of a topical cream applied 30–45 minutes prior to the procedure. Ice packs just before injecting also help to numb the area, thus making the procedure more comfortable.

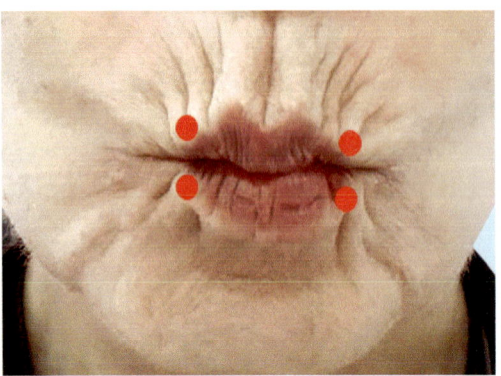

Fig. 6: Injection points recommendation 2.

Injections are given using 1 cc syringes with a 30 G or 32 G half inch needle. The injections are superficial, intradermal, raising blebs. Microdroplet technique is usually used, but another technique known as "linear threading" is also practiced.[10]

It is advised to start with low doses of 1–2 units per lip quadrant,[3] or 2–4 units divided equally over four injection sites on the upper lip, and 1–2 units divided equally over two injection sites in the lower lip. An expert consensus group recommends not more than 4 units in the upper lip.[11,12] Dosages required for Asians is less than those for Caucasians.[13] Additional doses, if required, may be given on a follow-up visit at 1–2 weeks. It is then that the 1 "outer orbicularis oris" is also addressed if required with 1–2 units **(Fig. 5)**.[8] With toxins with higher diffusion index like Dysport, even lower doses can be used.[2] Injections are made into the muscle, not lines.

PRECAUTIONS

Correct dosing and ensuring symmetry are the main points of concern, while injecting in this area. Record any pre-existing asymmetry at rest as well as while the patient phonates with "p" or "b" syllables. Treatment of smokers lines with conservative dosing leads to inadequate response while overdosing or incorrect positioning of the injection points leads to loss of mouth's functional competence, with inability to blow, whistle, phonate or even swish and spit.[8] Injecting too close to the oral commissures shall cause upper lip inversion and drooling as lip elevators are affected. Asymmetrical smile or lip ptosis may also result with incorrect injection points. Avoid injecting in the midline which shall lead to flattening of the cupid's bow.

POSTINJECTION INSTRUCTIONS

Postinjection avoid massage in this area as unnecessary diffusion may lead to side effects. Cool packs or ice may be used in case of bruising. Patients must avoid NSAIDs, for 72 hours post treatment.

USEFUL TIPS

- Record any asymmetry at rest and activity.
- Always mark the injection points.
- It is a good idea to either load four syringes with one unit each or load just one unit each time to ensure correct dosing.
- Ensure correct dilution, avoid excessive dilution which leads to increased diffusion and complications.
- Inject superficially creating blebs.
- Wait for a week before additional dosing.
- Deeper injections must be avoided in those with a longer naso-vermillion distance.

COMPLICATIONS

- Treatment of smoker's lines often leads to inadequate responses due to conservative dosing.
- Over dosing of the muscle can lead to a loss of the mouth's functional competence, thus the patient is unable to blow, whistle,

suck or pronounce the letters "p" or "b," or even swish and spit.[8]
- Injecting to close to the oral commissures can lead to inversion of the upper lip and even drooling due to the lip elevator muscles being affected. There may be an asymmetrical smile or even lateral ptosis of the lip.
- Injecting in the midline can lead to a flattening of the cupid's bow.
- Asymmetry can be there due to unequal number of units on either side.

REFERENCES

1. Wollina U. Perioral rejuvenation: restoration of attractiveness in aging females by minimally invasive procedures. Clin Interv Aging. 2013;8:1149-55.
2. Pinto CAS, Rebellato PRO, Schmitt JV, et al. Lip volumization using botulinum toxin. Surg Cosmet Dermatol 2017;9(1):24-8.
3. Carruthers J, Carruthers A. BOTOX use in the mid and lower face and neck. Semin Cutan Med Surg. 2001;20(2):85-92.
4. Coleman S, Grover R. The anatomy of the aging face: volume loss and changes in 3-dimensional topography. Aesthet Surg J. 2006;26(1S):S4-9.
5. Hotta TA. Understanding the perioral anatomy. Plast Surg Nurs. 2016;36(1):12-8.
6. Westbrook KE, Varcallo M. Anatomy, head and neck, facial muscles. Treasure Island (FL): StatPearls Publishing; 2019.
7. Sandoval SE, Cox JA, Koshy JC, et al. Facial fat compartments: a guide to filler placement. Semin Plast Surg. 2009;23(4):283-7.
8. Semchyshyn N, Sengelmann RD. Botulinum toxin A treatment of perioral rhytides. Dermatol Surg. 2003;29:490-5.
9. Trévidic P, Sykes J, Criollo-Lamilla G. Anatomy of the lower face and botulinum toxin injections. Plast Reconstr Surg. 2015;136(Suppl 5):84S-91S.
10. Higgins HW 2nd, Lee KC, Enzer Y. Neuromodulator threading: revisiting an approach to neurotoxin delivery. J Clin Aesthet Dermatol. 2014;7(6):38-41.
11. Ascher B, Talarico S, Cassuto D, et al. International consensus recommendations on the aesthetic usage of botulinum toxin type A (Speywood Unit)–Part II: wrinkles on the middle and lower face, neck and chest. J Eur Acad Dermatol Venereol. 2010;24(11):1285-95.
12. Kapoor KM, Chatrath V, Anand C, et al. Consensus recommendations for treatment strategies in indians using botulinum toxin and hyaluronic acid fillers. Plast Reconstr Surg Glob Open. 2017;5(12):e1574.
13. Dixit R. Midface indications. In: Sharad J, Vedamurthy M (Ed). Aesthetic dermatology: current perspectives, 1st edition. Mumbai: Jaypee Brothers Medical Publishers Pvt. Ltd; 2018. pp. 126-7.

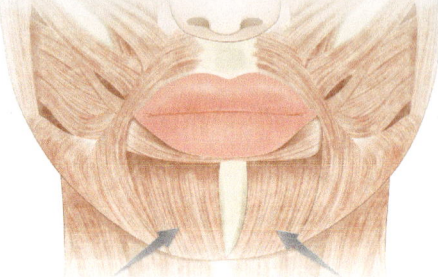

Gummy Smile—Botulinum Toxin

Malavika Kohli, Swati Mutha

INTRODUCTION

Smile is the most recognized expression in the world and is the cornerstone of social interaction. The value of attractive smile is undeniable.

Excessive gingival display (EGD) resulting in a "gummy smile" is a major esthetic concern with ramifications in an individual's personal and social life. A smile with more than 2 mm exposed gingiva is called gummy smile. It is one of the most common alterations among the population, with prevalence of 10.5–29% in which females predominate.[1,2]

TYPES

- Depending on part of Maxilla seen:[3]
  - Anterior
  - Mixed
  - Asymmetric
- Amount of gingival exposure (Goldstein classification)[4]
  - High
  - Low
  - Medium.

ETIOLOGY[5,6]/ANATOMY

The treatment of gummy smile primarily depends on the etiology. Hence, it is very important to find the cause of gummy smile after detailed clinical and radiological examination (if required). Gummy smile depends on:

- *The amount of gum tissue display:* Excess gum tissue can lead to gummy smile. It can be treated by periodontal surgery like gingivoplasty/crown lengthening.
- *The size and shape of the teeth:* Crown length (visible part of the tooth above gum line) up to 10 mm is normal. The ratio of crown width to length up to 75–85% is also considered as normal. Variations in the eruptive process can give rise to discrepancies in the normal proportions of teeth to gum tissues, which can result in shorter normal teeth and thereby gumminess of smile. Variation in eruption:
  - Anterior overeruption (excess overbite)
  - Altered active eruption (the teeth do not make it out of bone)
  - Altered passive eruption (gingiva does not recede as the person matures).

The tooth and gum tissue "complex" (wear and compensatory eruption): Excessive tooth wear can cause changes in the gum to tooth ratio. With wear and tear, teeth become incrementally shorter, this can cause compensatory eruption in which teeth actually erupt very slowly to compensate for the wear; it is body's way of maintaining a properly functioning bite with shorter teeth. As a result, the gumminess of the smile increases because the gums which are attached to the teeth move with them as they erupt. It can be corrected with orthodontic treatment to push the affected teeth back up into correct position.

- *The length and the degree of movement of the upper lip:* The average lip moves 6-8 mm from its normal resting position to a full smile. If the lip is hypermobile, meaning it rises way up, too much gum tissue may be revealed in the smile. Muscles involved in hypermobile upper lip—levator labii superioris, levator labii superioris alaeque nasi, levator anguli oris, and the zygomaticus muscles, individually, or combinations of them.[5,7] A person may have normal lip movement but just a short upper lip and therefore display more gum tissue than desired.
- *The vertical position of the upper jaw and teeth in relationship to the skull:* Vertical maxillary excess because the upper jaw (maxilla) is excessively long relative to the base of the skull to which it is attached. Treatment for this condition may include orthognathic surgery. If the teeth themselves hang down too much, they can sometimes be moved up orthodontically to make them less prominent.

TREATMENT

Strategy for Success

Correct diagnosis is key to solving a complex cosmetic concern. Gummy smiles exist for a variety of reasons which can be present together, and hence proper diagnosis is critical. There are various ways to treat a gummy smile depending on the cause. There is an adequate treatment for each etiology; two or more techniques can be combined.

- For gummy smile caused by excessive gingival tissue partially covering the anatomical crown of the teeth (which is also caused by altered passive eruption), a respective gingival surgery (gingivoplasty) is recommended.[8]
- *Teeth*: Depending on the kind of eruption, a dental surgeon can do the correction.
- *Vertical maxillary excess*: Orthognathic surgeries or laser-assisted lip repositioning surgery[9]—a minimally invasive alternative to orthognathic surgeries.
- *Hyperactive lip muscles*:
   - *Surgical options*: The containment of the elevator muscle of upper lip and wing of nose was used to treat gummy smile. This technique corrected the esthetic alterations of smile, reducing the upper lip elevation, resulting in smaller gingival display. It is an innovative and effective therapeutic option to obtain natural and harmonious smile.[10]
   - *Nonsurgical options*: Botulinum toxin (BT).

Lately, BT injection is considered an effective minimal invasive treatment of gummy smile. It is recommended in cases where gummy smile is caused by hyperactive lip muscles, resulting in localized reduction in elevator muscle activities and relaxes the pulling up action of the lip while smiling.[11] Muscles of facial expression responsible for the upper lip elevation and lateral retraction upon smiling are levator labii superioris, LLSAN, zygomaticus major, zygomaticus minor, and depressor septi. All of these muscles interact with the orbicularis oris muscle in the production of smile.[12]

The dosage of BT injection varies between male and female, depending on lip muscle volume. In general, males have larger muscle volume and require more units of BT to achieve the same result as female patients.[13] The injection point is located in the center of the triangle formed by levator labii superioris, LLSAN, and zygomaticus minor.

The effect of BT is seen within 1–2 weeks and usually lasts for 4–6 months. However, some authors conducted that several injections of BT could prolong the reduction of gingival exposure.[3,14]

Reason for this process is that the prolonged muscle paralysis that occurs after several injections can lately lead to partial muscle atrophy and permanent decrease in contraction ability, even after the disappearance of the toxic effect.[15]

It is important not to give injections before its effect has completely faded to avoid the formation of antibodies against the toxins which can lead to disappointing results later on.

- *Contraindications*: Pregnant or lactating women, neuromuscular patients. Patients on calcium channel blockers, cyclosporine and aminoglycosides drugs and patients with a history of hypersensitivity to Botox toxin or saline solution.[16]
- *Advantages*: It is less invasive, has reasonable cost, and requires less time despite its short-term effect, usually safe, no downtime.
- *Side effects*: Very rare and local. Pain, infection, inflammation, bruising, edema, loss of muscle strength, hematoma, and nerve palsy.
  - Improper technique may result in a asymmetric smile, collapse of oral commissure (sad look), long upper lip (joker smile), inferior lip protrusion, drooling and difficulty in smiling, speaking or eating which can be corrected with retouching.[3] Over administration can cause drooping or ptosis of the lip below gingival margin causing obstruction of visible teeth on full smile.[17,18] These side effects are avoidable but reversible, can take up to 6–8 weeks.

Botulinum Toxin Injection Technique

- *Step 1. Reconstitution*: Add 2.5 mL 0.9% normal saline solution to 100 units of vacuum-dried *Clostridium botulinum toxin type-A (BTx A)*.
- *Step 2. Site of injection*: By palpating the muscles during smiling and relaxing movements to ensure the accurate locations of injections and mark with a skin marker.
- *Step 3. Injection*: Pull out reconstituted BTx A in disposable 1 cc insulin syringe. The sites are cleaned and sterilized after topical anesthesia application. The injections are done on two points on each side. 4 units were injected on each side of the nasolabial fold, 1 cm lateral and below the nasal ala– **Yonsei point** 2. Two units were injected on each side of nasolabial fold, at the point of the greatest lateral contraction during the smile as shown in **Figure 1**. The depth of administration is intramuscular with the needle perpendicular to the skin surface and bevel facing upwards.

Postinjection instructions: Advise the patient not to lie down, exercise, or massage the injected area during the first 4 hour after the

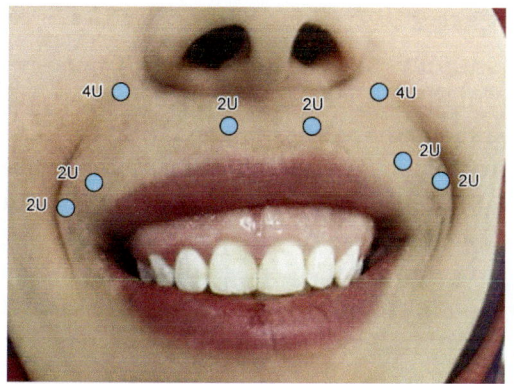

Fig. 1: The sites of injections of total 20 units of botulinum toxin.

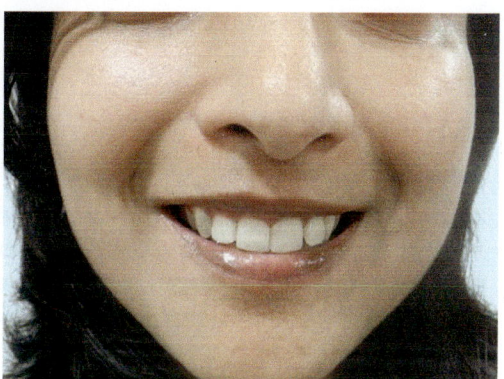

Fig. 2: Injecting fillers to hide the gum show by increasing the vertical height of the lip.

procedure. Apply an antibiotic cream on all injection sites.

Follow-up: After 1-2 weeks to see the result and if required more, few more units can be injected in the following sites, 2 units below the nose, two-thirds above the lip on each the ridge of the philtrum (orbicularis oris muscle) and another two units beside of nasolabial fold, besides the point of the greatest lateral contraction during the smile.

Review in 2 weeks and then at 3–4 months follow-up as the effect usually starts wearing off around 12–16 weeks. Hence, proper pre- and postprocedure counseling is required. Longevity of Btx A may be shortened in those with hyperkinetic peri oral muscles and also due to lesser units of Btx A.

Another Approach

Polo's opinion[19] states that the total dose of BT injection should be 10 U if the gingival exposure was more than 8.5 mm and the orbicularis oris muscle should not be injected.

Some authors[14,20,21] prefer to give low doses of BT initially then retouching, if needed, to avoid BT complications.

Fillers

In the case of a young patient with gum show of 1-2 mm, which could be due to a thin upper lip, injecting hyaluronic acid fillers can help to hide the gum show by increasing the vertical height of the lip **(Fig. 2)**.

The same may not be true in an older patient and other patient, where the gum show is due to overactive lip elevators. Here injection of BTX A will be required.

Inversion of the upper lip is due to overaction of the orbicularis oris muscle which can also lead to unwanted gum show on smiling. Often this is accompanied by a thin upper lip, in which case the gum show can be more pronounced. In such cases, injecting 0.25–1 units in the orbicularis oris at two points each side of the upper lip along the border will lead to eversion and therefore greater show of upper lip, thereby masking the upper lip. One can achieve 1 mm of correction with this. Further correction, if desired, will require a filler and the now relaxed orbicularis oris will allow better filler results.

Enough patients have obvious dental conditions that require dental work for smile correction before BTX A or filler can be injected for an esthetic finish. This would come in last.

CASE EXAMPLES

Case 1

This is a case of high lip line with altered active eruption. Clinical tooth length is shorter than anatomical tooth length. Altering the tissue levels and increasing tooth display will improve the appearance by improving tooth proportions. But there is increased lip mobility and the lip moves more than the normal 6-8 mm from position of rest. So, post dental treatment you are still left with a display more than 3-4 mm which remains a gummy smile. Needs either botulinum toxin to decrease mobility or lip repositioning surgery **(Figs. 3A and B)**.

Case 2

Gummy smile with altered passive eruption leading to poor tooth proportions and increased tissue display. Soft tissue recontouring helps improve tooth proportions and decrease appearance of gummy smile. But there is increased lip mobility in this case too, so gummy smile persists, needs botulinum toxin or lip repositioning for correction of gummy smile **(Figs. 4A and B)**.

Case 3

High lip line with compensatory eruption following tooth wear. Decreased tooth height due to wear. Restoring tooth proportions with soft and hard tissue treatment or intrusion improves the gummy smile. Lip movement

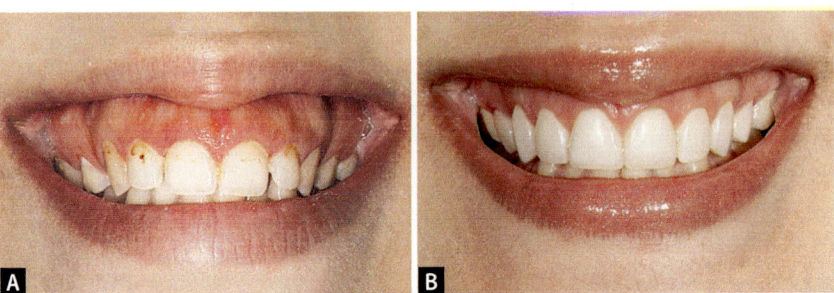

Figs. 3A and B: (A) Predental treatment; (B) Postdental treatment.

(*Courtesy*: Dr Saiesha Mistry)

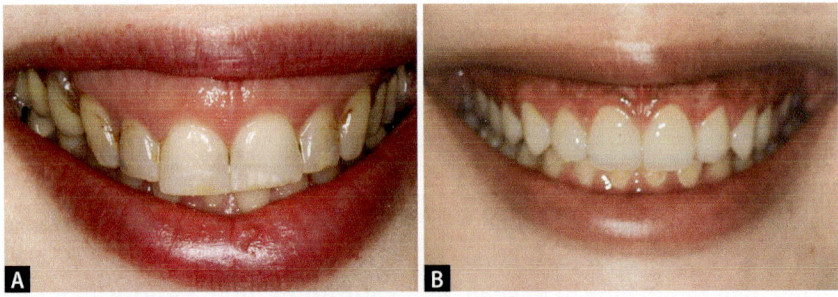

Figs. 4A and B: (A) Predental treatment; (B) Postdental treatment.

(*Courtesy*: Dr Saiesha Mistry)

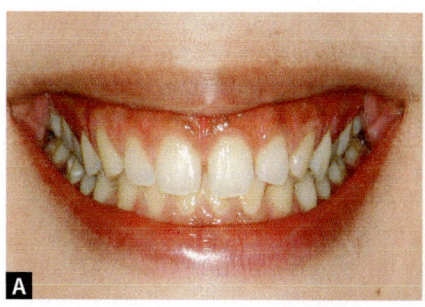 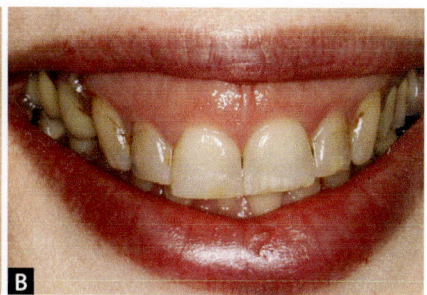

Figs. 5A and B: (A) Predental treatment; (B) Postdental treatment.

(*Courtesy*: Dr Saiesha Mistry)

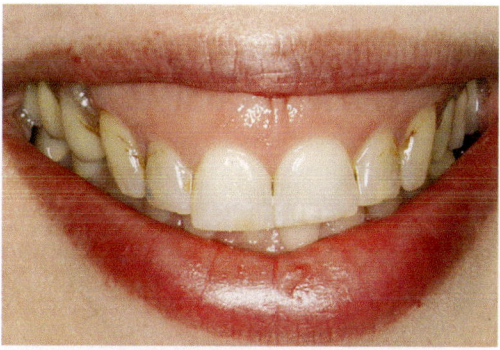

Fig. 6: Treatment of gummy smile due to vertical maxillary excess.

(*Courtesy*: Dr Saiesha Mistry)

more than 6–8 mm needs attention (**Figs. 5A and B**).

Case 4

Gummy smile due to vertical maxillary excess. Treatment would be a combination of dental surgical and plastic (**Fig. 6**).

USEFUL TIPS

- Treatment of gummy smile involves detailed analysis of smile and finding the etiology of gummy smile. Depending on etiology, the treatment plan should be strategized and discussed to give maximum and long lasting result.
- *Onabotulinum toxin* A provides a simple, effective, safe, minimally invasive, and cost-effective treatment for improving gummy smile caused due to hyperactive perioral muscles. It causes a significant improvement in smile esthetics with high patient satisfaction. The rule is to use a few units at each site. More can be added in touch up sessions on the next visits.
- Avoid correction of gummy smile in people who cannot tolerate weakening of their upper lip for professional reasons, e.g. saxophone players.

REFERENCES

1. Dong JK, Jin TH, Cho HW, et al. The esthetics of the smile: a review of some recent studies. Int J Prosthodont. 1999;12(1):9-19.
2. Peck S, Peck L, Kataja M. The gingival smile line. Angle Orthodont. 1992;62(2):91-100.
3. Mazzuco R, Hexsel D. Gummy smile and botulinum toxin: a new approach based on the gingival exposure area. J Am Acad Dermatol. 2010;63(6):1042-51.
4. Patel DP, Thakkar SA, Suthar JR. Adjunctive treatment of gummy smile using botulinum toxin type-A (case report). J Dent Med Sci. 2012;3(1):22-9.
5. Garber DA, Salama MA. The aesthetic smile: diagnosis and treatment. Periodontol 2000. 1996;11:18-28.

6. Levine RA, McGuire M. The diagnosis and treatment of the gummy smile. Compend Contin Educ Dent. 1997;18(8):757-62.
7. Silberberg N, Goldstein M, Smidt A. Excessive gingival display–etiology, diagnosis, and treatment modalities. Quintessence Int. 2009;40(10):809-18.
8. Wennström JL, Zucchelli G, Pini-Prato GP. Mucogingival therapy–periodontal plastic surgery. In: Lang NP, Lindhe J (Eds). Clinical Periodontology and Implant Dentistry, 5th edition. Oxford: Blackwell Munksgaard; 2008.
9. Farista S, Yeltiwar R, Kalakonda B, et al. Laser-assisted lip repositioning surgery: Novel approach to treat gummy smile. J Indian Soc Periodontol. 2017;21(2):164-8.
10. Storrer CL, Valverde FK, Santos FR, et al. Treatment of gummy smile: Gingival recontouring with the containment of the elevator muscle of the upper lip and wing of nose. A surgery innovation technique. J Indian Soc Periodontol. 2014;18(5):656-60.
11. Jaspers GWC, Pijpe J, Jansma J. The use of botulinum toxin type A in cosmetic facial procedures. Int J Oral Maxillofac Surg. 2011;40(2):127-33.
12. Dinker S, Anitha A, Sorake A, et al. Management of gummy smile with botulinum toxin type-A: A case report. J Int Oral Health. 2014;6(1):111-5.
13. Hwang WS, Hur MS, Hu KS, et al. Surface anatomy of the lip elevator muscles for the treatment of gummy smile using botulinum toxin. Angle Orthod. 2009;79(1):70-7.
14. Polo M. Botulinum toxin type A (Botox) for the neuromuscular correction of excessive gingival display on smiling (gummy smile). Am J Orthod Dentofacial Orthop. 2008;133(2):195-203.
15. Nasr MW, Jabbour SF, Sidaoui JA, et al. Botulinum toxin for the treatment of excessive gingival display: A systematic review. Aesthet Surg J. 2016;36(1):82-8.
16. Borodic G. Immunologic resistance after repeated botulinum toxin type a injections for facial rhytides. Ophthalmic Plast Reconstr Surg. 2006;22(3):239-40.
17. Niamtu J 3rd. Cosmetic oral and maxillofacial surgery options. J Am Dent Assoc. 2000;131(6):756-64.
18. Baş B, Ozan B, Muğlali M, et al. Treatment of masseteric hypertrophy with botulinum toxin: a report of two cases. Med Oral Patol Oral Cir Bucal. 2010;15(4):649-52.
19. Polo M. Commentary on: botulinum toxin for the treatment of excessive gingival display: a systematic review. Aesthet Surg J. 2016;36(1):89-92.
20. Carruthers A, Carruthers J, Flynn TC, et al. Dose-finding, safety, and tolerability study of botulinum toxin type B for the treatment of hyperfunctional glabellar lines. Dermatol Surg. 2007;33(1 Spec No):S60-8.
21. Kane MA. The effect of botulinum toxin injections on the nasolabial fold. Plast Reconstr Surg. 2003;112(Suppl 5):66S-72S.

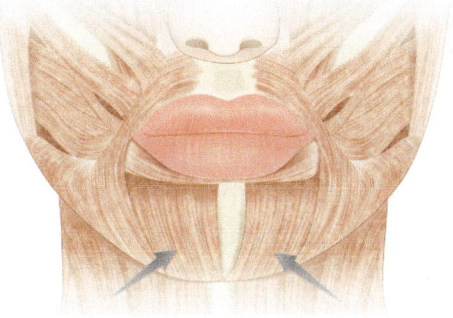

CHAPTER 35

Botulinum Toxin for Marionette Lines

Ishad Aggarwal

INTRODUCTION

Marionette line or melomental fold is the crease that forms between the oral commissure and the lateral mentum or the chin. It is a vertical fold that gives patient a sad face appearance. It is formed due to a variety of factors such as laxity of the mandibular ligament, resorption of the mandible, loss of deep fat pads, and over activity of the depressor anguli oris (DAO) muscle.[1] A validated photonumeric 5-point scale has been established to assess the severity of the marionette lines **(Table 1)**.

The treatment of marionette lines aims at restoring a youthful and happier look to the face. Generally, a combination of treatments is used, depending upon the severity of the marionette lines. These treatments are energy-based devices, fillers, and botulinum toxin.

The role of botulinum toxin in treatments of marionette lines is mostly never as a stand-alone procedure—it is most commonly used in combination with fillers. In this chapter, we shall discuss the relevant anatomy of the musculature involved in formation of the marionette lines and usage of botulinum toxin in improving the downwards turn of the oral commissures.

ANATOMY OF MARIONETTE LINES[1]

The sequence of layers in the region of marionette folds are skin, superficial fat compartment, fibers of the platysma muscle, deep fat compartment, DAO muscle, and the bone. For the purpose of this chapter, we will discuss the anatomy of the DAO muscle because it is responsible for causing the downturning of the oral commissures.

DEPRESSOR ANGULI ORIS MUSCLE[3,4]

Origin and insertion: It arises from the oblique line of the jaw where its fibers converge to be inserted into the angle of the mouth. At its origin, it fuses with the platysma, and at its insertion with the orbicularis oris and risorius muscle. On contraction, it depresses the corner of the mouth. It is innervated by the mandibular branch of the facial nerve.

Table 1: Grading of marionette lines.[2]

Grade	Description
Grade 1	No marionette lines or jowl dip
Grade 2	Slight turn down at the corners of the mouth
Grade 3	Moderate marionette lines, mild jowl dip
Grade 4	Severe marionette lines extending toward the chin, moderate jowl dip
Grade 5	Severe marionette lines almost reaching the chin, severe jowl dip

Its medial border overlaps with the depressor labii inferioris, and its lateral border is adjacent to the risorius, zygomaticus major, and platysma muscles.

Topography of Depressor Anguli Oris[4]

Topography of DAO was described by Choi YJ Et et al. in their paper. According to them the safest area for injecting DAO is in a fan shape area which can be marked as following.
- Identify and check the location of the modiolus by palpating the cheek. The modiolus is the mobile muscular mass located at the lateral border of the mouth corner, and is formed by a convergence of the muscle fibers from the DAO muscle and the zygomaticus major, orbicularis oris, risorius, buccinators, and levator anguli oris muscles.
- Draw a sagittal line passing through the modiolus.
- Draw an oblique line at an angle of 30° on the medial side of the modiolus.
- Draw an oblique line at an angle of 45° on lateral side of modiolus.

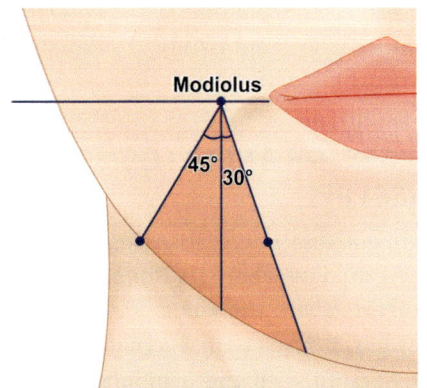

Fig. 1: Reference points for injection of botulinum toxin in the depressor anguli oris.

Depressor anguli oris is a fan shape muscle that lies between these two oblique lines. Inferior border of mandible can be considered to be the safest and most effective site for injecting DAO.

Injection Technique

Traditionally, the injection point for botulinum toxin for DAO has been taught as a point 1 cm lateral and inferior to the corner of the lip. The injection has to be given superficially and not more 2-4 units of botulinum neurotoxin A (BoNTA) is to be injected. The triangle detailed above can be used for confirmation of the safety of the chose injection point.

However, the injector must assess the muscle bulk and take note of any pre-existing asymmetry of lips at rest and during animation, and the same must be communicated to the patient beforehand.

Possible Complications[4]

Inadvertent wrongly placed injections is the most common complication of DAO injections with BoNTA. If the botulinum toxin affects the muscles surrounding the DAO, namely depressor labii inferioris medially and risorius and zygomaticus major laterally, the result is lip asymmetry and an asymmetrical smile, respectively.

ILLUSTRATED EXAMPLES

Case 1

This 54-year-old female came with drooping corners of the lips. 2 units of botulinum toxin were injected each side on the DAO. 2 weeks after the injections, the patient came back with visibly improved corners of the lips **(Fig. 2)**.

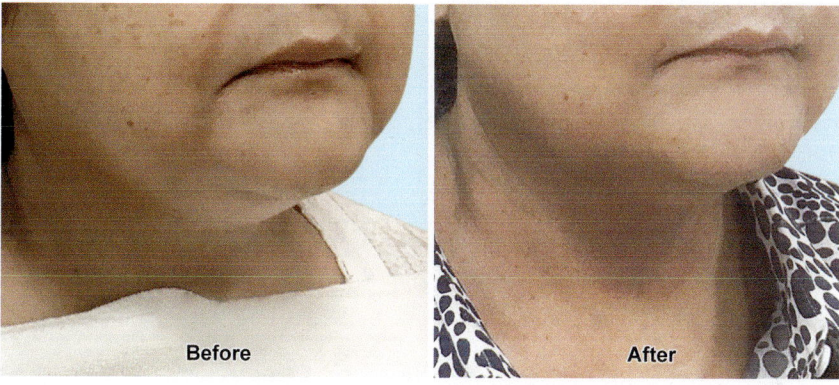

Fig. 2: Drooping corners of the lips.

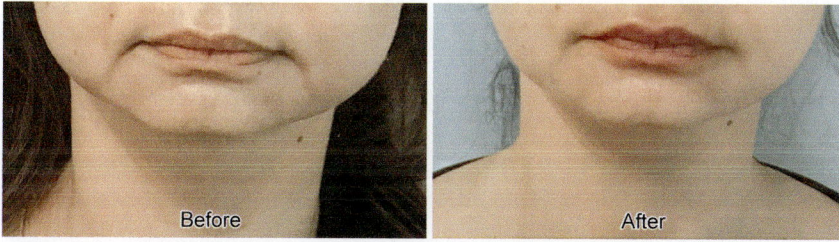

Fig. 3: Marionette lines and drooping corners of the lips.

Case 2

A 45-year-old female came with marionette lines and drooping corners of the lips. Juvéderm Ultraplus XC was used to fill the marionette lines and 2 units of botulinum toxin were injected in DAO each side. 2 weeks later, she presented with improved marionette lines and raised corners of the lips **(Fig. 3)**.

POSTINJECTION INSTRUCTIONS

The patients are advised not to lie down supine for a few hours after the injection. They are also asked to avoid massaging the area injected. A topical antibiotic formulation can be prescribed to be applied gently on the injection site for 4–5 days.

USEFUL TIPS

- Depressor anguli oris is the muscle, which is responsible for causing the downward turn of the oral commissures, which can make the face look sad and depressed.
- Cosmetic correction of drooping oral commissures can be done by injecting small doses of botulinum toxin into the DAO muscle.
- Depressor anguli oris is surrounded medially by depressor labii inferioris muscle and laterally by risorius; hence, knowledge of topography of DAO is vital to avoid inadvertent diffusion of the botulinum toxin into these muscles.

REFERENCES

1. Pessa JE, Rohrich RJ. The lips and chin. In: Pessa JE, Rohrich RJ (Eds). Facial Topography, Clinical Anatomy of the Face. Missouri: Quality Medical Publishing; 2012. pp. 251-91.
2. Carruthers A, Carruthers J, Hardas B, et al. A validated grading scale for marionette lines. Dermatol Surg. 2008;34(Suppl 2):S167-72.
3. Braz AV, Louvain D, Mukamal LV. Combined treatment with botulinum toxin and hyaluronic acid to correct unsightly lateral-chin depression. An Bras Dermatol. 2013;88(1):138-40.
4. Choi YJ, Kim JS, Gil YC, et al. Anatomical considerations regarding the location and boundary of the depressor anguli oris muscle with reference to botulinum toxin injection. Plast Reconstr Surg. 2014;134(5):917-21.

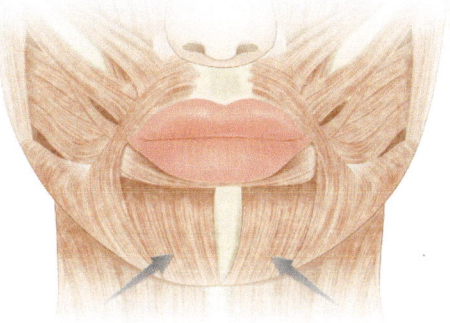

Dimpled Chin

Rajat Kandhari, Kritu Bhandari

INTRODUCTION

Although, an off label indication use of botulinum toxin type A (BoNTA) for addressing the dimpled chin is a frequently carried out procedure in clinical practice, and has been shown to be an effective treatment for moderate rhytides of the mentalis. Use of BoNTA for the mentalis muscle is frequently combined with injections into the depressor anguli oris (DAO) for the downturned corners of the mouth. The compact spatial arrangement of the muscles in the lower face requires that the injecting physician has a thorough understanding of the muscular anatomy in order to prevent undesirable adverse effects.[1] The use of BoNTA in the lower face is frequently combined with use of soft tissue fillers, resurfacing techniques, or invasive procedures such as rhytidectomy, implants, etc. for optimal outcomes.

ANATOMY OF THE MENTALIS MUSCLE

The mentalis is a short, stout, conical, and two-bellied muscle that originates deep to the depressor labii inferioris on the anterior aspect of the mandible on either side of the midline at the level of the incisive fossa and root of the lower lateral incisors. It travels downward, converging its two muscle bellies toward the midline to insert into the skin of the apex of the chin on either side of the frenulum of the lower lip.[2] Superiorly, the fibers of the mentalis mingle with some of the fibers of the orbicularis oris, whereas laterally they interdigitate with the fibers of the depressor labii inferioris **(Figs. 1A and B)**. Contraction of the mentalis muscle raises the chin, which causes wrinkles and dimpling, and assists in everting the lower lip. This expresses sadness, anger, disdain, or doubt.[2,3]

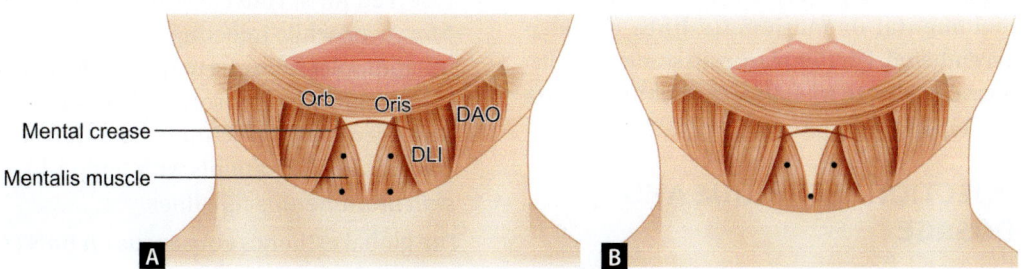

Figs. 1A and B: Suggested techniques for injection of Botox into the paired mentalis muscles to improve dimpled chin.

(DAO: depressor anguli oris; DLI: depressor labii inferioris)

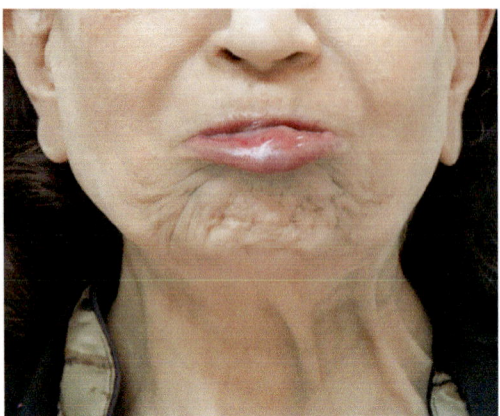

Fig. 2: Hyperkinetic depressor angulis oris, mentalis, and platysmal bands—an ideal candidate for injection in the lower face musculature.

The dimpled chin is often not noticed by the patient, until it has been pointed out to them by someone else. The appearance is much like a "golf ball" or an "orange peel" and is often referred to as a "golf ball" chin or "peau d'orange" appearance **(Fig. 2)**. The dimpled appearance of the chin is often accentuated with age, especially when the mentolabial crease becomes more pronounced. The wrinkling is a result of constant expression, the loss of collagen and subcutaneous fat as a result of aging, and/or cumulative photodamage.

In most individuals, when frowning in displeasure or projecting an expression of sadness, doubt, or disdain, the DAO contracts simultaneously with the mentalis, so the melomental or marionette lines are also accentuated. For this reason, in some patients, it is advisable to treat the DAO while treating the hyperkinetic mentalis.[4,5]

INJECTION TECHNIQUE AND DOSAGE

Injections are best done with the patient in the upright sitting or semirecumbent position. It is recommended to insert the needle (31 G, BD, ultra-fine, 4.0 units, 6 mm) perpendicular to the skin, to its full depth in the midline. Ice fomentation can help relieve any pain or discomfort to the patient if needed. For optimal outcomes, around 4–8 U of BoNTA may be injected into the mentalis, and the units at every point may vary based on the specific technique adopted.

There are various techniques that can be considered for treating the dimpled chin **(Figs. 3 and 4)**.[6]

- *Two-point technique*: This is the most commonly employed method and involves administering 2–4 units on either side of the midline may be administered directly into the two bellies of the mentalis. This technique is considered appropriate for people with a "squarish" chin or a vertical mental cleft.
- *Single-point technique*: 4–6 units into the mentalis at the apex of the mental protuberance. A midline injection approximately 0.5–1 cm above the lowermost point of the chin and no closer than 1.5 cm from the lower lip is ideal for injecting. This technique is appropriate for those with a pointed or narrow chin.
- *Diamond-shaped technique:* Four injection points in the shape of a diamond for equal distribution with 2 units administered at each of these points for a uniform distribution. This may be reserved for severe cases of wider chins. Moreover, while injecting neurotoxin in a microdroplet form one may consider using this technique (personal observation). The microdroplet technique may be used particularly for patients with "crepe-like" skin or numerous fine lines.

The global esthetics consensus on BoNTA recommends the use of 1–4 injection points on either side of the midline with 2–3 units at each injection point.[7]

Chapter 36: Dimpled Chin

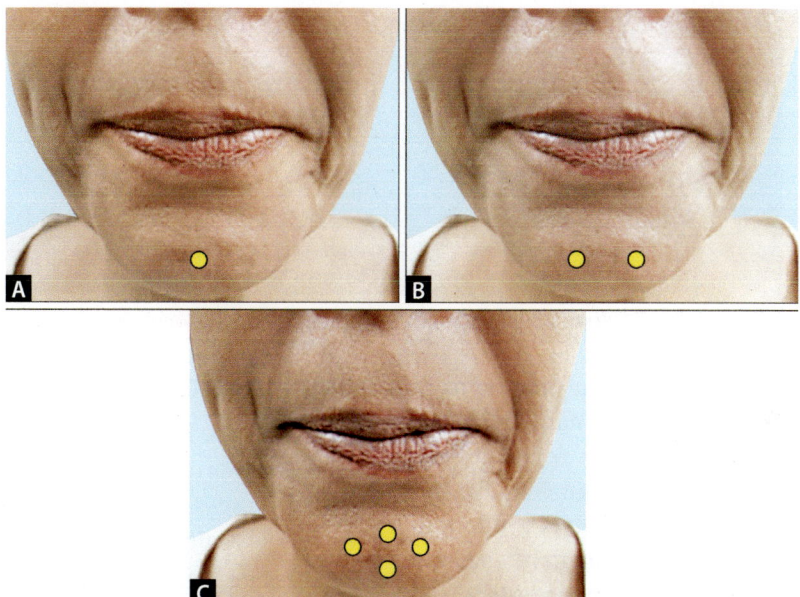

Figs. 3A to C: Techniques of treating the mentalis muscle. (A) Single-point technique; (B) Two-point technique; and (C) Diamond-shaped technique.

(*Courtesy:* Dr Rajat Kandhari)

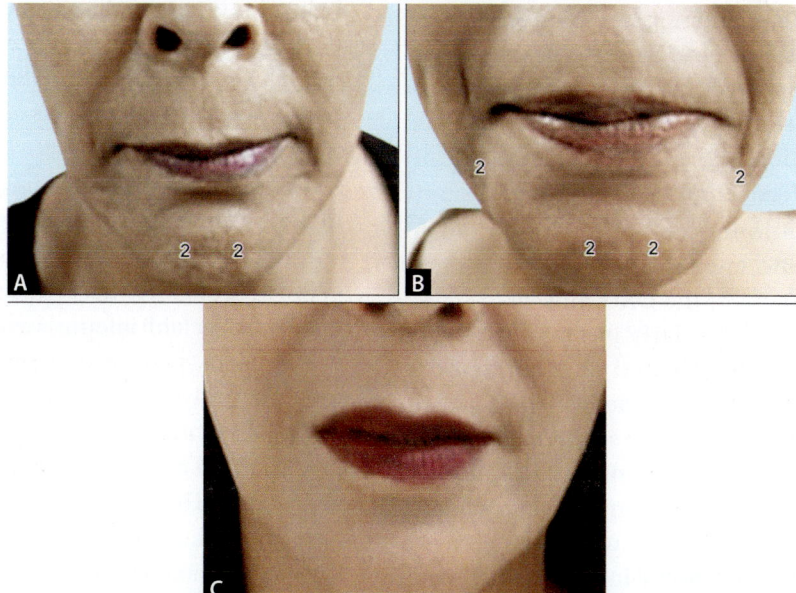

Figs. 4A to C: (A) Treatment of the mentalis with the two-point technique; (B) Treatment of the depressor anguli oris (DAO) along with the mentalis with 2 units on either side; (C) After treatment of the mentalis and DAO.

(*Courtesy:* Dr Rajat Kandhari)

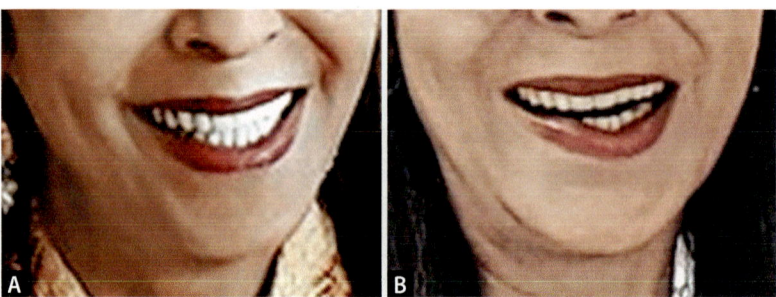

Figs. 5A and B: (A) Normal smile preinjection; (B) Asymmetry 2 weeks postinjection.

Relaxing the mentalis not only helps in reducing the puckered appearance of the chin but also diminishes the appearance of the deep transverse labiomental crease and slightly raises the lower lip. It is prudent to inject below the transverse mental crease and as close as possible to the lower border of the body of the mandible. Further, high-volume injections, improper technique, and vigorous massage postinjection can cause diffusion of the neurotoxin into the orbicularis oris, depressor labii inferioris, or both leading to unwanted side effects. The onset of asymmetry in the lip due to diffusion into the depressor labii inferioris typically occurs 2 weeks postinjection and may last for up to 3–4 months **(Figs. 5A and B)**.

As mentioned above treatment of a hyperkinetic mentalis is often combined with treatment of the DAO muscle (2 units either side) particularly in patients where it can be easily palpated or identified on expression. Moreover, a deeply placed filler administered in the same session or 2 weeks later, along with the use of BoNTA helps in rejuvenation of the chin and appears to offer gratifying and sustained overall outcomes. This is particularly useful in cases with a deep transverse labiomental crease or in cases with "crepe like" skin or fine lines in the lower face.

COMPLICATIONS

Complications while treating the hyperkinetic mentalis essentially arise due to improper technique, excessive dosing, and/or vigorous massage postinjection.[1]

- *Excessive dosing/high volumes*: Over enthusiastic treatment of the mentalis can result in immobilizing the muscle resulting in difficulty in approximating the lower lip tightly against the teeth. Patients typically complain of food accumulating in this space while eating, involuntary dripping from the lower lip when drinking, or drooling from the corners of the mouth when at rest.
- *Improper technique:* Injections very close to the lower lip or high up close to mental crease may result in injections diffusion of the neurotoxin to the adjacent fibers of the depressor labii inferioris or orbicularis oris muscle, resulting in relaxation of the tight oral sphincter, reduction of lip competence, mouth asymmetry, lower lip ptosis, and a reduction in buccal motor movements. The patient in these cases may also experience difficulty in articulating certain letters or words.
- *Vigorous massage postinjection:* This will also result in the neurotoxin migrating to

the adjacent muscles causing undesirable sphincter incompetence and associated side effects as mentioned above. Patients should be forewarned regarding this prior to injection.

USEFUL TIPS

- Most patients are unaware of the existence of the dimpled chin until it has pointed to them by someone else.
- 4–8 U of BoNTA is usually sufficient to relax the mentalis muscle.
- Inject below the transverse mental crease and as close as possible to the lower border of the body of the mandible.
- High-volume injections/improper technique can cause diffusion of the toxin into the orbicularis oris or depressor labii inferioris leading to motor dysfunction of the lower lip/sphincter incompetence.
- Immobilizing the mentalis with a high dose of low-volume toxin can prevent the lower lip from approximating tightly against the teeth—problems with drinking and articulating.
- Injections of the mentalis muscle are frequently combined with soft tissue fillers for more optimal outcomes.

REFERENCES

1. Benedetto AV. Cosmetic uses of botulinum toxin A in the lower face, neck and upper chest. Botulinum Toxin in Clinical Dermatology. United States: Taylor & Francis; 2006.
2. Emer J, Waldorf HA. Neurotoxin update and review, Part 2: The art. Cosmetic Dermatology. 2010;23(10):474-80.
3. Carruthers J, Fagien S, Matarasso SL, et al. Consensus recommendation on the use of botulinum toxin type A in facial aesthetics. Plast Reconst Surg. 2004;114 (Suppl 6):1S-22S.
4. Shetty MK; IADVL Dermatosurgey Task Force. Guidelines on the use of botulinum toxin type A. Indian J Dermatol Venereol Leprol. 2008;74 (Suppl):S13-22.
5. Beer K, Yohn M, Closter J. A double-blinded placebo-controlled study of Botox for the treatment of subjects with chin rhytids. J Drugs Dermatol. 2005;4(4):417-22.
6. Arsiwala S, Kandhari R. Botulinum toxin for the midface, lower face and neck. In: Mysore V (Ed.) ACS (I) Textbook on Cutaneous and Aesthetic Surgery. New Delhi: Jaypee Brothers Medical Publishers; 2017. p. 742.
7. Sundaram H, Signorini M, Liew S, et al. Global aesthetics consensus: Botulinum toxin type A—evidence-based review, emerging concepts, and consensus recommendations for aesthetic use, including updates on complications. Plastic Reconstructive Surg. 2016;137(3):518e-29e.

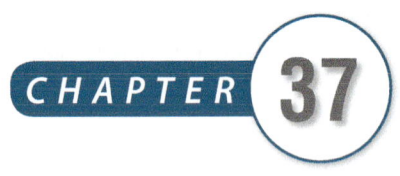
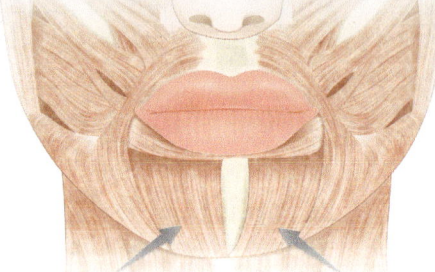

Botulinum Toxin in Platysmal Bands

Sudha Vani Damarla, Manogna Vellala

INTRODUCTION

The platysma is a superficial muscle which originates at the chest and inserts into the mandibular border.[1] Along with the depressor anguralis oris, the depressor labii, and the mentalis, the platysma acts as a depressor muscle.[2] With age and use, the platysma is responsible for the development of neck bands, which are accentuated by aging of the overlying skin. Platysma also worsens jowls by providing a downward pull. This blurs and then obscures the sharp angle of the jaw, leading to a loss of a youthful countenance.

RELEVANT ANATOMY

The platysma originates from the pectoralis and deltoid fascia over the upper chest and inserts into the mentum; the periosteum of the ramus of the mandible; and the orbicularis oris, depressor anguralis oris, and risorius muscles.[3] Its anterior fibers from both sides may cross each other at the midline and may form various patterns of decussation. In some cases, the fibers may even separate completely.[4,5] When the upper and lower portions of the platysma contract, they pull the skin to the center of the muscle. This is the cause of horizontal neck bands. The platysma is supplied by the cervical motor branch of the facial nerve.

In the young, the platysma is covered by a layer of subcutaneous fat. With age, the fat layer is lost and the fibrous strands of the muscle become more prominent. Furthermore, the resting tone of the platysma increases with age and this is another factor responsible for the senescent appearance of the neck with age. The reason for the increased tone is attributed to be due to compensatory hypertrophy as the platysma supports the deeper neck structures. Decreased neck extension with advancing age could also be a contributory factor.

The platysmal tone can be demonstrated by asking the patient to grimace (**Figs. 1A and B**).

INJECTION TECHNIQUES

Botulinum toxin injections were traditionally used for neck tightening and jaw recontouring by means of direct injection into the platysmal bands.[6] The quantity of toxin used, however, was very high.

The "Nefertiti lift," was a technique described by Levy. In this technique, injection is done into the upper part of the platysmal band and horizontal injections are given along the mandible.[7,8] This leads to jawline recontouring by release of the platysma's downward pull.

The limitation of this technique is that it fails to address the anterior platysmal fibers.

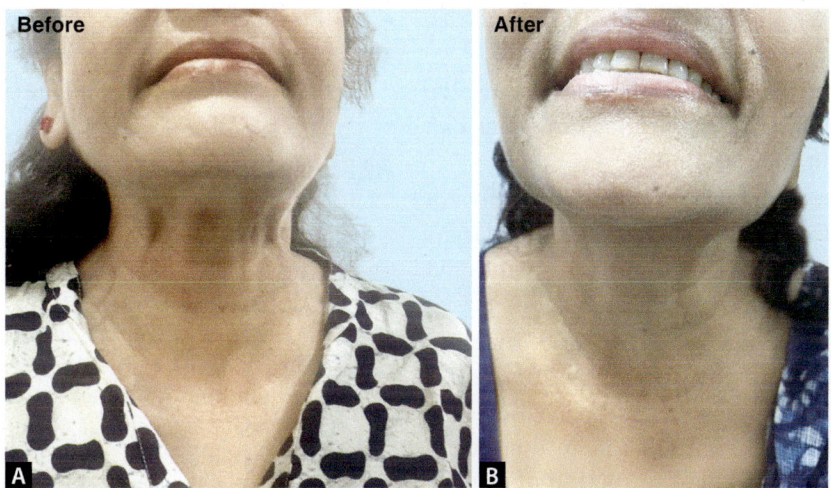

Figs. 1A and B: (A) Before botulinum toxin injection, (B) After 30 units of injection.

This may lead to anterior wrinkling and loss of anterior contour of the neck.

To address these shortfalls, a few adaptations such as using a single injection site with 20U to 30U onabotulinumtoxinA per side[9] were developed. The microbotox technique developed by Dr Woffles consists of treating the entire neck with minute intradermal doses of BoNT-A, with a total dose of 60–80 onabotulinumtoxinA.[10]

The platysma needs to be activated by asking the patient to grimace. This permits visualization of the muscle. The anatomy of the muscle in each patient should be taken into consideration before injecting. The technique varies in patients with diffuse muscle and those with numerous bands.

For patients in whom the muscle is diffuse, the injection should likewise be diffuse and should be spaced at a distance of between 1.5 cm and 2 cm across the neck in a line. Care should be taken to place the needle in the superficial dermis. Around 2–2.5 units should be injected at each point.

If the bands of the muscle are discrete, each band should be held individually and the needle should be inserted directly into the muscle. Around 1–1.5 cm spacing should be given between injections and each band should receive 2.5 units of the toxin.

To manage horizontal neck lines, 1–2 units of botox are injected into the deep dermis at a spacing of 1–2 cm. This technique was described by Carruthers et al.[11]

The maximum dose should not exceed 40 units.

PRECAUTIONS

If the toxin is mistakenly injected into the strap muscles of the neck, it may lead to dysphagia and, in rare cases, may necessitate the use of a feeding tube. The risk of dysphagia is higher if more than 40 units are injected. A sensation of heaviness was described in one patient in a study by De Almeida et al. In the same study, unilateral retraction of the lower lip was observed due to slight weakness of the depressor labii inferioris (DLI). This was, however, not perceived by the patients.[12]

Due to unopposed action, excessive contraction of the upper face muscles can be seen in a few cases.

Higher doses of toxin can lead to diffusion through the platysma and may reach the larynx and also the neck flexors (sternocleidomastoid muscle).

Care should be taken to avoid injection into the strap muscles (the small, flat muscles inferior to the hyoid bone including the sternohyoid, omohyoid, sternothyroid, thyrohyoid). To avoid retraction of mouth, injection should be made 1 cm posterior to junction of nasolabial fold and mandible and direction of injection should be posterior. The total dose should not exceed 20 units on either side. In case of retraction of lip by injection into DLI, injection of contralateral side can correct the appearance.[7] In case of individuals with high degree of laxity of skin and prolapse of fat, botulinum toxin injection into the platysma may not produce the desired results. These patients should be counseled in advance.

POSTINJECTION INSTRUCTIONS

Standard post botulinum toxin injection instructions are given to the patient. The patient should be followed up after 2 weeks and response should be assessed. Touch ups can be done if required at this juncture.

USEFUL TIPS

- Injection of botulinum toxin into the platysma causes improvement in the contour of the aging neckline.
- The use of low doses can minimize complications and maximize the benefits of the injection.
- A thorough knowledge of the anatomy of the muscle and inter-individual variations is essential for performing the procedure.

REFERENCES

1. Hwang K, Kim JY, Lim JH. Anatomy of the platysma muscle. J Craniofac Surg. 2017;28(2):539-42.
2. Coleman SR, Grover R. The anatomy of the aging face: volume loss and changes in 3-dimensional topography. Aesthet Surg J. 2006;26(1S):S4-9.
3. Fagien S, Raspaldo H. Facial rejuvenation with botulinum neurotoxin: an anatomical and experiential perspective. J Cosm Laser Ther. 2007;9 (Suppl 1):23-31.
4. Finn JC, Cox SE. Practical botulinum toxin anatomy. In: Carruthers A, Carruthers J (Eds). Botulinum Toxin. London, United Kingdom: Elsevier-Saunders; 2005. pp. 19-30.
5. Hoefflin SM. Anatomy of the platysma and lip depressor muscles a simplified mnemonic approach. Dermatol Surg. 1998;24(11):1225-31.
6. Brandt FS, Bellman B. Cosmetic use of botulinum A exotoxin for the aging neck. Dermatol Surg. 1998;24(11):1232-4.
7. Levy P. The "Nefertiti lift": a new technique for specific re-contouring of the jawline. J Cosm Laser Ther. 2007;9(4):249-52.
8. Levy PM. Neurotoxins: current concepts in cosmetic use on the face and neck-jawline contouring/platysma bands/necklace lines. Plast Reconstr Surg. 2015;136(Suppl 5):80S-3S.
9. Carruthers J, Trindade de Almeida AR. Platysma and Nefertiti lift. In: Carruthers J, Carruthers A (Eds). Procedures in Cosmetic Dermatology: Botulinum Toxin, 4th edition. London, United Kingdom: Elsevier-Saunders; 2017.
10. Wu WT. Microbotox of the lower face and neck: evolution of a personal technique and its clinical effects. Plast Reconstr Surg. 2015;136 (Suppl 5):92S-100S.
11. Carruthers J, Carruthers A. Botulinum toxin A in the mid and lower face and neck. Dermatol Clin. 2004;22(2):151-8.
12. de Almeida ART, Romiti A, Carruthers JDA. The facial platysma and its underappreciated role in lower face dynamics and contour. Dermatol Surg. 2017;43(8):1042-9.

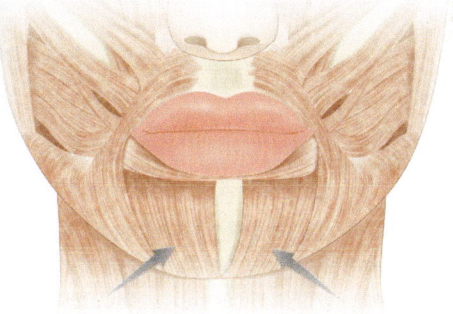

CHAPTER 38

Nefertiti Lift

Bhavesh K Swarnkar

INTRODUCTION

The main determining factors of the aging neck are the presence of submental fat, loss of definition of the mandibular border and neck angle, flaccidity and poor quality of the skin as well as horizontal lines and vertical bands of the platysma muscle. These bands are mainly determined by hyperkinetic activity and loss of muscle tone.[1] This hyperkinetic activity of the platysma muscle and its interfaces as well as its connections with adjacent oral muscles, combined with the function of the depressor anguli oris (DAO), lead to marked bands and depressed oral commissures, which are also aspects commonly associated with aging.[2]

Despite the explosion of noninvasive cosmetic treatment options for the face, the modalities available to improve neck appearance have been limited. Brandt and Bellman first documented use of botulinum toxin (BTX) for the treatment of lower face and neck.[3,4] Nefertiti lift refers to the use of botulinum toxin to improve jawline definition. It reduces jowling and improves horizontal lines on neck by relaxing the platysma which is a major depressor of the lower face.[5] The technique is indicated for patients with horizontal and vertical platysma muscle bands and with downturned oral commissures, without excessive skin laxity or submental lipodystrophy. Patients with unrealistic expectations regarding results are to be excluded from the treatment.[5]

ANATOMY

The platysma is a broad muscle, originating in the pectoral and deltoid area from the fascia, covering the pectoralis major and deltoid muscle. Its posterior fibers are inserted into the DAO and risorius muscles as well as into the lateral portion of the orbicularis oris muscle. The anterior fibers are inserted into the periosteum of the medial portion of the mandibular border. These fibers interface those of the masseter, buccinator, and DAO. Superficial platysmal fibers can insert directly into masseter, risorius, and DAO. It is mainly these anterior portions that are responsible for the formation of platysmal bands when muscular contraction occurs.[6] The platysma depresses the lower jaw and pulls the lower lip, and corners of the mouth sideways and down, partially opening the mouth. Banding occurs with aging and change in the submental spaces.[7,8] When the platysma muscle tenses, it lifts the neck out (accentuating platysmal bands) and lowers the eyelids and midface (accentuating the malar and nasolabial folds) and the mandible (making the neck shorter and wider), making it the major muscle responsible for the emotive response of surprise. Clinically, the actions created by the platysma clearly demonstrate a significant facial component.[1]

Anatomical Variations

In 75%, the medial fibers in the submental area interdigitate with the contralateral platysma muscle for up to 1–2 cm below the chin. In 15%, the muscle fibers interdigitate all the way down to the thyroid cartilage, and in 10% the medial platysmal fibers do not interdigitate.[9]

Blood supply of platysma is through a branch of external carotid artery.

The platysma is the most superficial muscular layer of the face and is innervated by the cervical branch of the facial nerve. This branch of the facial nerve courses deep to the superior aspect of the platysma inferior to the mandible.[10]

Injection Technique

Prior to injection, each patient has to be assessed to determine whether treatment would be effective. Patient has to sit straight in front of examiner and asked to pull down hard on platysma muscle as shown in **Figures 1 A and B**.[11] This can also be done by asking patient to sound alphabet E. Disappearance of the mandibular border with this action indicates the potential for successful treatment.

With the patient in the supine position, the injections are administered utilizing a thin needle (30 G ½ inch) attached to an insulin-type syringe. The procedure is usually performed without anesthesia though a topical anesthetic may be used in patients who are more sensitive to pain. Application of cold compresses before and shortly after injection provides further pain relief and reduces bruising.

Approximately 2–3 units are injected along the mandibular border and in the upper part of the posterior platysmal band for a total of 15–20 units on each side as shown in **Figures 1A and B**. In each case, the patient is asked to contract the platysmal muscle and injected on the marked points. Patient needs to follow up after 2 weeks for reassessment. Touch-ups can be given at the follow-up, if required. The average duration of the effect is 4–6 months. The best results are observed in younger patients who have greater muscular strength and no significant laxity or submental lipodystrophy. Kane reported some objective

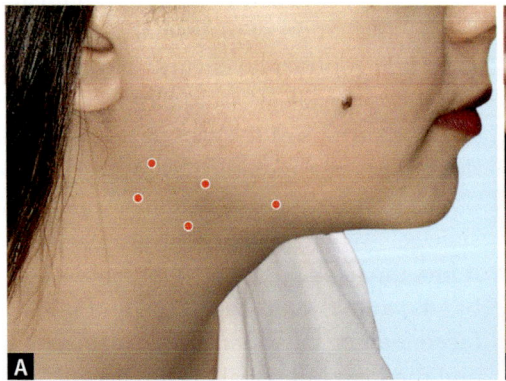
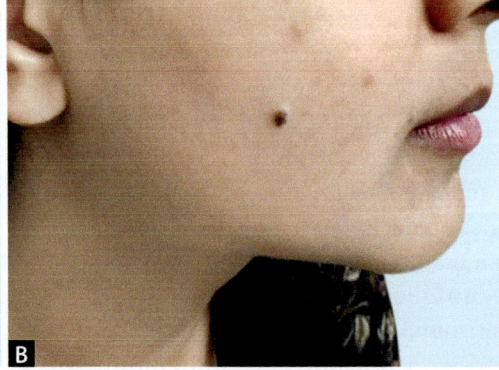

Figs. 1A and B: (A) Pretreatment picture showing points of injection for botulinum toxin 2 units on each point; (B) Improvement in the form of well-defined jaw line and lift of angle of mouth after 14 days.

improvement in neck contouring in 44 patients injected with increasing dose up to 20 units on each side.[12] Tangential injections of BTX produce longest and most effective results than perpendicular injections because the BTX is nicely spread in adjacent area.[13]

RESULTS

The results obtained, namely the attenuation of the platysmal bands and elevation and redefinition of the angle of the mouth, become visible within 2 or 3 days following the injection and remain stable for a variable period of time. The effect is longer lasting in the neck region (4 months on average). Although the results can be better appreciated during movements of expression and facial animation, they can also be seen in the face and neck at rest.[14]

PRECAUTIONS

Apart from the known side effects of botulinum toxin, there are certain specific side effects like early experience of dysphagia and excess muscular contraction in the upper face which can be achieved by using lower doses, avoid injecting too deep under the mandible posterior to the nasolabial folds. Undesired muscle weakening of neck is also reported which might be due to diffusion or migration of the toxin in the muscles or surrounding the injection site. Apart from these there are reversible adverse reactions observed such as transient edema and ecchymoses, hematoma formation, muscle soreness or neck discomfort, and headache. Many patient experiences mild neck weakness for a period of 1–2 weeks.[15]

POSTINJECTION INSTRUCTIONS

Patient is advised to not to massage the treated area for next 2-3 days.

Neck movement would help in dissipation of botulinum in the muscle in a uniform pattern. Movements like neck extension and flexion, and grimacing would be good exercise for the same.

USEFUL TIPS

Proper selection of the patient in very important for successful results.

A detailed communication regarding patients expectations and expected outcome is very important.

REFERENCES

1. de Castro CC. The anatomy of the platysma muscle. Plast Reconstr Surg. 1980;66(5):680-3.
2. Perkins SW, Sandel HD. Anatomic considerations, analysis, and the aging process of the perioral region. Facial Plast Surg Clin North Am. 2007;15(4):403-7.
3. Brandt FS, Bellman B. Cosmetic use of botulinum A toxin for aging neck. Dermatol Surg. 1998;24(11):1232-4.
4. Wise JB, Greco T. Injectable treatments for the aging face. Facial plat Surg. 2006;22(2):140-6.
5. Carruthers J, Fagien S, Matarasso SL, et al. Consensus recommendations on the use of botulinum toxin type a in facial aesthetics. Plast Reconstr Surg. 2004;114(Suppl 6):1S-22S.
6. Thiel W. Photographic Atlas of practical anatomy, 2nd ed. Heidelberg: Springer; 2005.
7. Levy PM. The "Nefertiti lift": a new technique for specific re-contouring of the jawline. J Cosmet Laser Ther. 2007;9(4):249-52.
8. Sommer B, Sattler G. Botulinum Toxin in Aesthetic Medicine, Vol VIII. Berlin: Blackwell Wissenschafts-Verlag; 2001.
9. Hoerter JE, Patel BC, StatPearls (2019). Anatomy, Head and Neck, Platysma. [online] Available from: https://www.ncbi.nlm.nih.gov/books/NBK545294/ [Last accessed on December, 2019].
10. Huettner F, Rueda S, Ozturk CN, et al. The relationship of the marginal mandibular nerve to the mandibular osseocutaneous ligament and lesser ligaments of the lower face. Aesthet Surg J. 2015;35(2):111-20.

11. Lavy PM. Case report, Nefertiti lift: A new technique for specific recontouring of jaw line. J. Cosmet Laser Ther. 2007,9:249-52.
12. Kane MA. Nonsurgical treatment of platysmal band with injection of botulinum toxin A. Plast Reconstr Surg. 1999;103(2):653-63.
13. Fulton JE. Botulinum toxin. The newport beads experiment. Dermatol Surg. 1998;24(11):1219-24.
14. Goldman A, Wollina U. Elevation of the corner of the mouth using botulinum toxin type A. J Cutan Aesthet Surg. 2010;3(3):145-50.
15. Gassia V, Beylot C, Béchaux S, et al. Botulinum toxin injection techniques in the lower third and middle of the face, the neck and the décolleté: the "Nefertiti lift". Ann Dermatol Venereol. 2009;136(Suppl 4):S111-8.

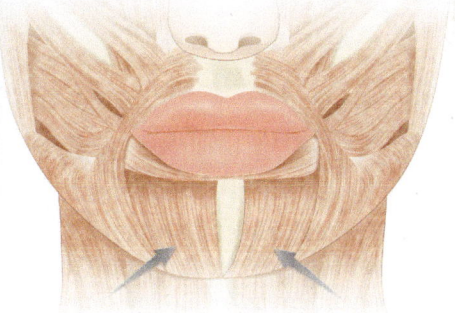

CHAPTER 39

Botulinum Toxin in Masseteric Hypertrophy

Sudha Vani Damarla, Manogna Vellala

INTRODUCTION

Botulinum toxin was initially used for the management of bruxism to relax the masseter.[1] The improvement in appearance following these injections has led to widespread use of the toxin for esthetic reasons to improve the contour of the jaw.

Masseteric hypertrophy is an uncommon condition, as it can alter the contour of the face causing square jaw or box-shaped appearance and it can be unilateral or bilateral.[2] It is more common in adolescence and early adulthood and the mean age of the patients in a study was found to be 30 years.[3] The etiology of this condition is unknown. Stress, chronic bruxism, and microtrauma have all been implicated in the etiology of masseteric hypertrophy.

ANATOMY

The masseter is a masticatory muscle with a thick, approximately quadrilateral structure. The masseter has two portions, superficial and deep of which the superficial is bigger.

The superficial portion of the masseter originates from the zygomatic process of the maxilla and the anterior two-thirds of the lower portion of the zygomatic arch. It inserts into the lower half of the lateral surface of the mandible. The deep portion of the masseter originates from the posterior third of the lower border and the medial surface of the zygomatic arch. It inserts into the upper half of the ramus of the mandible. The masseter is innervated by the masseteric nerve which is a branch from the anterior division of the mandibular nerve. It functions as an elevator and retractor of the mandible. It is interesting to note that the hypertrophy of the masseter is not true work hypertrophy but follows a pattern of compensatory enlargement due to change in type of muscle fiber and hence the term hypertrophy might be a misnomer. It is more common in Pacific Asians owing to characteristic facial anatomy and dietary habits.[4] In one study utilizing computed tomography the normal thickness of the masseter muscle was found to be 0.8 cm but in cases of hypertrophy it was found to be 1.3 cm.[5]

INJECTION TECHNIQUE

Clinically, this condition presents with unilateral or bilateral swelling with a soft tissue mass noted at the angle of the mandible. This mass becomes more prominent on clenching the muscle. An imaginary line should be drawn joining the tragus to the corner of the mouth. This forms the upper margin. The lower margin is formed by the bony border of the mandible. The anterior and posterior margins are demarcated by the anterior and posterior margins of the masseter muscle, by asking the patient to clench his or her jaw.[6]

This area enclosed by these lines forms the "zone" of the injection. The injection points are placed 1 cm from the borders of the zone.

The number of injections and units to be used vary depending on the size of the muscle. Three to five points are chosen based on the size of the muscle, however three points injection technique is much more commonly used with 25–30 units on each side. This is sufficient for the vast majority of cases in India. It is essential to keep in mind that the injection should be deep enough as opposed to medium depth.

The patient should be asked to clench his teeth while the needle is being inserted into the muscle, following which he or she can be asked to relax. The toxin can be pushed into the muscle while it is relaxed.

Unlike other sites, botulinum toxin exerts its effects in masseter hypertrophy by causing disuse atrophy. For this reason, the results of the procedure appear initially after 2 weeks and peak is seen around 2–3 months.[7,8] This is in contrast to traditional treatments where results are seen within 2–3 days and peak at 2 weeks.

COMPLICATIONS

Superficial injection can reach the risorius muscle and can lead to an asymmetric smile. Temporary weakness in chewing can be seen postinjection but this returns to normal within 21 days.[9] If the cheek of the patient is sunken prior to the procedure, it may become more pronounced after the injection. Sagging jowls become more prominent after the injection.

Medium depth injection may not reach all the fibers of the muscle and this causes a peculiar appearance during chewing food. Hematoma formation can occur. Failure to maintain the upper boundary of the zone may lead to injury to the Stensen's duct. Injection into marginal mandibular and buccal branches of facial nerve may lead to alteration of smile. Common side effects like headache and dry mouth are usually self-limiting.

PRECAUTIONS

Patient selection is paramount in optimizing results. Patients with sunken cheeks should be offered additional modality of treatment like a filler in addition to the botulinum toxin injection. For patients with sagging jowls, a thread lift should be offered in addition to the injection.

Adequate depth of injection minimizes the risk of complications such as asymmetrical smile and abnormal appearance during chewing.

Aspiration of the syringe was performed to avoid intravenous injection. Injection points should be spaced 1 cm inside the borders of the zone in order to prevent the toxin from reaching the other facial muscles.

Twenty-five to thirty units per side may be required in females. Males may require 10 units more of the injection. By adhering to the upper border of the zone and placing the injection at least 1 cm away from the line drawn from the tragus to the corner of the mouth, injury to Stensen's duct can be avoided.

Safety of botulinum toxin injections in pregnancy or lactation has not been established. Drugs known to potentiate neuromuscular blockade (aminoglycosides) should be avoided. Single large doses of greater than 500 mouse units of botulinum may produce botulism.

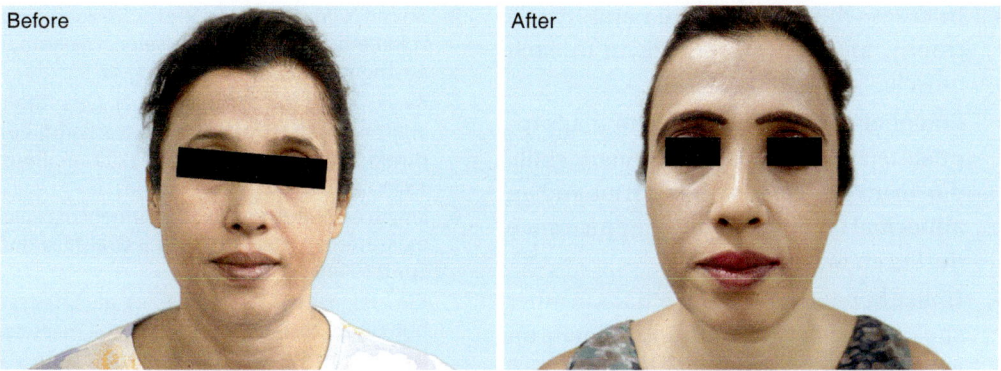

Fig. 1: Before and After 30 units of Botulinum injection.

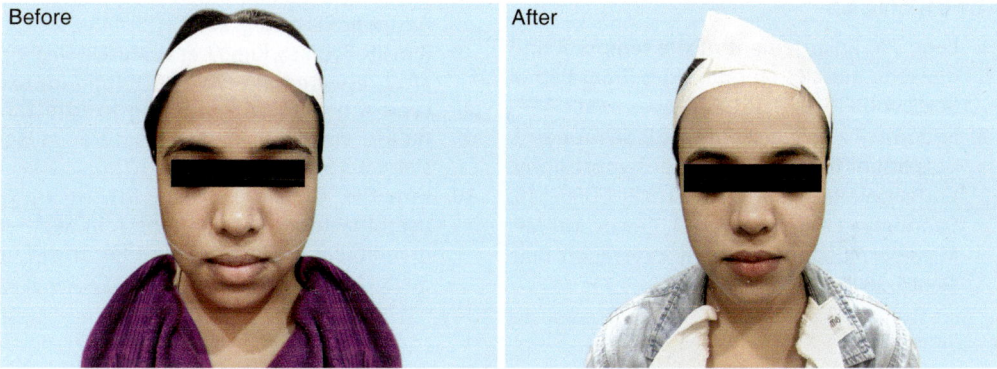

Fig. 2: Before and After Botulinum injection.
(*Courtesy*: Dr. Soma Sarkar)

POSTINJECTION INSTRUCTIONS

In case of masseteric hypertrophy, the delayed onset of action should be explained to the patient. The patient should be followed up after 2 weeks. The treatment may be repeated at 1–3 monthly intervals. The treatment lasts up to 6 months but in cases where care is taken to avoid excess jaw clenching the results can last even up to 1–2 years.[10]

USEFUL TIPS

- The masseter has two portions, superficial and deep.
- Injections into the masseter should always be given deep into the muscle.
- A zone with the anterior and posterior borders formed by the borders of the muscle, inferior border demarcated by the mandible and an upper border formed by a line joining the tragus to the corner of the mouth should be delineated for injection. Injections should be given a minimum of 1 cm within the borders of the zones.
- Where there is asymmetry, start with 25 U given in the hypertrophied muscle and 10 U given to the contralateral side to prevent shifting hyperfunction to the opposite side.

- In cases where there is bilateral hypertrophy, an equal dose is given to each muscle.
- Potential complications due to inappropriate technique include asymmetric smile due to involvement of the risorius and an abnormal "chipmunk-like" appearance during chewing.
- Unlike botulinum toxin injections in other sites, the effects of botulinum toxin on masseteric hypertrophy appear late and last longer.

REFERENCES

1. Legg JW. Enlargement of the temporal and masseter muscles on both sides. Trans Pathol Soc (Lond). 1880;31:361-6.
2. Fedorowicz Z, van Zuuren EJ, Schoones J. Botulinum toxin for masseter hypertrophy. Cochrane Database Syst Rev. 2013;(9):CD007510.
3. Sannomya EK, Gonçalves M, Cavalcanti MP. Masseter muscle hypertrophy: case report. Braz Dent J. 2006;17(4):347-50.
4. Jin Park Y, Woo Jo Y, Bang SI, et al. Radiofrequency volumetric reduction for masseteric hypertrophy. Aesthetic Plast Surg. 2007;31(1):42-52.
5. Xu JA, Yuasa K, Yoshiura K, et al. Quantitative analysis of masticatory muscles using computed tomography. Dentomaxillofac Radiol. 1994;23(3):154-8.
6. Smyth AG. Botulinum toxin treatment of bilateral masseteric hypertrophy. Br J Oral Maxillofac Surg. 1994;32(1):29-33.
7. Kim HJ, Yum KW, Lee SS, et al. Effects of botulinum toxin type A on bilateral masseteric hypertrophy evaluated with computed tomographic measurement. Dermatol Surg. 2003;29(5):484-9.
8. Yu CC, Chen PK, Chen YR. Botulinum toxin A for lower facial contouring: A prospective study. Aesthetic Plast Surg. 2007;31(5):445-51.
9. Kim KS, Byun YS, Kim YJ, et al. Muscle weakness after repeated injection of botulinum toxin type A evaluated according to bite force measurement of human masseter muscle. Dermatol Surg. 2009;35(12):1902-6.
10. Kim NH, Chung JH, Park RH, et al. The use of botulinum toxin type A in aesthetic mandibular contouring. Plast Reconstr Surg. 2005;115(3):919-30.

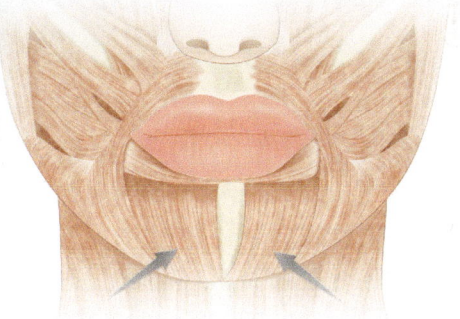
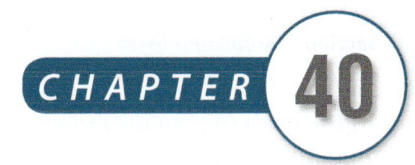

Complications of Botulinum Toxin and their Management

Sheilly Kapoor, Komal Sharma

INTRODUCTION

A review of the spectrum of possible complications with esthetic Botox applications is important with increased demand and larger numbers of physicians offering Botox injections. Only botulinum toxin type A is currently approved for cosmetic use. OnabotulinumtoxinA (BoNTA-ONA; Botox/Botox Cosmetic, Allergan Inc., Irvine, CA, USA), abobotulinumtoxinA (BoNTA-ABO; Dysport, Medicis Aesthetics Inc., Scottsdale, AZ, USA) and incobotulinumtoxinA (BoNTA-INCO; Xeomin, Merz Aesthetics, Inc., Franksville, WI, USA) are injectable neurotoxins that have been approved by the United States Food and Drug Administration (FDA) for esthetic purposes (glabellar lines) since 2002, 2009, and 2011, respectively.[1]

SAFETY PROFILE AND DRUG INTERACTIONS

The excellent safety profile of Botox is illustrated by the reversible, short-term, and localized effects of Botox in the observed complications. No reports of life-threatening allergic or urticarial reactions have been reported with facial Botox applications.[2] Each vial of Botox contains 100 units of Botox, 0.9 mg of sodium chloride, and 0.5 mg of human albumin.[3] Clinically, the standard unit based on the lethal dose (LD 50) of botulinum type A toxin in 50% of test mice serves as an important unit of measurement and reference.[4] The lethal dose for a 70-kg human is estimated to be around 2,800 units. Not surprisingly, there have been no reports of deaths from esthetic Botox injections.[5]

Aminoglycosides (gentamycin), cyclosporine, and D-penicillamine can potentiate the effects of Botox.[6-9] On the other hand, *aminoquinolone*s, such as chloroquine and hydroxychloroquine, have inhibitory effect on Botox activity by intracellular interaction within the cell.[10]

The quantities of Botox used in esthetic cases are usually too small to cause significant drug interactions.[3,6,11]

SYSTEMIC SIDE EFFECTS

Despite the efficacy of Botox in the treatment of myriad neurologic and cosmetic conditions, it may carry some risk of severe adverse effects which may be the result of local or systemic spreading of the drug. The classic presentation of systemic food-borne botulism includes a flaccid descending paralysis, clear sensorium, and no fever.[12] In severe cases, there is respiratory failure and death. There is a rare case report of a 22-years old man who received Botox for axillary hyperhidrosis and after

2 weeks most of generalized complications of botulinum toxin appeared. Pyridostigmine could relieve symptoms of the patient.[13]

Systemic Botox exposure is evidenced by antibody development against various components of botulinum toxin complex. Decreased Botox efficacy is the main negative clinical consequence of Botox-induced antibodies. Although, unlikely to be seen in esthetic treatments, these Botox-resistant patients require shorter intervals between injections and higher doses per treatment session.[14]

CONTRAINDICATIONS

Botox is contraindicated in individuals who have known hypersensitivity or allergy to botulinum toxin A or human albumin. In those with neuromuscular disorders, such as myasthenia gravis, multiple sclerosis, and Eaton-Lambert syndrome, Botox injections may potentially worsen symptoms of the existing disease state.[15] Pregnant women and nursing mothers should not be treated (US FDA Category C drug).[16] Those older than 75 years are treated more conservatively as a cautionary move owing to comorbidities and polypharmacy in the elderly.[6]

COMPLICATIONS

A careful medical history of the patient and exhaustive clinical examination remain the foremost essential. Detailed pretreatment counseling can significantly increase patient satisfaction. It is essential to understand the patient's desires and expectations. It is essential to establish realistic goals and agreed upon with the patient. Complications are minimized by good injection technique, accurate understanding of underlying facial anatomy, and appropriate site-specific dosing of Botox.

Nonmuscular Etiology Complications (Table 1)

Mild *bruising* was reported in 11–25% of patients who received Botox injections.[17,18] Patients who are on prescriptive blood thinners like aspirin and anticoagulants such as warfarin should be advised to stop these drugs (if medically advisable) 3–4 days before injections. Patients on nonsteroidal anti-inflammatory drugs, vitamin E supplements, herbal remedies like ginseng, ginkgo, and high doses of garlic may also experience higher rates of bruising.

Table 1: Complications of non-muscular etiology.	
Complication	**Management**
Bruising	• Prior icing • Injecting intradermally • Use of a fresh needle every 4 pricks • Immediate digital pressure if vessel punctured
Pain	• Prior icing • Use of topical anesthesia
Hypoesthesia	Temporary and self-resolving
Cutaneous infections	Maintaining aseptic precautions
Dry skin and flakiness	Topical moisturizers
Headache	Oral pain killers

Measures to reduce injection site bruising include use of 30-gauge needles, changing the needle after every three to four injections, icing the injection site before injection, and injecting intradermally. Still, if a vessel gets punctured, immediate digital pressure on the injection site will minimize subsequent bruising.

Injection site *pain* can be reduced by using topical anesthetic cream and icing the treatment site immediately before injection. Injection site temporary *hypoesthesia* may be due to localized edema and trauma.

Cutaneous *infections* are a potential complication following injections if proper aseptic precautions are not followed. It is also advisable to avoid injections adjacent to active acne lesions. A number of cases of iatrogenic mycobacterial infection have been reported through contaminated needles, syringes, drugs or instruments.[19]

Dry skin and subsequent flakiness in some patients may be due to decreased sweat gland activity.[20]

A minority of patients receiving Botox injection may complain of transient *headaches*. It is hypothesized that headaches may result from the needle hitting the periosteum, deep muscle hematomas or toxin-related muscle spasms immediately postinjection.[5]

Muscle Paralysis-related Complications (Table 2)

Patients present with localized functional or esthetic deficits after Botox injections.

- *Periorbital complications:* Although periorbital injections can be safely used in most patients, placing periorbital injections outside a recommended "orbital zone" can help minimize complications **(Fig. 1)**. It is recommended that injections should be placed 1 cm above the supraorbital rim superiorly, outside

Table 2: Complications of muscular etiology.

Periorbital complications	• Lid ptosis • Ectropion • Strabismus • Pseudo-herniation of infraorbital fat
Brow malposition	• Brow ptosis • Lateral brow elevation (spoking) • Brow asymmetry
Perioral complications	• Upper lip ptosis • Lower lip ptosis • Inability to smile • Lip weakness
Cervical complications	• Dysphagia • Hoarseness of voice • Neck weakness
Masseter injection complications	• Headache • Smile limitation • Paradoxical bulging • Sunken cheeks • Sagging
Hyperhidrosis injections complications	• Hand weakness • Decreased fine motor skills

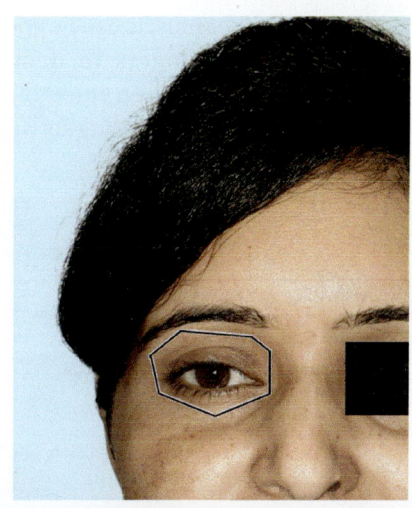

Fig. 1: Depicting outline of the safe "orbital zone." Owing to safety concerns, reducing treatment doses and placing periorbital injections outside a recommended "orbital zone" is helpful in minimizing periorbital complications.

the infraorbital rim inferiorly and laterally and 1 cm lateral to the lateral canthus. Intradermal injections are helpful in decreasing Botox spread, inadvertent intravascular delivery, and injection of deeper muscles and structures.[5] Injecting too low on the third CF injection point can cause diffusion into the zygomaticus muscle and an asymmetrical smile.

- *Lid ptosis:* Lid ptosis can manifest within 48 hours to a week after injections **(Fig. 2)** and usually resolves within 2–6 weeks.[21] Upper eyelid ptosis was noted in an average of 6.5% patients based on pooled data from five published studies.[5,22] Ptosis of the upper eyelid occurs from effects of diffused Botox on the levator palpebrae superioris muscle during injections of the orbicularis oculi, corrugators supercilii, and procerus muscles.[23] Elderly and patients who have pre-existing lid ptosis are particularly at risk of this complication.

  The corrugator muscle can be grasped between two fingers to decrease regional spread when injecting the glabellar area[24] and placing corrugator injections at least 1 cm above the level of the supraorbital ridge. In place of conventional injections where risk of eyelid and brow ptosis is there due to attenuation of lower fibers of frontalis muscle, a modified injection technique may reduce complications. In this technique, needle depth is passed through the muscle sheath from the nasal side of brow tip upward and lateral on the eyebrow length and the toxin is injected while gradually removing the needle tip from the muscle.[25] Smaller injection volumes can logically reduce solution spread. Besides being of temporary nature, lid ptosis responds well to several alpha-adrenergic agonist ophthalmic eye drops. Apraclonidine 0.5%, naphazoline, and phenylephrine 2.5% two drops, two to three times a day stimulate Mueller's muscles and help elevate the ptotic eyelid (typical 2 mm of lid elevation achieved).[5,22]

- *Ectropion:* Toxin injections placed around the lower eyelid can compromise orbicularis oculi function and may result in ectropion, especially in an older patient.

  The "snap test" or "lower lid extraction test" are useful tools in assessing lower lid tone before giving periorbital injections. Violation of the boundaries of "orbital zone" can significantly increase the risk of complications.

  The treatment of postinjection ectropion includes prevention of exposure keratitis and corneal damage. This can be achieved by using topical lubricating drops, lid taping, and ocular moisture chambers.[5]

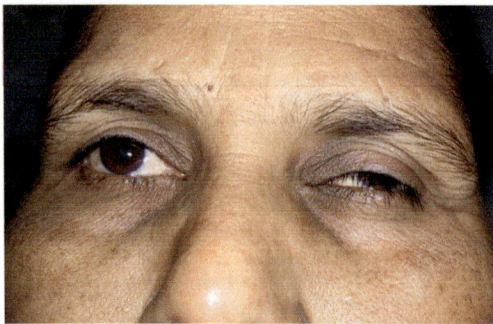

Fig. 2: Depicting eyelid ptosis that can occur due to diffusion of botulinum toxin into levator palpebrae superioris muscle and compromising its function.

- *Strabismus:* Transient strabismus has been observed in lateral periorbital injections (for crow's feet) and after nasalis muscle injections (for "bunny scrunch" lines). Diplopia can occur due to Botox diffusion into ocular muscles (lateral rectus weakness that results from crow's feet area injection and medial rectus palsy from injection for bunny scrunch lines).[26]

  Prompt consultation with an ophthalmologist can help in accurate diagnosis and a temporary strabismus treatment plan. Eye patching or the application of Fresnel membrane prism to eyeglasses can allay the diplopia until recovery.[27]

- *Pseudoherniation of infraorbital fat pads:* Injections in the inferior orbital, inferolateral canthal, and high malar regions can lead to toxin diffusion into orbicularis oculi muscle. The orbicularis oculi muscle and the orbital septum, provide a sling-like support that reduces the appearance of orbital fat pads.[28] Decreased tone of orbicularis oculi muscle fibers in this region causes pseudoherniation of infraorbital fat pads.

  To avoid this complication, it is best to avoid infraorbital injections in patients who are at risk for this complication.

- **Brow malposition:** The paralysis of the frontalis muscle reduces horizontal forehead lines but leads to lowered brow position in most patients. The contradictory goals of rhytid effacement and avoidance of brow ptosis can be achieved by conservative treatment of the medial forehead and by not treating or undertreating the lateral forehead. In some

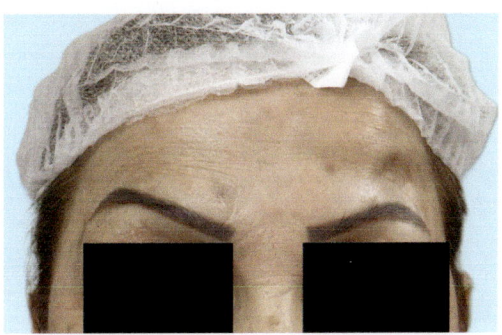

Fig. 3: Depicting excessive lateral brow elevation. If botulinum toxin treatment areas are limited to the glabella and middle one-third of the forehead, it can lead to "spoking" of eyebrows or "joker face" type of brow arching.

cases, the differential elevation of lateral brow in comparison with the paralyzed medial brow due to lateral frontalis muscle hyperactivity can result in a "sinister" or "joker face" type of brow arching **(Fig. 3)**. Patients who have low set brows are more likely to be happier with an elevated brow position along with some residual forehead creases, than a flat forehead with a crowded eyelid appearance.

Eighty percent of middle-aged women have asymmetric brow position.[29]

Brow asymmetry can become exaggerated by, or sometimes directly attributable to Botox injections. This can be easily amended with additional "fine tuning" injections after 2 weeks.

- *Perioral complications:* The unacceptably high frequency of upper lip ptosis combined with the inability to smile, has led most practitioners to address deep melolabial folds with treatment modalities other than Botox.[30]

  Medial mentalis muscle injections for correction of chin dimpling or peau d'orange skin can sometimes paralyze

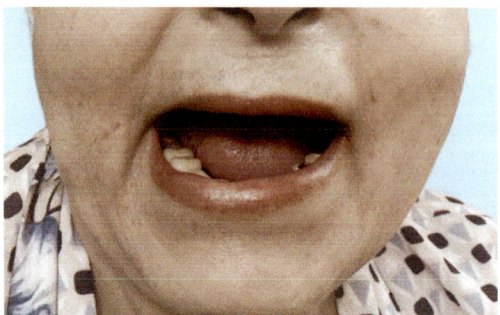

Fig. 4: Depicting lower lip droop and weakness. Correction of chin dimpling can be achieved by medial mentalis muscle injections. Overly lateral placement of injections for correction of chin dimpling by injecting medial mentalis muscle can sometimes paralyze the depressor labii muscles.

the depressor labii muscles, if placed too laterally. This results in a lower lip droop and weakness **(Fig. 4)**.

Subtle elevation of the oral *commissure* can be achieved by injecting depressor anguli oris muscle. Depressor anguli oris is located laterally over the mandible, best felt while clenching the teeth. Lower lip dysfunction can occur if the injections are placed too medially causing toxin diffusion into the depressor labii muscles.

Perioral injections aimed at softening of radial perioral lines can also cause lip weakness. To avoid lip dysfunction, injections are placed 5 mm apart and total perioral injection doses are kept to a minimum (upper lip—6 units and lower lip—4 units).

Botox lip treatments are best avoided in scuba divers, wind instrument players, and professional vocalists where complete oral competence is necessary.

Periorbital injections have been reported as a rare cause for upper lip ptosis in several cases, presumably from Botox diffusion into, and weakening of, the zygomaticus major muscle.[5]

- *Cervical complications:* Botox injections placed into the neck for treating fine cervical lines and vertical platysmal bands in larger doses (>50 units) increases the risk for temporary dysphagia and rarely hoarseness. An attenuated platysmal layer, especially in older patients, increases the possibility of direct Botox injections or localized diffusion into the sternocleidomastoid (SCM) and strap muscles, causing neck weakness and dysphagia.[21,31,32]

In a study by Matarasso and colleagues, out of 1,500 patients treated with Botox injections for platysmal bands, 10% of the patients reported a mild and transient cervical discomfort 2–5 days postinjection, 1% reported neck weakness upon head elevation, while only one patient (0.067%) experienced clinically significant dysphagia.

In most cases, the dysphagia is mild and transient.[18] If severe dysphagia is noted, a temporary change to a soft diet or pureed foods may be instituted and emotional support provided until full recovery occurs.

- *Masseter injection complications:* Toxin injections for masseter hypertrophy have a high efficacy and safety profile, but the risks of a variety of side effects or complications remain. In a study, of the 2,036 treatments, a temporary mastication force decrease was reported after 611 (30%), bruising after 51 (2.5%), headaches after 12 (0.58%), smile limitation after 3 (0.15%), paradoxical bulging after 10 (0.49%), sunken cheeks (subzygomatic volume loss) after 9 (0.44%), and sagging after 4 (0.20%).[33]

- *Lack of facial animation:* Overzealous toxin treatments may induce an expressionless, mask-like face. The goal should be to create a balance between wrinkle correction and patient's need for facial expression. Individuals who are in professions where there is a greater need for facial animation like actors, broadcasters and those who need to communicate with children should be treated with caution. The patient should be aware and convinced with physician's strategy for a balanced Botox treatment.[5]

- *Hand weakness:* Treatment of palmoplantar hyperhidrosis with toxin injections can sometimes result in temporary hand weakness with reduction in fine motor skills lasting several weeks. To prevent this, injections should be placed superficially with appropriate dosing (up to 50 units each palm) and spacing (1 cm apart).

SUMMARY

In spite of simplicity of this procedure, complications can still occur even with an astute and experienced injector. Taking all due precautions does help in minimizing complications. When complications do occur, early recognition of complications and prevention of long-term sequelae is the goal, though they are almost always reversible and short lived.[1] Educating the patient, supporting emotionally, and, if needed, intervening medically can help minimize the impact of any complications on the patient.

REFERENCES

1. Levy LL, Emer JJ. Complications of minimally invasive cosmetic procedures: Prevention and management. J Cutan Aesthet Surg. 2012;5(2):121-32.
2. Kwak CH, Hanna PA, Jankovic J. Botulinum toxin in the treatment of tics. Arch Neurol. 2000;57(8):1190-3.
3. Product Information Package Insert. (71390US12J). Irvine, California: Allergan Inc.; 2002.
4. Hatheway CG. Immunology of botulinum toxin. New York: Marcel-Dekker; 1993.
5. Vartanian AJ, Dayan SH. Complications of botulinum toxin A use in facial rejuvenation. Facial Plast Surg Clin N Am. 2003;11:483-92.
6. Mosby's Drug Consult, 13th edition. St. Louis (MO): Mosby; 2003.
7. Blitzer A, Binder WJ, Boyd JB, et al. Management of facial lines and wrinkles. Philadelphia: Lippincott Williams & Wilkins; 2000.
8. Physicians Desk Reference, 56th edition. Montvale (NJ): Thompson Medical Economics; 2002.
9. Wang YC, Burr DH, Korthals GJ, et al. Acute toxicity of aminoglycosides antibiotics as an aid to detecting botulism. Appl Environ Microbiol. 1984;48:951-5.
10. Simpson LL. The interaction between aminoquinolines and presynaptically acting neurotoxins. J Pharmacol Exp Ther. 1982;222:43-8.
11. Aoki KR. Pharmacology and immunology of botulinum toxin serotypes. J Neurol. 2001;248(Suppl 1):3-107.
12. Arnon SS. Clinical botulism. In: Brin MF, Jankovic J, Hallett M (Eds). Scientific and therapeutic aspects of botulinum toxin. Philadelphia: Lippincott Williams & Williams; 2002. pp. 145-50.
13. Rouientan A, Alizadeh Otaghvar H, Mahmoudvand H, et al. Rare complication of botox injection: A case report. World J Plast Surg. 2019;8(1):116-9.
14. Jankovic J. Botulinum toxin: clinical implications of antigenicity and immunoresistance. In: Brin MF, Jankovic J, Hallet M (Eds). Scientific and Therapeutic Aspects of Botulinum Toxin. Philadelphia: Lippincott Williams & Williams; 2002. pp. 409-15.
15. Huang W, Foster JA, Rogachefsky AS. Pharmacology of botulinum toxin. J Am Acad Dermatol. 2000;43(2):249-59.
16. Jankovic N, Brin MF. Therapeutic uses of botulinum toxin. N Engl J Med. 1991;324(17):1186-93.
17. Lowe NJ, Lask G, Yamauchi P, et al. Bilateral, double-blind, randomized comparison of 3 doses of botulinum toxin type A and placebo in patient with crow's feet. J Am Acad Dermatol. 2002;47(6):834-40.

18. Matarasso A, Matarasso SL, Brandt FS, et al. Botulinum toxin for the management of platysmal bands. Plast Reconstr Surg. 1999;103(2):645-52.
19. Saeb-Lima M, Solis-Arreola GV, Fernandez-Flores A. Mycobacterial infection after cosmetic procedure with botulinum toxin A. J Clin Diagn Res. 2015;9(4):WD01-2.
20. Bulstrode NW, Grobelaar AO. Long-term prospective follow-up of botulinum toxin treatment for facial rhytids. Aesthetic Plast Surg. 2002;26(5):356-9.
21. Matarasso SL. Complications of botulinum A exotoxin for hyperfunctional lines. Dermatol Surg. 1998;24(11):1249-54.
22. Carruthers JA, Lowe NJ, Menter MA, et al. A multicenter, double-blind, randomized, placebo-controlled study of the efficacy and safety of botulinum toxin type 490. J Am Acad Dermatol. 2002;46(6):840-9
23. Scott AB. Botulism toxin injection of extra ocular muscles as an alternative to strabismus surgery. Trans Ophthalmol Soc. 1981;87:1044-9.
24. Binder WJ, Blitzer A, Brin MF. Treatment of hyperfunctional lines of the face with botulinum toxin A. Dermatol Surg. 1998;24(11):1198-205.
25. Karbassi E, Nakhaee N, Zamanian M. The efficacy and complications of a new technique of Abobotulinum-toxin A (Dysport) injection in patients with glabellar lines. J Cosmet Dermatol. 2018;00:1-4.
26. Garcia A, Fulton JE Jr. Cosmetic denervation of the muscles of facial expression with botulinum toxin. A dose-response study. Dermatol Surg. 1996;22:39-43.
27. Carruthers JDA, Carruthers A. Botulinum toxin and laser resurfacing for lines around the eyes. In: Blitzer WJ, Binder WJ, Boyd JB, Carruthers A (Eds). Management of Facial Lines and Wrinkles. Philadelphia: Lippincott Williams & Wilkins; 2000. pp. 315-32.
28. Paloma V, Samper A. A complication with aesthetic use of Botox: herniation of the orbital fat. Plast Reconstr Surg. 2001;107(5):1315-6.
29. Matarasso A, Terino EO. Forehead-brow rhytidoplasty: reassessing the goals. Plast Reconstruct Surg. 1994;93(7):1378-89.
30. Blitzer A, Binder WJ. Current practices in the use of botulinum toxin A in the management of facial lines and wrinkles. Facial Plast Surg Clin North Am. 2001;9(3):395-404.
31. Kessler KR, Skutta M, Benecke R. Long-term treatment of cervical dystonia with botulinum toxin: efficacy, safety, and antibody frequency. German Dystonia Study Group. J Neurol. 1999;246: 265-74.
32. Brandt FS, Bellman B. Cosmetic use of botulinum A exotoxin for the aging neck. Dermatol Surg. 1998;24:232-4.
33. Peng HLP, Peng JH. Complications of botulinum toxin injection for masseter hypertrophy: Incidence rate from 2036 treatments and summary of causes and preventions. J Cosmet Dermatol. 2018;17(1):33-8.

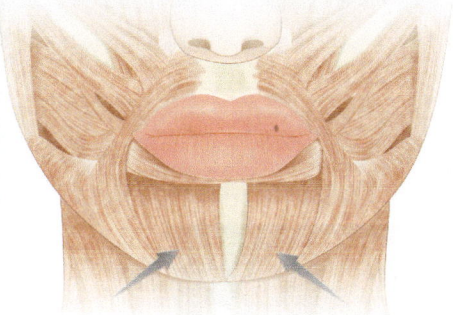

CHAPTER 41

Botulinum Toxin in Men

Rajat Kandhari

INTRODUCTION

Men appear to be a rampantly-growing segment of the facial esthetic industry. Not only is there increased awareness of minimally invasive cosmetic procedures and more disposable per capita income, males want to look good, youthful, energetic, exude confidence, and dynamism. Amongst the esthetic procedures commonly performed in men, botulinum toxin seems to be at the forefront, recording a 9% increase in the number of procedures performed in 2010 and growing ever since. Moreover, the ability of botulinum toxin to deliver quick, reproducible results with a minimal downtime make it a popular treatment option amongst male patients.[1] Despite this rapid growth, men have been a neglected group in majority of the literature focusing on facial esthetics.

ANATOMICAL CONSIDERATIONS

Men and women demonstrate distinct differences in their facial anatomy,[2,3] and it is pertinent that the injecting physician understands these differences, in order to provide optimal outcomes for their patients. The anatomical differences are discussed below:

- *The bony skeleton*: Men have larger skulls, prominent supraorbital ridges,[4,5] "low set" eyebrows, and flatter foreheads compared to females.[6] Further, males also demonstrate a wider, more projected glabella,[7] a broader chin,[8] and a prominent jawline **(Fig. 1)**.[9] Recent data also suggest that men have greater facial movement,[10] age earlier and demonstrate severe rhytides as compared to women.[11]
- *Facial skin and subcutaneous tissue*: Men have thicker skin, increased density of sweat and sebaceous glands, and more muscle mass.[2,12-14]
- *Facial vasculature:* Males usually possess a heavy vascular network on the face which lends support to the beard hair, and this is turn may result in postinjection hematoma formation more commonly.[15-17]

The distinct differences in anatomy, heavier muscle mass, thicker skin, and demonstration of more severe wrinkles in the male population, suggest that, the injector may in fact need to alter his/her dosing and number of injection points in this subset of the population, to a higher dose/more injection points as compared to females in order to deliver optimal results.

CURRENT STATUS OF THE USE OF BOTULINUM TOXIN TYPE A IN MALE PATIENTS

- *Growing popularity and scarcity of data*: Minimally invasive esthetic procedures

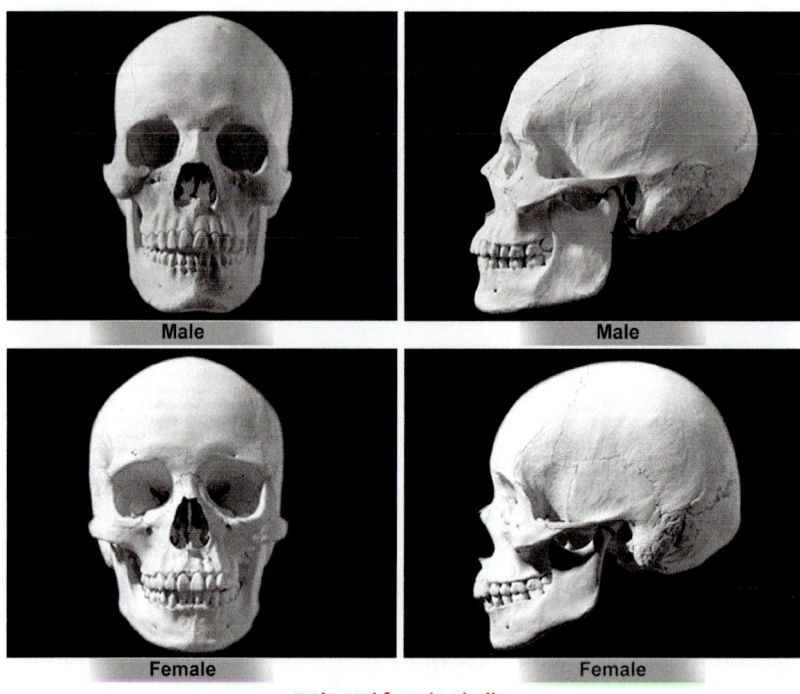

male and female skulls
(scanned from White 1031:321)

Fig. 1: Male skull demonstrating an overall larger size, large forehead with prominent supraorbital ridges, wide glabella, square orbit and a prominent mandible.

performed in men have demonstrated an exponential growth of 273%[18] with botulinum toxin type A (BoNT A) procedures revealing a 300% growth since the year 2000. Moreover, lateral canthal lines appear to be an area, men are keen on addressing.[19] Despite the aforementioned data, there is still a lack of awareness and education amongst men regarding these procedures leading to low conversion rates for these procedures in clinical esthetic practices.[20] The treatment approach for men and women varies and it is important that the injecting physician familiarizes oneself with aforementioned gender differences and tailor treatment plans accordingly. Currently, there is a glaring lack of good quality literature discussing the use of BoNT A exclusively in men.

- *The issues with dosing and gender specific differences:* Quantification of facial rhytides in men and women using a 3D-fringe projection method and validated assessment scales, have clearly demonstrated that facial wrinkles affect men significantly earlier and more strongly than women.[21] In the current literature, most of the phase 3 placebo-controlled, randomized and multicentric clinical trials define fixed or definite doses for the use of onabotulinumtoxinA, without considering gender differences, e.g. 20 U for glabellar frown lines, 20 U for forehead lines[22] and 24 U for crow's feet.[23] Secondly, there is scarcity of clinical data evaluating the use of BoNT A specifically in men, only two studies take into account sex-based dosing adjustments, and both these studies are

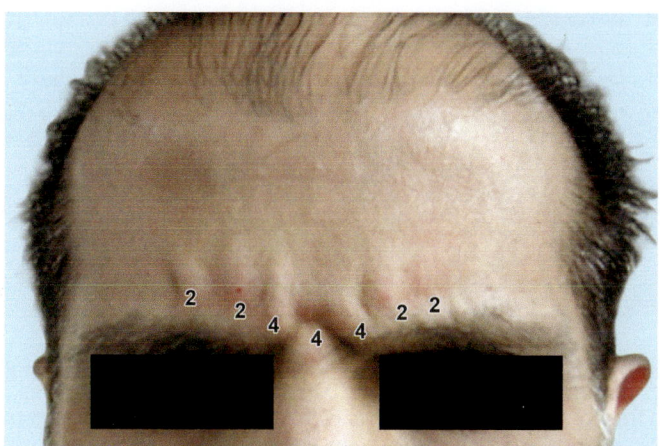

Fig. 2: 7-point injection strategy for glabellar frown lines in males with longer corrugators.

on abobotulinumtoxinA.[24,25] The studies concluded that men require higher doses of neurotoxin (50 U of abobotulinumtoxin A or more for glabellar frown lines) and may be less responsive to lower doses as compared to women. Further, there were no differences in the adverse effect profiles in both studies with higher doses in males. To add to the confusion, many of the present consensus recommendations do not necessarily give due consideration to gender differences, and instead suggest a dosing range for a particular indication. Studies demonstrating the use of BoNT A exclusively in males suggest a higher dosing, twice the typical dose used in women for glabellar frown lines, with a starting dose of at least 40 units.[26]

INJECTION TECHNIQUES
Glabellar Frown Lines

Despite the requirement in men for higher dosing, there seems to be a trend toward decreased dosing for the glabellar lines in different recommendations between 2004 and 2018. Forty five percent (5 out of 11) of the recommendations suggest a 5–7-point injection strategy while injecting the glabellar complex, and it is usually the males who may require more injection sites compared to the standard 5-point injection of the glabellar complex due to a higher muscle mass **(Fig. 2)**. The dose at each of the points would depend upon the severity of the rhytides and has not been clearly elucidated in any of the guidelines. Typically, it is the tail of the corrugator supercilii muscle, which lies superficially and may be injected in an intradermal fashion, while the rest of the complex (the belly of the corrugator and the procerus) is injected intramuscularly.

Majority of the recommendations suggest an average dosing below 30 units of BoNT A with a 5-point injection technique **(Figs. 3A and B)**.

Lateral Canthal Lines

As mentioned above, improvement of the lateral canthal lines is the most commonly requested indication by males.[20] Crow's feet are typically injected using a 2–5 injection point strategy, administering 2–4 units per site. At this area, one must strive to raise a bleb while injecting with the needle pointing

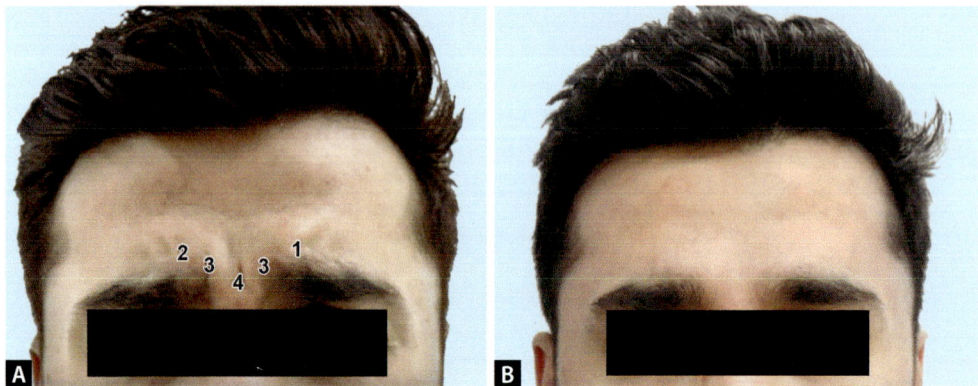

Figs. 3A and B: (A) Treatment of glabellar frown lines with 13 units of onabotulinumtoxinA; (B) Softening of lines post treatment with a 5 point injection strategy.

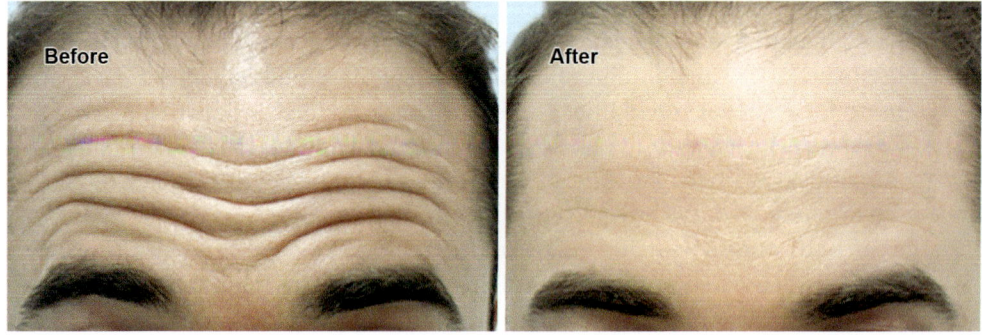

Fig. 4: Treatment horizontal forehead lines with neurotoxin in a male patient.

away from the globe and the thumb of the nondominant hand at the orbital rim. The injections may be spaced out 1–1.5 cm apart. Some experts suggest that higher amounts (1–2 units higher) of onabotulinumtoxin A are required to treat crow's feet in men.[27,28] The average dose for lateral canthal lines is between 20 U and 25 U of BoNT A for both sides.

Horizontal Forehead Lines

Post 2004, most of the recommendations suggest a lower dosing of the frontalis muscle than previously suggested. The lower dosing allows for preserving some lines and movement of the frontalis muscle, which is desirable in men. As mentioned above, due to their higher muscle mass the frontalis muscle in men may require a higher dosing as compared to women. The injection technique would be the usual, although the frontalis in men may require a greater number of injection points, and treatment of the lateral aspect of the frontalis frequently. The average dosing would be 10–20 U **(Fig. 4)**.

Few modifications in the treatment of men that have been suggested in the recent literature **(Table 1)**.[29]

Table 1: Suggested modifications in onabotulinumtoxin A treatment of the male face.

Indication	Modifications
Glabellar frown lines	• 50–100% increase in the usual FDA-approved dosing of 20 U of onabotulinumtoxinA • 7-point injection technique may be employed for longer corrugators/to address the lateral frontalis to avoid "spocking" • A longer procerus muscle may warrant 2 injection points in the superior and inferior parts of the muscle belly
Lateral canthal lines	• 10–25% increase in usual dosing
Horizontal forehead lines	• Approximately 10–25% increase in the usual dosing • Males have larger foreheads and may require more injection sites • The lateral fibers of the frontalis should be treated to avoid the "spock effect" • The superior aspect of the frontalis should not be missed especially in men with receding hairlines to avoid the "shower cap" effect

Source: Green JB, Keaney TC. Aesthetic treatment with Botulinum Toxin: approaches specific to men. Dermatol Surg. 2017;43:S153-6.

CONCLUSION

Men are frequenting esthetic clinics worldwide, more often than before. Surprisingly, even after a decade of BoNT A approval for cosmetic indications by the US FDA, data on its use in male patients is scarce. Dose ranging studies and consensus guidelines specific to the male gender are the need of the hour. This will enable physicians worldwide to achieve better treatment outcomes in this particular subset of the population.

USEFUL TIPS

- Men have distinct anatomical differences as compared to women, more muscle mass and more wrinkles, and usually require higher dosing for optimal outcomes.
- The injector may modify his/her dosing and the number of injection points in the male patient in order to provide favorable results.
- There is an urgent need for recommendations in dosing with differing doses for men and women.

REFERENCES

1. American Society of Plastic Surgeons. (2010). Men Fuel Rebound in Cosmetic Surgery. [online] Available from: https://www.plasticsurgery.org/news/press-releases/men-fuel-rebound-in-cosmetic-surgery [Last accessed on December, 2016].
2. Keaney T. Male aesthetics. Skin Therapy Lett. 2015;20(2):5-7.
3. Keaney TC. Aging in the male face: intrinsic and extrinsic factors. Dermatol Surg. 2016;42(7):797-803.
4. Krogman WM. Sexing skeletal remains. In: Krogman WM (Ed). The Human Skeleton in Forensic Medicine. Springfield, IL: Charles C. Thomas; 1973. pp. 112.
5. Garvin HM, Ruff CB. Sexual dimorphism in skeletal browridge and chin morphologies determined using a new quantitative method. Am J Phys Anthropol. 2012;147(4):661-70.
6. Whitaker LA, Morales L Jr, Farkas LG. Aesthetic surgery of the supraorbital ridge and forehead structures. Plast Reconstr Surg. 1986;78(1):23-32.
7. Russell MD, Brown T, Garn SM, et al. The Supraorbital Torus: "A Most Remarkable Peculiarity" [and Comments and Replies]. Curr Anthropol. 1985;26(3):337-60.
8. Thayer ZM, Dobson SD. Sexual dimorphism in chin shape: implications for adaptive hypotheses. Am J Phys Anthropol. 2010;143(3):417-25.

9. Donnelly SM, Hens SM, Rogers NL, et al. Technical note: a blind test of mandibular ramus flexure as a morphologic indicator of sexual dimorphism in the human skeleton. Am J Physical Anthropol. 1998;107(3):363-6.
10. Weeden JC, Trotman CA, Faraway JJ. Three-dimensional analysis of facial movement in normal adults: influence of sex and facial shape. Angle Orthod. 2001;71(2);132-40.
11. Tsukahara K, Hotta M, Osanai O, et al. Gender-dependent differences in degree of facial wrinkles. Skin Res Technol. 2013;19(1):e65-71.
12. Codinha S. Facial soft tissue thicknesses for the Portuguese adult population. Forensic Sci Int. 2009;184(1):80-e1-7.
13. Cha KS. Soft-tissue thickness of South Korean adults with normal facial profiles. Korean J Orthod. 2013;43(4):178-85.
14. Wysong A, Joseph T, Kim D, et al. Quantifying soft tissue loss in facial aging: a study in women using magnetic resonance imaging. Dermatol Surg. 2013;39(12):1895-902.
15. Moretti G, Ellis RA, Mescon H. Vascular Patterns in the Skin of the Face. J Invest Dermatol 1959;33(3):103-12.
16. Mayrovitz HN, Regan MB. Gender differences in facial skin blood perfusion during basal and heated conditions determined by laser Doppler flowmetry. Microvasc Res. 1993;45(2):211-8.
17. Baker DC, Stefani WA, Chiu ES. Reducing the incidence of hematoma requiring surgical evacuation following male rhytidectomy: a 30-year review of 985 cases. Plast Reconstr Surg. 2005;116(7):1973-85.
18. Farhadian JA, Bloom BS, Brauer JA. Male aesthetics: a review of facial anatomy and pertinent clinical implications. J Drugs Dermatol. 2015;14(9):1029-34.
19. American Society of Plastic Surgery (2015). New Statistics Reflect the Changing Face of Plastic Surgery. [online] Available from: https://www.plasticsurgery.org/news/press-releases/new-statistics-reflect-the-changing-face-of-plastic-surgery [Last accessed on December, 2019].
20. Jagdeo J, Keaney T, Narurkar V, et al. Facial treatment preferences among aesthetically oriented men. Dermatol Surg. 2016;42(10):1155-63.
21. Flynn TC, Carruthers A, Carruthers J, et al. Validated assessment scales for the upper face. Dermatol Surg. 2012;38(2 Spec No.):309-19.
22. Fagien S, Cohen JL, Coleman W, et al. Forehead line treatment with onabotulinumtoxinA in subjects with forehead and glabellar facial rhytids: A phase 3 study. Dermatol Surg. 2017;43:S274-84.
23. Moers-Carpi M, Carruthers J, Fagien S, et al. Efficacy and safety of onabotulinumtoxinA for treating crow's feet lines alone or in combination with glabellar lines: a multicenter, randomized, controlled trial. Dermatol Surg. 2015;41(1):102-12.
24. Brandt F, Swanson N, Baumann L, et al. Randomized, placebo-controlled study of a new botulinum toxin type a for treatment of glabellar lines: efficacy and safety. Dermatol Surg. 2009;35(12):1893-901.
25. Kane MA, Brandt F, Rohrich RJ, et al. Evaluation of variable-dose treatment with a new US botulinum toxin type A (Dysport) for correction of moderate to severe glabellar lines: results from a phase III, randomized, double-blind, placebo-controlled study. Plast Reconstr Surg. 2009;124(5):1619-29.
26. Carruthers A, Carruthers J. Prospective, double-blind, randomized, parallel-group, dose-ranging study of botulinum toxin type A in men with glabellar rhytids. Dermatol Surg. 2005;31(10):1297-303.
27. Carruthers J, Glogau RG, Blitzer A. Advances in facial rejuvenation: botulinum toxin type A, hyaluronic acid dermal fillers, and combination therapies—consensus recommendations. Plast Reconstr Surg. 2008;121(Suppl 5):5S-30S.
28. Carruthers J, Fagien S, Matarasso SL. Consensus recommendations on the use of botulinum toxin type A in facial aesthetics. Plast Reconstr Surg. 2004;114(Suppl 6):1S-22S.
29. Green JB, Keaney TC. Aesthetic treatment with botulinum toxin: approaches specific to men. Dermatol Surg. 2017; 43(Suppl 2):S153-6.

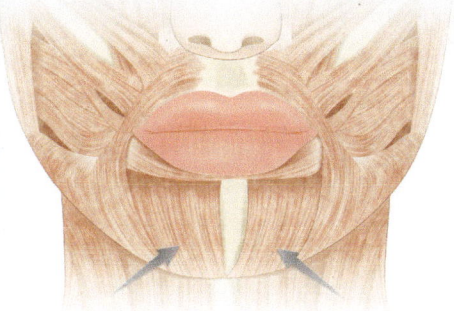

Microdosing in Botulinum Toxin

Rajat Kandhari, Ishmeet Kaur

INTRODUCTION

Experience with the use of botulinum toxin in the nineties saw physicians injecting too much neurotoxin in the traditional dosing (2.5 mL saline–100 units of neurotoxin) particularly for the forehead which led to complaints by patients of having a "frozen" forehead, inability to move the forehead, "unnatural" appearance, and stiff eyebrows. Moreover, large volumes and excessive dosing led to a "shiny forehead" appearance which was essentially due to the diffusion of the botulinum toxin back to the skin from the muscle.

Microbotox (also known as *mesobotox*) is a technique developed by Dr Woffles Wu in the year 2000, which involves uniformly placed, intradermal, and microdroplets of botulinum toxin type A to target the superficial fibers of facial muscles that have their insertion into undersurface of dermis thus attenuating the visible rhytids and providing a lifting and tightening effect.[1,2] Since the technique spares the deeper fibers, it allows for a rested appearance with preservation of muscle movement. Further, microbotox also helps decrease sweat and sebum production thereby improving skin texture.[3,4] Dr Wu developed the technique using onabotulinum toxin type A (Botox; Allergan Pharmaceuticals Ireland, Westport, County Mayo, Ireland) and hence the term microbotox came into being. It was later tried and found successful on other parts of the face including infraorbital, lower face, and neck and even in combination with traditional dilutions of Botox. It has also demonstrated benefit in conditions such as hyperhidrosis and acne.[1,2,5,7]

HOW IS MICROBOTOX DIFFERENT FROM TRADITIONAL DILUTIONS OF BOTULINUM TOXIN?—THE MECHANISM OF ACTION

The basic mechanism of action of microbotox is same as that of botulinum toxin, i.e. by inhibiting the release of neurotransmitter, acetyl choline from the nerve ending which induces muscle weakness/paralysis.[1,2] However, their action varies in terms of depth and intensity of muscle weakness. **Figures 1A and B** compares the difference between the level of action, diffusion, and cosmetic effects of traditional Botox and microbotox.[1,8,9]

- *Microbotox acts on superficial muscle fibers:* Microbotox acts on the superficial layer of facial muscles that are attached to the undersurface of the dermis. The higher dilution and low concentration of neurotoxin help in preserving the function of the deeper muscle fibers thereby imparting a natural appearance. The fine lines and wrinkles are reduced

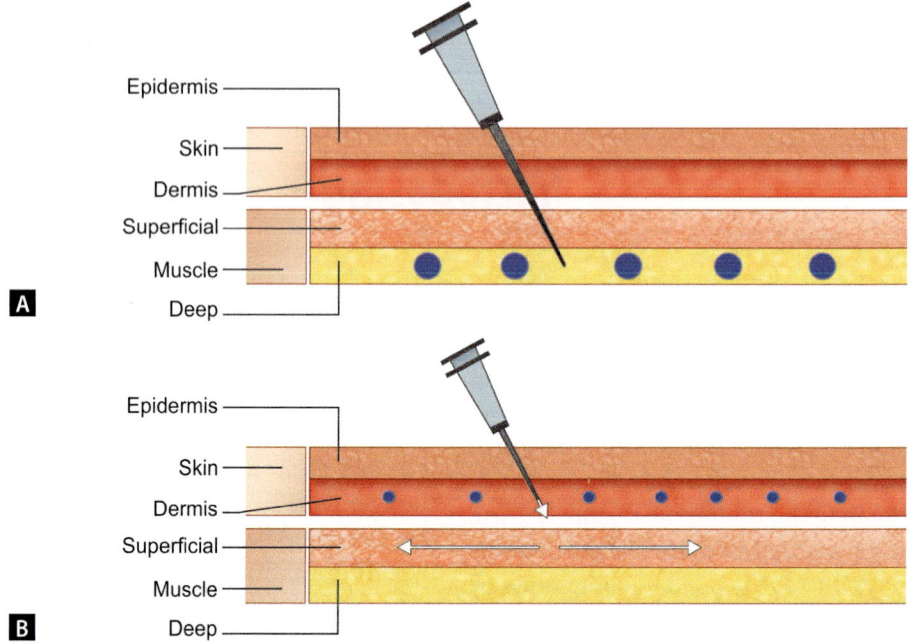

Figs. 1A and B: (A) Conventional technique of administration of botulinum toxin into the deeper fibers of the muscle; (B) Microbotox technique wherein the neurotoxin is administered intradermal, finding its way to the superficial muscle fibers and sparing the deeper muscle fibers.

by weakening the facial muscles and not inducing their complete paralysis. It has a beneficial role in forehead or under-eye regions where traditional botulinum toxin dosage and droplet size often lead to a stiff immovable forehead or masked appearance.[1,2,8]

- *Decrease in sweat and sebum production:* By inducing bulk atrophy of the sweat and sebaceous glands, microbotox has the tendency to decrease sweat and sebaceous gland activity thus improving the texture and giving luster to the skin.[1-4,10]

The objective of microbotox is not to allow diffusion of the toxin into the entire muscle to paralyze it completely. The duration of the effect of microbotox typically lasts for 3–4 months and in some cases up to 6 months.[1,2]

DILUTION AND INJECTION TECHNIQUE

- *Dilution:* There are different ways of preparing your microbotox solution **(Fig. 2)**. A frequently administered method is to dilute 100 units of onabotulinum toxin type A (Botox; Allergan Pharmaceuticals Ireland, Westport, County Mayo, Ireland) with 10 mL of normal saline. This gives 10 units of Botox per mL or 4 markings of a standard 40-unit insulin syringe corresponding to 1 unit of Botox. One may use 1–5 such syringes depending upon the indication to be addressed.

Alternatively, Dr Wu suggested that for most parts of the face such as the glabellar, crow's-feet, forehead, and infraorbital regions, the concentration of microbotox

100 units in 10 mL normal saline	100 units in 5 mL normal saline	100 units in 2.5 mL normal saline	Abobotulinumtoxin
• 1 unit = 0.25 mL • 4 units = 1 mL	• 1 unit = 0.5 mL • 2 units = 1 mL • 4 units = 2 mL	• Standard dilution • The dose used is according to the are being injected as depicted in table 1	• 500 units vial is reconstituted with 2.5 mL NS • 70 units /mL (0.35 mL) is diluted further with 0.65 mL in a 1 cc syringe

Fig. 2: Differing dilution techniques for preparing a solution for microbotox.

Table 1: Regionwise onabotulinumtoxinA administration.		
Region	**Dilution**	**Comments**
Forehead	24/28 units, i.e. 0.6–0.7 mL of standard dilution Botox topped up with saline = 24 U in 1 mL solution	If traditional Botox has been given to the glabellar, eyebrow, and central forehead regions to create a brow lift, then 16 U is sufficient just for the lateral forehead alone
Under eye	8–12 units in 1 mL of solution	Small margin for error—with too little BTX, the result is negligible. With too much administered, you are at risk of complications
Neck and jawline	24 U–2 syringes in 1 mL solution	May require a 3rd syringe depending upon severity of lines. Great technique for fine lines and creases on the neck

used is 20 units in 1 mL of solution. This is equivalent to reconstituting a 100 unit vial of Botox with 5.0 mL saline and then directly drawing out 1 mL of the solution into the syringe. Further, one may find it more convenient to use a standard dilution of onabotulinum toxin type A (2.5 mL saline–100 units of Botox) and then further diluting it with lidocaine/normal saline. The amount of standard solution or the number of units of Botox which are further diluted is dictated by the indication to be addressed. For example, 24 units, i.e. 0.6–0.7 mL of standard dilution Botox is further topped up with saline providing 24 U in 1 mL solution while treating the forehead. The exact dilutions according to the areas to be addressed have been enumerated **(Table 1)**.

In case, abobotulinumtoxin A (Dysport; Ipsen Ltd, Berks, United Kingdom) is being used by the injector a 500 unit vial is reconstituted with normal saline with a final concentration of 70 units per mL.[7]

- *Injection technique:* To reduce pain, prior application of topical anesthetics, vibration, or cooling devices can be utilized. The loaded syringe is then used for injection using a 30- or 32-G needle. With the bevel pointed downward and parallel to the skin, the needle is advanced very slowly into the skin and then pressure is applied to the plunger until a small blanched bleb appears in the skin. A resistance should be felt on pressing the plunger, if the solution is easily injected, the solution is probably too deep or intramuscular.

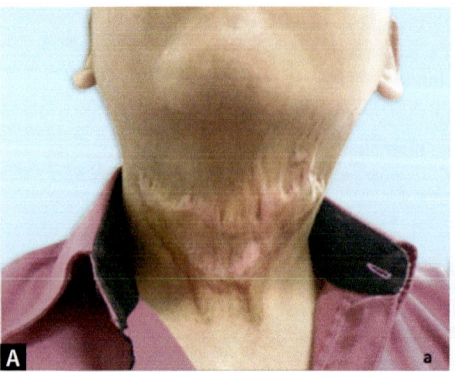
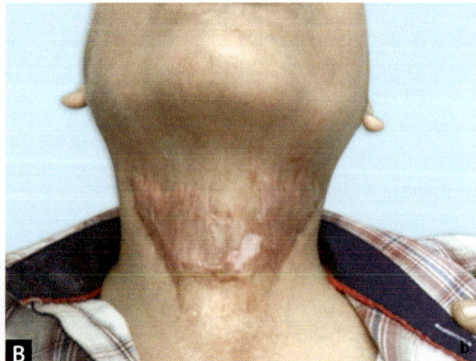

Figs. 3A and B: (A) Keloid on the neck post burn leading to contracture; (B) Significant softening and improvement in range of motion post 24 units microbotox with intralesional triamcinolone acetonide 40 mg/mL in a single session.

About 0.05 mL or 2 units in numerous small droplets (10–20) or 0.01 mL of the solution should be injected per point at 0.8–1.0 cm intervals into the dermis or the interface between the dermis and the superficial surface of the facial muscles in a grid-like fashion. Nappage technique is usually not recommended, as the amount of botulinum toxin A (BTXA) cannot be really quantified with this method, and lot of product can be lost between the punctures.[1-2]

The injection technique requires mastering over time, as delivery of uniform microdroplets consistently is the key to an effective treatment. All air bubbles must be carefully removed from the syringe prior to injection as this may compromise the injection accuracy.

INDICATIONS

Microbotox may be used for the following indications, although it is particularly effective in treating neck and lower face rhytids.[1-3,5,11-14]

- Dynamic forehead lines
- Glabellar lines
- Lateral canthal lines
- Lower face
- Neck lines (platysmal bands)
- Open pores
- Acne and acne scars
- Keloids **(Figs. 3A and B)**
- Hyperhidrosis.

For treatment of the upper face, microbotox may be used alone or in combination with traditional botulinum toxin dilution particularly in women desiring an eyebrow lift. The technique involves treating the glabellar complex, the central forehead and the tail of the brow with conventional botulinum toxin dilution (2.5 mL saline–100 units of Botox), while the rest of the frontalis muscle is treated with 20 units of Botox in 1 mL of solution **(Fig. 4)**. One should underinject the lateral forehead to avoid any lowering of the eyebrow or sensation of heaviness.

Only those experienced with the use of microbotox should use it in the under-eye region or the midface as the margin of error here is minimal and requires the droplet size to be tiny and delivered in a uniform manner. Too little of the neurotoxin may lead to negligible effect while too much may lead to diffusion

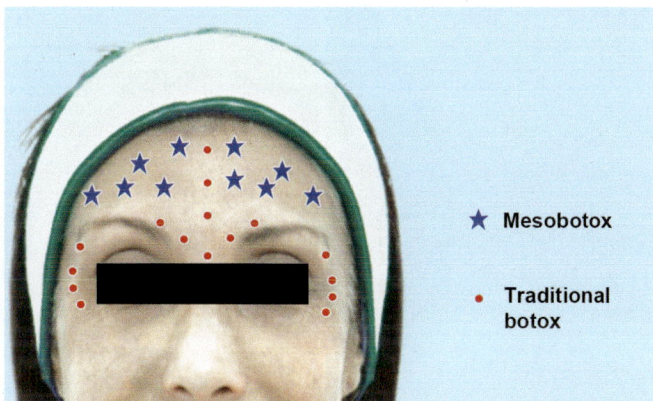

Fig. 4: Technique for a brow lift with a combination of microbotox and conventional botulinum toxin.

of the toxin to deeper muscle fibers and undesirable adverse effects in the midface.

Microbotox decreases sweat and sebaceous gland activity (mediated through both cholinergic and noradrenergic receptors) and they become atrophic. This results in the skin envelope shrinking and giving the patient a feeling of the skin becoming tighter and a "mini lift" feel. For the above reason microbotox is also used for the treatment of acne and open pores. Treatment for open pores may be combined with microneedling radiofrequency for more optimal outcomes.

In the lower face and neck, usually 1 mL of solution containing 28 U is used per side (total of 56 U) to reduce superficial platysma activity and achieve better cervicomental and jawline contouring. In patients with thin necks, a dilution of 20 units per mL solution is sufficient. In patients with visibly thicker necks or deep horizontal neck lines, a concentration of 28 units per mL solution gives better results.[1,2,7] In the authors experience, the microbotox technique is particularly useful for the lower face and neck, where it may be combined with conventional dosing of botulinum toxin. The conventional dilution of Botox is used to debulk the masseter muscle and for the vertical platysmal bands, whereas the microbotox technique is essentially used to provide a sheen or tightness to the skin on the neck, particularly in patients with fine horizontal neck lines and "crepe like skin" on the neck **(Figs. 5A and B)**. Further, energy-based devices may be combined to the treatment protocol in order to provide more optimal or long-lasting results. Approximately 100–150 injections are delivered over the entire anterior neck in an area bounded by a line drawn 5 cm above the mandibular border superiorly, a vertical line 1 cm posterior to the depressor anguli oris medially, the anterior border of the sternocleidomastoid muscle posteriorly, and the upper border of the clavicle inferiorly **(Fig. 6)**.[7]

CONTRAINDICATIONS

Despite lower dose and volume of microbotox, the contraindications are similar to those of standard Botox technique and include:
- History of allergic reaction to the toxin/human albumin
- Pregnancy (category C)
- Lactation

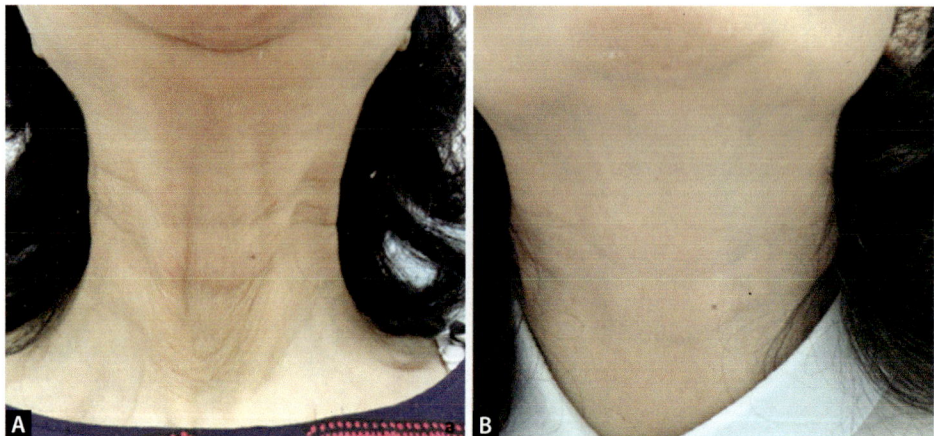

Figs. 5A and B: (A) Preinjection crepe like skin in the neck: (B) Postadministration of the microbotox technique for the neck—42 units of onabotulinumtoxin A in a microbotox solution.

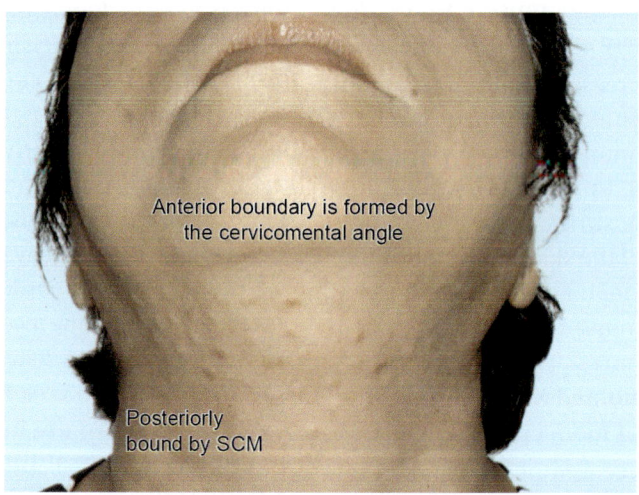

Fig. 6: The boundaries for injection of the neck region with the microbotox technique are bounded by a line 5 cm above the mandibular border superiorly, a vertical line 1 cm posterior to the depressor anguli oris medially, the anterior border of the sternocleidomastoid muscle (SCM) posteriorly, the cervicomental angle anteriorly and the upper border of the clavicle inferiorly.

- Patients with pre-existing neuromuscular conditions (myasthenia gravis and eaton lambert syndrome)
- Patients using medication that could potentiate the effect of botulinum (aminoglycoside antibiotics, penicillamine, quinine, etc.)
- Unrealistic expectations.

ADVERSE EFFECTS

The adverse effects seen with microbotox are less dramatic and less frequent than the standard Botox technique. Serious complications of classical neurotoxin injections for the treatment of platysma's bands, such as dysphagia, respiratory impairment, and speech difficulty are usually not seen.[2,13]

Most complications have been reported to arise from mistakes with droplet size and depth of injection. If the injections are delivered subdermally and the droplet size is larger than what has been recommended, the microbotox will diffuse into the thickness of the underlying muscle creating total paralysis. This results in the following:

- A stiff immovable brow when delivered to the forehead region. In the lateral forehead, this may cause a sensation of heaviness and a brow ptosis. One should be particularly judicious in the use of neurotoxin in this area and should document any pre-existing brow or lid ptosis.
- Diffusion into the sternocleidomastoid muscle leads to weakness in movement of the neck.
- Diffusion into the depressor anguli oris, risorius, or depressor labii inferioris while using microbotox in the lower face can cause asymmetry of the face and a lopsided smile.[2]
- Diffusion into the orbicularis oculi particularly in patients with pre-existing skin laxity results in enhanced eye bags or festooning, lid laxity, a swollen waterlogged appearance, and the "inanimate lower eyelid." Avoid overinjecting this area in patients with a sluggish "snap test" as it is easy to develop complications.

Due to a lower neurotoxin concentration, these complications usually subside within 2–3 weeks.[2] Another, common problem encountered with the use of microbotox is the relatively short duration of action as compared to the standard botulinum toxin dosing. Patients may require more frequent sessions to maintain the results of treatment. Many patients find the treatment uncomfortable due to the discomfort associated with multiple injection points and the nature of the injections. However, using topical anesthesia prior to treatment or using lidocaine to dilute the neurotoxin is usually sufficient to overcome this problem.

CONCLUSION

Microbotox technique can be considered a simple, relatively safe, and effective treatment technique used for facial and neck rejuvenation. The ability for microbotox to preserve muscle movement and provide "natural looking" results makes it a desirable treatment option for patients and physicians. However, presently data on the use of microbotox, defined protocols, and studies for different indications are scarce, and only a single consensus recommendation advocates the use of microdroplet botulinum toxin dosing for certain areas.[15] Until data to define protocols and guidelines for the use of microbotox are available, the practicing physician may be judicious with its use.

USEFUL TIPS

- The microbotox technique requires mastering—The key lies in delivery of superficial, uniform sized, droplets in the dermis for the best outcomes.
- The amount or dilution of botulinum toxin is crucial as too little will result in inadequate results and an unhappy patient and too much will result in a large droplet size which would be delivered in the wrong plane resulting in undesirable outcomes.
- A luer lock syringe always works better as the standard insulin syringe (31 G) results in frequent leakage/wastage of the solution.

REFERENCES

1. Wu WTL. Facial rejuvenation without facelifts—personal strategies. Hong Kong: Regional Conference in Dermotological Laser and Facial Cosmetic Surgery; 2002.
2. Tamura B. Microbotox, Mesobotox, botulinum toxin microdroplets. In: Tamura B (Ed). botulinum Toxins, Fillers and Related Substances, Clinical Approaches and Procedures in Cosmetic Dermatology, 4th edition. Switzerland: Springer International Publishing; 2019.
3. Rose AE, Goldberg DJ. Safety and efficacy of intradermal injection of botulinum toxin for the treatment of oily skin. Dermatol Surg. 2013;39:443-8.
4. Shah AR. Use of intradermal botulinum toxin to reduce sebum production and facial pore size. J Drugs Dermatol. 2008;7(9):847-50.
5. Steinsapir KD, Rootman D, Wulc A, et al. Cosmetic microdroplet botulinum toxin A. Forehead lift: a new treatment paradigm. Ophthalmic Plast Reconstr Surg. 2015;31(4):263-8.
6. Awaida CJ, Jabbour SF, Rayess YA, et al. Evaluation of the microbotox technique: an algorithmic approach for lower face and neck rejuvenation and a crossover clinical trial. Plast Reconstr Surg. 2018;142(3):640-9.
7. Liew S. Discussion: Microbotox of the lower face and neck: evolution of a personal technique and its clinical effects. Plast Reconstr Surg. 2015;136(Suppl 5):101S-3S.
8. Hsu TS, Dover JS, Arndt KA. Effect of volume and concentration on the diffusion of botulinum exotoxin A. Arch Dermatol. 2004;140:1351-4.
9. Trindade de Almeida AR, Marques E, de Almeida J, et al. Pilot study comparing the diffusion of two formulations of botulinum toxin type A in patients with forehead hyperhidrosis. Dermatol Surg. 2007;33:S37-43.
10. Li ZJ, Park SB, Sohn KC, et al. Regulation of lipid production by acetylcholine signalling in human sebaceous glands. J Dermatol Sci. 2013;72:116-22.
11. Glogau RG. Botulinum A neurotoxin for axillary hyperhidrosis. No sweat Botox. Dermatol Surg. 1998;24:817-9.
12. Wu WT. Skin resurfacing with MIcrobotox and the treatment of keloids. In: Benedetto AV (Ed). Botulinum Toxins in Clinical Aesthetic Practice, 2nd edition. New York: Informa Healthcare; 2011. pp. 190-205.
13. Borodic GE, Joseph M, Fay L, et al. Botulinum A toxin for the treatment of spasmodic torticollis: dysphagia and regional toxin spread. Head Neck. 1990;12:392-9.
14. Wu WT. Facial sculpting and facial slimming with neurotoxins. In: Sundine M, Connell B (Eds). Aesthetic Rejuvenation of the Face, 1st edition. Stuttgart, Germany: Thieme Publishers; 2015.
15. Sundaram H, Signorini M, Liew S, et al. Global aesthetics consensus: botulinum toxin type A—evidence-based review, emerging concepts, and consensus recommendations for aesthetic use, including updates on complications. Plast Reconstr Surg. 2016;137(3):518-29.

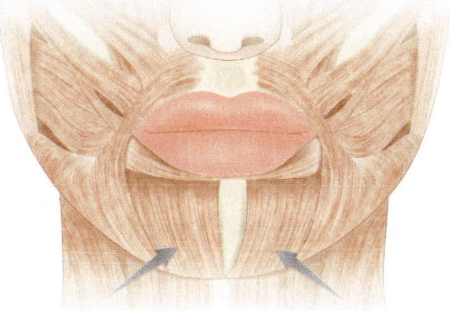

CHAPTER 43

Neurotoxin Resistance

Vivek Nair, Rashmi Sarkar

INTRODUCTION

With increasing use of botulinum toxin (BTx) there have been numerous case reports of patients who do not respond to BTx. The vast majority of these reports have been from the noncosmetic use of BTx. However, cosmetic use of BTx has also shown nonresponders and it is important for dermatologists to be aware of this phenomenon. In this chapter we will take a brief look at the issue and strategies to tackle it.

BOTULINUM TOXIN STRUCTURE

Botulinum toxin is produced by the anaerobic, spore-forming, rod-shaped bacterium, Clostridium botulinum which is present abundantly in the soil. The botulinum toxin complex contains a 150 kD neurotoxin complexed with up to six additional proteins. The neurotoxin is cleaved by clostridial proteases into a heavy chain (~100 kD) and a light chain (~50 kD).[1] This activates the toxin; the 100 kD fraction binds to glycoprotein receptors on presynaptic nerve membranes and the 50 kD fragment is then endocytosed where it inhibits the SNARE complex which blocks the release of the neurotransmitter acetylcholine, causing dose-dependent weakening of the target muscle.[2]

There are seven immunologically distinct serotypes of botulinum toxin (A to G), of which types A and B are used clinically. Of these, only Type A is used for cosmetic indications. Three types of BTx type A are available for clinic use—Botox (onabotulinumtoxinA; Allergan, Inc., Ireland), Dysport (abobotulinumtoxinA; Ipsen Ltd, UK), and Xeomin (incobotulinumtoxinA; Merz Pharmaceuticals GmbH, Germany). A fourth, daxibotulinumtoxinA, is under phase III clinic trials currently. It has shown lower immunogenicity and longer duration of action in phase II trials.[3]

The core neurotoxin is typically accompanied by nontoxic accessory proteins (NAPs), comprised of hemagglutinin (50 kD) and nonhemagglutinin proteins (130 kD), that associate with the core neurotoxin to help stabilize it and prevent degradation.[1,4] These proteins have the capacity to induce an immune response in the body. Of these, the hemagglutinin (Hn-33) is the most immunogenic.[5]

BOTULINUM TOXIN RESISTANCE

Resistance to BTx can be of two types—primary nonresponse (PNR) in which patient shows no improvement with the first and all subsequent injections of BTx, and secondary nonresponse

(SNR), in which a patient has shown benefit from at least one BTx injection in the past but loses clinical response over subsequent treatments. The loss of response may be partial or complete.[6]

True PNR is very rare and many cases labeled as such may be cases where there have been technical errors in injection such as injecting the wrong muscle, inactive toxin, inadequate dosing, and in some cases pre-existing antibodies. Such antibodies may be present in special populations such as the US military who were given a pentavalent vaccine for strains A-E during the Gulf War.[6] There has also been some speculation about cross reaction with the tetanus toxoid vaccine due to a 50% homogeneity between the two toxins.[7] Another theory for PNR was genetic alterations in the binding sites for BTx but a recent genomic study found no such mutations in either BTx binding or cleavage proteins.[8]

Secondary nonresponse is defined as an absence of clinical response after at least two consecutive injections in a patient who was BTx responsive earlier.[6] This is a phenomenon reported mainly in neurology literature possibly on account of the much larger doses used, frequent booster doses (reinjection within 6 weeks), certain formulations of BTx like rimabotulinumtoxinB which are more immunogenic, and shorter injection intervals.[9,10] One of the main causes of SNR is the development of neutralizing antibodies (NAb) which prevent the action of BTx. This ranges from 0.2% to 3.6% for BTxA (with the lowest rates being for incobotulinum toxin due to lack of NAP), and 18% to 42.4% for BTxB in the neurology literature.[6] For cosmetic indications, the incidence of BTx antibodies is extremely low, probably on account of the much lower dose requirement compared to neurology patients for most indications.

The few studies that have been done show incidence rates of 0–0.19% of antibody formation.[11-16] Still the phenomenon of SNR has been reported for cosmetic indications such as glabellar injections, facial rhytides, and masseteric hypertrophy.[17-19] Most of these cases, however, are not reported in a clinical setting and the few that are reported, especially from resource poor countries, cannot be worked up properly due to lack of research laboratories that perform the BTx antibody tests. So, the exact incidence remains unknown as of now.

BOTULINUM TOXIN ANTIBODIES

Antibodies to BTx can be broadly classified as neutralizing (NAb) and non-neutralizing (NNAb). The former target the core neurotoxin, particularly the binding site of the heavy chain and thereby inhibit neurotoxin action. The latter target the accessory proteins or sites on the core neurotoxin which are nonessential; these do not affect neurotoxin efficacy.[6] These may actually block access to the core neurotoxin and reduce the incidence of NAb.[7] There may be a genetic predisposition to BTx antibody formation due to differences in the major histocompatibility genes (MHC).[20] Antibodies to BTx are serotype specific and do not block other serotypes of BTx.[21]

One of the main challenges is the detection of these antibodies in a clinical setting. **Table 1** summarizes the tests available currently and all of these are complicated requiring specialized research laboratories. A simple bed side test which can show the presence of NAb is the need of the hour.

The gold standard among the tests are the mouse protection assay (MPA) and the mouse hemidiaphragm assay (MHDA), and the latter was used in a study which showed that over

Table 1: Tests to detect botulinum toxin antibodies.[7]		
In-vitro assays	**Bioassays**	**Clinical assays**
Enzyme-linked immunosorbent assays (ELISA)	Mouse protection assay (MPA)	Unilateral brow injection (UBI)
Western blot assay (WBA)	Mouse hemidiaphragm assay (MHDA)	Frontalis antibody test (FAT)
Radioimmunoprecipitation Assay (RIPA)		Extensor digitorum brevis assay (EDB)
Synaptosome inhibition assay (SIA)		Sternocleidomastoid test (SCM)
		Sudomotor/Ninhydrin sweat test (SST)

55.5% of SNR cases did not have NAb.[22] So what causes treatment failure in these cases? The answer to this question remains to be conclusively found but technical errors may play a significant role.

In-vitro assays have the advantage of high sensitivity but cannot differentiate NAb from NNAb and therefore, do not correlate with clinical response. Bioassays, on the other hand, have very high specificity and can differentiate NAb and NNAb but have a sensitivity of <50%. Given these characteristics it makes sense to use in-vitro assays as screening tests followed by the more cumbersome bioassays for confirmation. Clinical assays offer the most direct evaluation of response as well as obviate the need for research laboratories; here muscles on one side serve as the control for muscles on the other side to evaluate response after only one side is injected (UBI and FAT). These have very little practical relevance in the cosmetic patient though due to low acceptability of the cosmetic stigmata during the period of the test (2–4 weeks). Extensor digitorum brevis assay (EDB) and sternocleidomastoid test (SCM) are electromyographic tests of injected muscles and SST is a sweat test based on the anticholinergic property of BTx.

Various studies have tried to look for predisposing factors to BTx antibody formation. These suggest that antibody formation is positively correlated with cumulative dose of BTx injected. This would explain why the phenomenon of SNR is higher in neurology patients where the cumulative doses are much higher than in cosmetic indications. Another factor showing a positive association with antibody formation is giving "booster" doses of BTx as well as high dosing frequency. Booster is defined as any follow-up toxin given within 6 weeks of the original injection to improve result.[23] Accessory protein loads plays an important part in antibody formation. The original formulation of Botox had a protein load five times that of the Botox formulation available after 1997 and the incidence of antibody formation to the former was six times higher than the former.[24] Inactive toxin is another factor favoring antibody formation. This refers to the amount of undissociated core neurotoxin (150 kD) present in the injected toxin; this is inactive but still immunogenic. BTxA is about 95% activated during manufacturing and thus, has a lower immunogenic potential than BTxB where 25–30% of the toxin remains inactive.[25]

STRATEGIES TO COMBAT BOTULINUM TOXIN RESISTANCE

Neutralizing antibodies can decrease with time. One study showed patients achieving a Nab negative status after a mean duration of 30 months (ranging from 10 months to 78 months), while another showed that over half the patients studied over 6 years showed a drop in their Nab titers.[26,27] Unfortunately, patients usually promptly make new NAb on re-exposure to the original toxin.[28] In some patients of partial SNR due to NAb, it is possible to restore response by updosing BTx—doses four times higher than standard may be required.[29]

Another strategy to combat resistance is to switch a toxin-containing complexing protein (e.g. Botox, Dysport) to one without these proteins (e.g. Xeomin). One must wait for a complete drop in the NAb titers before reinitiating treatment with the new toxin.[28] Plasmapheresis has been used to hasten the removal of the NAb; this is of limited application in elective toxin use for cosmetic indications.[21]

As stated earlier in the chapter, BTx antibodies are serotype specific. Hence, changing BTxA to BTxB can offer temporary efficacy; again this applied more to neurology than to cosmetic indications since BTxB is not approved for the latter. Any such benefit is temporary because of the very high immunogenicity of BTxB.

Toxin with a higher component of inactive toxin is more immunogenic. Therefore, strict manufacturing and cold chain practices must be ensured to make sure the proportion of inactive toxin remains low.[30] Incobotulinumtoxin, in addition to being the least immunogenic BTx, is also stable at room temperature; thereby, removing the fallibility of the cold chain from the equation. Reconstituted toxin loses its potency gradually, even when stored at 2–8°C, and should be used within 2 weeks to ensure consistent results. Not doing so may be a cause of clinical failure which might incorrectly be labeled an antibody associated nonresponse.

USEFUL TIPS

- There are seven immunologically distinct serotypes of botulinum toxin (A to G), of which types A and B are used clinically. Of these, only Type A is used for cosmetic indications.
- The core neurotoxin is typically accompanied by NAPs. These proteins have the capacity to induce an immune response in the body.
- Resistance to BTx can be of two types— PNR and SNR. True PNR is very rare.
- Secondary nonresponse is defined as an absence of clinical response after at least two consecutive injections in a patient who was BTx responsive earlier.
- About half of these cases of SNR are caused due to NAbs.
- Antibodies to BTx can be broadly classified as neutralizing (NAb) and non-neutralizing (NNAb). The former target the core neurotoxin, thereby inhibit neurotoxin action. The latter target the accessory proteins; these do not affect neurotoxin efficacy.
- Strategy to combat BTx antibodies is to wait for them to decrease with time and then replace the BTx formulation with incobotulinumtoxinA (Xeomin). Updosing with the original BTx formulation is another option but these patients eventually stop responding to even the higher doses.

- It is essential to eliminate the technical causes of BTx nonresponse before considering the role of neutralizing antibodies.

REFERENCES

1. Kukreja RV, Singh BR. Comparative role of neurotoxin-associated proteins in the structural stability and endopeptidase activity of botulinum neurotoxin complex types A and E. Biochemistry. 2007;46(49):14316-24.
2. Dong M, Yeh F, Tepp WH, et al. SV2 is the protein receptor for botulinum neurotoxin A. Science. 2006;312(5773):592-6.
3. Jankovic J, Truong D, Patel AT, et al. Injectable daxibotulinumtoxinA in cervical dystonia: A phase 2 dose-escalation multicenter study. Mov Disord Clin Pract. 2018;5(3):273-82.
4. Brandau DT, Joshi SB, Smalter AM, et al. Stability of the Clostridium botulinum type A neurotoxin complex: an empirical phase diagram based approach. Mol Pharm. 2007;4(4):571-82.
5. Kukreja R, Chang TW, Cai S, et al. Immunological characterization of the subunits of type A botulinum neurotoxin and different components of its associated proteins. Toxicon. 2009;53(6):616-24.
6. Bellows S, Jankovic J. Immunogenicity associated with botulinum toxin treatment. Toxins (Basel). 2019;11(9):491.
7. Naumann M, Boo LM, Ackerman AH, et al. Immunogenicity of botulinum toxins. J Neural Transm (Vienna). 2013;120(2):275-90.
8. Pirazzini M, Carle S, Barth H, et al. Primary resistance of human patients to botulinum neurotoxins A and B. Ann Clin Transl Neurol. 2018;5:971-5.
9. Dressler D, Saberi FA. Safety of botulinum toxin short interval therapy using incobotulinumtoxin A. J Neural Transm (Vienna). 2017;124(4):437-40.
10. Atassi MZ, Dolimbek BZ, Jankovic J, et al. Molecular recognition of botulinum neurotoxin B heavy chain by human antibodies from cervical dystonia patients that develop immunoresistance to toxin treatment. Mol Immunol. 2008;45(15):3878-88.
11. Kawashima M, Harii K. An open-label, randomized, 64-week study repeating 10- and 20-U doses of botulinum toxin type A for treatment of glabellar lines in Japanese subjects. Int J Dermatol. 2009;48(7):768-76.
12. DYSPORT® [Package Insert]; Ipsen Biopharmaceuticals, Inc.: Basking Ridge, NJ, USA, 2016.
13. Monheit GD, Cohen JL; Reloxin Investigational Group. Long-term safety of repeated administrations of a new formulation of botulinum toxin type A in the treatment of glabellar lines: interim analysis from an open-label extension study. J Am Acad Dermatol. 2009;61(3):421-5.
14. Moy R, Maas, C, Monheit G, et al; Reloxin Investigational Group. Long-term safety and efficacy of a new botulinum toxin type A in treating glabellar lines. Arch Facial Plast Surg. 2009;11(2):77-83.
15. Imhof M, Kühne U. A phase III study of incobotulinumtoxinA in the treatment of glabellar frown lines. J Clin Aesthet Dermatol. 2011;4:28-34.
16. Glaser DA, Pariser DM, Hebert AA, et al. A prospective, nonrandomized, open-label study of the efficacy and safety of onabotulinumtoxinA in adolescents with primary axillary hyperhidrosis. Pediatr Dermatol. 2015;32:609-17.
17. Stengel G, Bee EK. Antibody-induced secondary treatment failure in a patient treated with botulinum toxin type A for glabellar frown lines. Clin Interv Aging. 2011;6:281.
18. Borodic G. Immunologic resistance after repeated botulinum toxin type A injections for facial rhytides. Ophthalmic Plast Reconstr Surg. 2006;22(3):239-40.
19. Lee SK. Antibody-induced failure of botulinum toxin type A therapy in a patient with masseteric hypertrophy. Dermatol Surg. 2007;33(1 Spec No.):S105-10.
20. Oshima M, Deitiker P, Hastings-Ison T, et al. Antibody responses to botulinum neurotoxin type A of toxin-treated spastic equinus children with cerebral palsy: A randomized clinical trial comparing two injection schedules. J Neuroimmunol. 2017;306:31-9.
21. Dressler D. Clinical presentation and management of antibody-induced failure of botulinum

toxin therapy. Mov Disord. 2004;19(Suppl 8): S92-100.
22. Lange O, Bigalke H, Dengler R, et al. Neutralizing antibodies and secondary therapy failure after treatment with botulinum toxin type A: much ado about nothing? Clin Neuropharmacol. 2009;32:213-8.
23. Kessler KR, Skutta M, Benecke R. Long-term treatment of cervical dystonia with botulinum toxin A: efficacy, safety, and antibody frequency. German Dystonia Study Group. J Neurol. 1999;246(4):265-74.
24. Jankovic J, Vuong KD, Ahsan J. Comparison of efficacy and immunogenicity of original versus current botulinum toxin in cervical dystonia. Neurology. 2003;60:1186-8.
25. Callaway JE. Botulinum toxin type B (Myobloc): Pharmacology and biochemistry. Clin Dermatol. 2004;22(1):23-8.
26. Sankhla C, Jankovic J, Duane D. Variability of the immunologic and clinical response in dystonic patients immunoresistant to botulinum toxin injections. Mov Disord. 1998;13(1):150-4.
27. Dressler D, Bigalke H. Botulinum toxin antibody type a titres after cessation of botulinum toxin therapy. Mov Disord. 2002;17:170-3.
28. Dressler D, Pan L, Adib Saberi F. Antibody-induced failure of botulinum toxin therapy: re-start with low-antigenicity drugs offers a new treatment opportunity. J Neural Transm (Vienna). 2018;125(10):1481-6.
29. Dressler D, Münchau A, Bhatia KP, et al. Antibody-induced botulinum toxin therapy failure: can it be overcome by increased botulinum toxin doses? Eur Neurol. 2002;47:118-21.
30. Dressler D, Hallett M. Immunological aspects of Botox, Dysport and Myobloc/NeuroBloc. Eur J Neurol. 2006;13 (Suppl 1):11-5.

Index

Page numbers followed by *f* refer to figure, *b* refer to box and *t* refer to table

A

Ablation, mid dermis depth of 173
Ablative fractional laser 174
    concept of 171
Abobotulinum toxin type A 179, 267
Abscess
    aseptic 156
    formation 146
Abundant blood supply 141
Accelerate hyaluronic acid absorption 124
Acetonide 262*f*
Acne 262
    scars 78, 262
Acyclovir 68
Alar-facial groove 119*f*
Allergan infraorbital hollows scale descriptors 100*t*
Allergic reaction 146
    history of 263
Allograft 6
Alveolar artery, inferior 48
Aminoglycosides 242, 245
    antibiotics 264
Aminoquinolones 245
Anaerobic 267
Anesthesia 72
    topical 72, 73
    types of 72
Angle's classification 129
Angular artery 46*f*, 47, 47*f*, 110
Apraclonidine 248
Arteplast 5
Aspirin 136
Autograft 6
Autoimmune diseases 67
Avascular necrosis 146
Average caucasian face 137

B

Bacterium, rod-shaped 267
Basic filler injection techniques 76*f*
Basic injection technique 75, 119*f*
Biofilm reaction 156, 157
Biscarbodiimide 11
Bleeding disorders 67
Blunt tipped metal cannula 76*f*
Bolus injection 135
    technique 144
Bone 161
Bony prominence 153
Bony skeleton 253
Bony volume, loss of 107
Botox
    injection of 188, 229*f*
    lip treatments 250
    sign 202*f*, 204
Botulinum injection 243*f*
Botulinum toxin 132*f*, 147*f*, 160, 171, 184, 186, 187, 197, 202, 218, 221*f*, 225, 226*f*, 234, 238*f*, 241, 248*f*, 253, 260*f*
    antibodies 268, 269*t*
    applications of 191
    brow lift 187
    combination of 165
    conventional 263*f*
    dilution of 265
    effects of 239
    injection 131, 184*f*, 195, 205, 234, 235*f*, 236
        safety of 242
        technique of 220, 204*f*
    microdosing in 259
    resistance 267, 270
    serotypes of 267, 270
    structure 267

traditional dilutions of 259
treatment 249f
type A 179, 180t
    indication use of 229
    use of 208, 237, 253, 267
Broad muscle 237
Broad muscular layer 171
Brow 23, 198f
    arching, joker face type of 249f
    asymmetry 247
    injection, unilateral 269
    lift 77, 197
    malposition 247, 249
    position 197
    ptosis 189, 189f, 197, 247
    region, injections in 27
    tail of 262
Bruising 146, 157, 246
    mild 246
Buccal fat 44
    pad 39f, 82
Bunny lines 202, 202f, 205f, 208f, 209
    injections 211
        points for 210f
Butanediol diglycidyl ether 10, 16

C

Cadaver dissection 33f
Calcium hydroxylapatite 5
Canine fossa 160
Cannula 75, 125
    depth of 96f
    entry point 102f
    technique 96
    type 131
Central retinal artery occlusion 122
Cervical complications 247, 250
Cervicomental angle 59
Cheek 51, 77
    anteromedial 103
    volume, assessment of 62f
Chemical
    peels with fillers 162
    structure 9
Chin 20, 21, 42, 51, 58
    area 135
    augmentation 128

correlation of 63f, 131
dimpled 229, 230
elongation of 131
fat compartments 45
projecting aspect of 128
sagittal section of 129f
size of 136
superficial fat compartments 45f
with toxins, combination treatment of 131
Chloroquine 245
Clostridial proteases 267
Clostridium botulinum 267
Columellar artery 46, 46f
Complex modulus G 17
Compressor naris 209
Concentration 11
Congenital small ear lobes 149
Congestion, venous 156
Contact cooling device 74f
Core neurotoxin 268–270
Coronoid process 133
Corrugator supercilii 24, 30f, 197
    muscle 24f, 197
Cosmetic
    deterioration 160
    injectables
        procedure 68b
        use of 67b
    intervention 182
    procedures 143f
Crosshatching 75
Cross-linking 16
    types of 11f
Crow's feet 166, 191
    lines 193f
        injection pattern 191, 192f, 193f
    treatment of 191
Crown length 218
Cupid's bow 43f, 144
    enhancement, technique for 145f
Cyclosporine 245

D

da Vinci's golden ratio 137
Deep dermis 172f
Deep fat pads 161
Deep fatty layer running 116

Deep temporal
   arteries 48
   fascia 80
      deep layer of 82
      superficial layer of 82
   fat pad 82
Deformity, severe 104
Deltoid fascia 234
Deoxycholate 164
   injections 165
Depressor
   anguli oris 36, 45, 46, 46f, 123, 134, 140, 147, 226f, 227, 229, 264f
      botulinum toxin injection of 147f
      function of 237
      muscle 225
      topography of 226
      treatment of 231f
   labii inferioris 36, 45, 46, 128, 140
   septi 36, 203, 209, 219
   supercilii 25
Dermal atrophy 153
Dermal fillers 1, 4, 10, 150f, 154, 154t
   augmentation 131
   classification of 3, 4t, 6t
   facial anatomy for 23
   injections 75
   rank 154
Dermal graft 6
Dermis 161
Dermosubcutaneous junction 172f, 173
Diamond-shaped technique 230, 231f
Diepoxyoctane 16
Dilator naris muscle 211f
Dilution and injection technique 260
Divinyl sulfone 11
Dorsal nasal artery 33f, 100
Dorsum, surface of 150
D-penicillamine 245
Drug molecules, size of 175
Dry
   skin 246, 247
   vermillion 43f
Dynamic forehead lines 262
Dynamism 253
Dysphagia 247, 264
   risk of 235

E

Earlobe
   and décolletage 149
   repair, technique for 151
Eaton Lambert syndrome 264
Ecchymosis 157
Ectropion 247, 248
Edema 156
Elastic and collagen fibers, loss of 213
Elastic modulus 17
Enzyme-linked immunosorbent assays 269
Epidermis 160, 161
Esthetic
   balance 197
   consultation 68
   enhancement 3
   procedures 166
      combination of 168
      sequence of 166
   rejuvenation 85
   utility, report of 186
Euclid's elements 52
Extensor digitorum brevis assay 269
Extracellular polymeric substance 157
Eyebrow 50, 92, 92f, 95, 95f, 182, 197
   asymmetrical 200
   center 96
   downward, pulls medial end of 209
   fat pad, anatomy of 91f
   head 96
   injection of 96t
   reshaping of 186
   tail 96
   unit, assessment of 94
Eyelids 30
   check position of 187
   ptosis 194, 248f

F

Face
   anatomy of 133f
   arteries of 45, 48
   cosmetic enhancement of 160
   different zones of 63f
   esthetic unit of 208
   fat compartments of 32f

layers of 161*t*
ligaments of 40, 41*f*
lower third of 133
middle third of 51
muscles of 25*f*, 129*f*
muscular anatomy of 204*f*
proportions 138*f*
regions of 35*f*
upper one-third of 50
Facial
  aging 133
  analysis 138
  animation, lack of 250
  artery 45, 46*f*, 47*f*, 122, 134
    anatomical location of 135*f*
    branches of 215
    course of 46*f*
  assessment 50, 59, 61
    highlights of 50
  esthetic industry 253
  expressions, muscles of 161
  massage 122
  muscles, superficial fibers of 259
  nerve 39, 40*f*
    buccal branches of 242
    frontal branch of 29
    temporal branch of 28*f*
  profiles, types of 130*f*
  proportions and angles 57
  rhytides, quantification of 254
  shapes 50*f*
  skin 173, 253
  vasculature 253
  zone 20
Famciclovir 68
Fanning 75
Fascial anatomy 80*t*, 82*t*
Fat 6
  pads, loss of 213
Fibers, arrangement of 43*f*
Fibrous retinacular cutis ligaments 161
Fillers 160, 165, 221
  Belotero range of 19
  classification of 3
  clumping of 156
  combination of threads of 164
  complications 154
    classification of 154, 156*t*
  desirable feature of 20
  for lower face
    chin 128
    jawline 133
    lip augmentation 137
    marionette lines 123
  for midface
    areas and scars 149
    cheeks 107
    nasolabial folds 118
    tear trough and infraorbital areas 98
    tear-trough and nose 112
  for upper face
    eyebrow 90
    forehead and temporal region 79
    temples 85
    upper eyelid 94
  inappropriate placement of 156
  injection 26
    around 116
    techniques 75
    tower technique of 124*f*
  juvéderm range of 110*f*
  migration of 156
  procedures 154
  selection 16, 19
    guidelines for 20*t*
  treatment, pre-requisites for 70
  use of 16
Filling temple region, cannula approach for 87*f*
Fine lines 19, 20
Firm pressure 206
Fitzpatrick wrinkle scale, modified 118
Fluctuant mass 156
Food and Drug Administration 3, 10
Foraminae 133
Forehead 23, 50, 78, 79, 81, 82, 261
  and eyebrow
    positions 198
    region, muscles of 24
  and face, superficial fat compartments of 38*f*
  botulinum toxin, effect of 189*t*
  central 262
  depressors of 186

height 54, 186
 injection techniques for 187*t*
 lines 186
  correction of 188
 nerves of 26
 treatment of 186
 vessels nerves of 26
Fractional carbon dioxide laser 173, 173*f*
Fractional CO$_2$ laser 175
Fractional laser
 assisted botulinum toxin delivery 171
 channels 172
Frankfurt plane 57, 58*f*
Frontalis 186
 antibody test 269
 muscle 23*f*, 24, 24*f*, 26*f*, 30*f*, 197
  paralysis of 249
Frown lines 182
Frozen forehead 259
FxCO$_2$ treatment, pass of 173

G

Gels
 hardness 12
 physical properties of 16
Gentamycin 245
Gingival display, excessive 218
Gingival exposure, amount of 218
Ginkgo 246
Glabella 78, 186
 dermis of 209
Glabellar arterial branches 26
Glabellar complex 166
Glabellar frown lines 255, 257
 treatment of 256*f*
Glabellar rhytides 182
Glycosaminoglycans 6
Golden ratio, concept of 51, 51*f*
Goldstein classification 218
Golf ball 230
Granuloma 146
 bilateral 155*f*
 formation 156, 185
Greater facial movement 253
Gum tissue display, amount of 218

Gummy smile 218, 219
 botulinum toxin injection for 148*f*
 treatment of 223, 223*f*

H

Hand fillers, technique for 149
Hand weakness 247, 251
Headache 246
 transient 247
Hemagglutinin 267
Hematoma 157
 formation 242
Herbal remedies like ginseng 246
Herpes simplex virus 67, 156
Heterograft 6
High-intensity focused ultrasound 164
High-volume injections/improper technique 233
Hinderer's lines 55, 559, 108*f*
Hirmand's classification 100*t*
Horizontal facial thirds 52, 53*f*
Horizontal forehead lines 256, 257
Horizontal neck bands, causes of 234
Human papilloma virus 67
Hyalase 147
Hyaluron 9
Hyaluronic acid 3, 9, 11, 14, 16, 20, 92*f*, 154, 160
 chemical structure of 10*f*
 consisting of 141
 dermal fillers 132
  properties of 10
 distribution of 9
 fillers 14, 16, 92*f*, 103*f*, 138*f*, 150*f*
  properties of 9
  use of 101
 functions of 9
 molecule 9
 properties of 10
Hyaluronidase 126, 147
Hydroxychloroquine 245
Hyperactive lip muscles 219
Hyperhidrosis 262
 indication 174
 injections complications 247
Hyperkinetic activity 237
Hyperkinetic depressor angulis oris 230*f*

Hyperkinetic mentalis 232
Hypertrophic scarring 185
Hypoesthesia 246
    temporary 247
Hypoplastic maxilla 119f

I

Iatrogenic blindness 88
Ideal brow 90
Ideal lip
    filler 141
    proportions 138f
Inanimate lower eyelid 265
Incobotulinum toxin type A 179
Infections 146, 156, 157
    cutaneous 246, 247
Inferior alveolar branches 133
Inferior labial artery 45
Inflammatory nodule 155f
Inflammatory skin diseases 67
Infraorbital artery 48
Infraorbital fat 30
    pads, pseudoherniation of 247, 249
Infraorbital foramen 110
Infraorbital margin 114
Infraorbital nerve 73f
Infraorbital region 98
Infratrochlear artery 47f
Injectable anesthetics 72
Injected muscles, electromyographic tests of 269
Injection
    lipolysis 164, 165
    method of 132
    procedure of 132
    site pain 247
    techniques 76, 81, 87, 90, 186
Insulin syringe 182, 265
Intense pulsed light 163
Internal maxillary artery 47, 48
Intra-arterial injection 119
Intradermal injection 126
Intralesional triamcinolone 158, 262f
Intraorbital fat, herniation of 99
Intravascular complication 83f, 114f
Intravascular injection 96, 114f, 116
In-vitro assays 269

Iodine starch test 174f
    results of 174f

J

Jaw, angle of 234
Jawline 42, 51, 77, 136, 166
    contour 169f
    in females 134
    in males 134
Jowl and submandibular fat compartments 44f
Jowling 237
    correction of 45
Juvéderm ultra 18, 104
Juvederm ultraplus 18, 104
Juvéderm voluma 18, 120

K

Keloids 262
    predisposition 67
Koebner response 67

L

Labiomental fold 58
Lacrimal portion 191
Lactation 67, 263
Laser-assisted drug delivery 171
Lasers 163
Lateral brow
    elevation 247
    lift 199
Lateral canthal lines 191, 255, 257, 262
Lateral corrugators 183
Lateral nasal artery 46
Lemperle scale 118
Lethal dose 245
Levator anguli oris 36
Levator labii superioris 30, 36, 140, 203, 219
    alaeque nasi 36, 99, 147, 203, 209
Levator palpebra superioris 186
    muscle 248f
    role of 186
Lid
    laxity 194
    ptosis 200, 247, 248

Linear retrograde technique 92*f*
Linear threading 75
Lips 20, 42, 51, 77, 137, 147, 213
    anatomy of 139*f*
    assessment 137
    augmentation 62, 148
        procedures 137
    chin relationship 59
    contouring 145
    correlation of 63*f*
    drooping corners of 227*f*, 227*t*
    lines 213
    marionette lines 166
    moving 138
    muscles of 36, 139
    vertical height of 221*f*
    weakness 247
Lipstick lines 213
Local anesthesia, eutectic mixture of 141
Loose areolar tissue layer 80
Lower buccal branch 40
Lower eyelid 191, 195
    injection techniques for 195
Lower face 20, 21, 42, 61, 62*f*, 166, 262
    aging curves of 44*f*
    and neck 263
        treatment of 237
    central 123
    fat compartments in 43
    muscles of 36, 42
    sequence of treatments in 167
    treatment plan for 167
Lower jaw
    position of 130*f*
    zones in 134*f*
Lower lip 137
    droop and weakness 250*f*
    ptosis 247
Lower temporal
    compartment 86*f*
    region, structures of 82*t*
Low-viscosity 152
Luer lock syringe 265
Lumpiness 126, 146
Lumps 138
    formation 126

M

Main arterial blood supply 116
Major histocompatibility genes 268
Malar body 56*f*
Malar projection 112
Malar septum, structure of 33*f*
Mandible 214
    angle of 133
    bone 133
    ramus of 133
Mandibular border 237
Mandibular branch 40
Mandibular ligament 41, 130, 160
Mandibular prognathism 129
Marginal mandibular nerve 46*f*
Marionette lines 77, 225
    grading of 225*t*
    grading scale 124*t*
    severity of 225
    treatment of 225
Masseter
    deep layer of 82
    hypertrophy 62
    injection complications 247, 250
    muscle 43
    originates, superficial portion of 241
    superficial layer of 82
Masseteric hypertrophy 241, 243, 244
    etiology of 241
Maxilla 214, 219
    frontal process of 209
    part of 218
    skeletal resorption of 213
    soft tissue protrusion of 59*f*
Medial brow lift 198
Medial mentalis muscle injections 250*f*
Medial platysmal fibers 238
Melomental fold 126, 225
Mental crease, dermal fillers in 132
Mental nerve 73*f*
Mentalis 140
    moderate rhytides of 229
    muscle 37, 128, 131, 229, 229*f*, 231*f*, 250*f*
        anatomy of 229
        hypertrophy of 129
        injection of 233
    treatment of 231*f*

Mesobotox 259
Microbotox 262
    action of 259
    acts on superficial muscle fibers 259
    objective of 260
    solution 264f
    technique 263, 265
        postadministration of 264f
    volume of 263
Microgenia 128
Microneedling radiofrequency 263
Midcheek groove 34f
Midface 21, 35, 107f, 166
    assessment 61f
    augmentation 109f, 113f
    concerns 167
    fat compartments of 37
    filler 125
        injections 126f
    muscles of 36
    planes 55
    rejuvenation 61
    sequence of treatments in 167
    volumization 126
Mid-pupillary line 99, 114, 183
Minimally invasive esthetic procedures 253
Minors' iodine starch test 173
Modiolus, anterior portion of 214
Moisturizers, topical 246
Motor nerve innervation 139
Mouse hemidiaphragm assay 268, 269
Mouse protection assay 268, 269
Mouth
    left angle of 155f
    retraction of 236
Mueller's muscles 248
Multiple microablative columns 171
Muscle
    anatomy of 209t
    deeper fibers of 260f
    functions of 209t
    main 203, 214
    masticatory 241
    paralysis-related complications 247
    tone, loss of 213, 237
Myasthenia gravis 264

N

Naphazoline 248
Nasal
    bone 209
    cartilage 209
    dorsum hyperhidrosis 211
    flutter 211, 212
    hyperhidrosis 212
    septum, cartilaginous 209
    tip
        elevation of 210, 211f
        injection 212
        projection 57, 57f, 57t
Nasalis 203
    muscle 36
Nasofrontal angle 58f
Nasoglabellar lines 202, 206, 208f, 209
    causes of 203
Nasojugal groove 34f, 98, 99, 101, 104f
Nasolabial angle 57, 57f, 116
Nasolabial filler, complications of 155f
Nasolabial fold 20, 77, 113f, 118
    junction of 236
Nasomaxillary angles 59f
Natural lip symmetry 138
Neck
    and jawline 261
    angle 237
    lines 262
    movement 239
    rejuvenation 171
    weakness 247
Needle 75
    type 131
Neural structures 110
Neuromuscular disease, history of 67
Neurotoxin
    diffusion of 232
    injections, classical 264
    preparations 179
    resistance 267
Neutralizing antibodies 270
    development of 268
    role of 271
Ninhydrin sweat test 269
Nodulation 126
Nodules 156

Nonanimal stabilized hyaluronic acid, evolution of 10
Nonbarbed threads and barbed threads, types of 164t
Nonhemagglutinin proteins 267
Nonsteroidal anti-inflammatory drug 82, 111, 136
Nonsurgical skin tightening devices 163
Nontoxic accessory proteins 267
Normal smile preinjection 232f
Nose 20, 21, 51, 56, 77, 115, 208
    augmentation 115f
    chin evaluation 59
    correlation of 63f
    dorsum of 116
    lifting upper lip and wing of 209
    lip-chin line 60f
    muscles of 209f
    part of 203
    width 55

O

Omega-3 fatty acid 136
Omohyoid 236
Onabotulinum toxin 173, 180, 223, 257t, 264f
    type A 179, 259
Ophthalmic artery 100
    branch of 26, 47f
Optical coherent tomography imaging 173f
Oral commissure 43f, 250
Oral muscles, adjacent 237
Oral pain killers 246
Orange peel 230
Orbicularis
    muscle 30
    oculi 31, 198
        muscle 30, 30f, 32f, 98
    oris 37, 140, 147, 214t
        muscle 43f, 139, 213
    retaining
        element 40
        ligament 25, 31, 31f, 99, 113
Orbit 30
Orbital rim 99
Orbital septum 99, 200
Orbital zone 247, 248
Overeruption, anterior 218

P

Pain 156, 246
Palatal necrosis 88

Palmar hyperhidrosis 173, 174
    severe bilateral 174f
Palmar sweating, severe 174f
Palmoplantar skin, anatomical section of 172
Palpable nodules 115, 116
Palpebromalar groove 99, 102, 103f
Papulopustular lesions 157
Paradoxical bulging 247
Parotid
    duct 39f
    gland hypertrophy 62
Parotidomasseteric ligament 42
Peau D'orange 230
Penicillamine 264
Pentavalent vaccine 268
Perform stretch test 187
Periocular rejuvenation 61, 61f
Perioral area 213
    blood supply of 215f
    muscles of 214f
Perioral blood vasculature 140f
Perioral complications 247, 249
Perioral muscles 140f
Perioral region 166
    bony structure of 214
Perioral rhytides 213
Periorbital arteries 33f
Periorbital complications 247
Periorbital injections 247f, 250
Periorbital veins 33f
Periosteum 82
Phenylephrine 248
Philtral ridge 43f
Philtrum 43f
    columns 145
Phosphatidylcholine 164, 165
Platysma 134
    muscle
        hyperkinetic activity of 237
        tenses 237
    originates 234
Platysmal auricular ligament 42
Platysmal bands 234, 239, 262
    formation of 237
Plump cheeks 112
Plumping 143
    lip, technique for 144f

Polyacrylamide hydrogel 5
Polyalkylimide gel 6
Poly-l-lactic acid 4
Polymethyl methacrylate 5
Polyvinylpyrrolidone-silicone suspension 5
Postdental treatment 223f
Posterior mandibular curve 44f
Postfiller administration, complications of 103
Postinflammatory hyperpigmentation 155f
    risk of 174
Postinjection instructions 82, 88, 97, 212
Powell and Humphreys' esthetic angles 59f
Predental treatment 223f
Pregnancy 67, 263
Prejowl sulcus 77
Preseptal skin 94f
Pretarsal skin 94ff
Prezygomatic space 31, 32f
Primary axillary hyperhidrosis treatment, use of 171
Procerus muscle 25, 203f
Prominent lid-cheek junction 99
Propionibacterium acnes 67
Pterion 29

Q
Quinine 264

R
Radioimmunoprecipitation assay 269
Ramus, processes of 133
Reduce pain 261
Reidel's plane 63
Respiratory impairment 264
Restylane 18, 104
Retaining ligaments 87, 161
Retinal artery embolus 122
Retrognathia 128
Retro-orbicularis oculi fat 91f, 95
Rheological parameters 17
Rheological properties 17, 20
Rheology 17
Rickett's esthetic line 129f, 132, 138f
Riedel line 60f
Risorius muscle 36
Risus sardonicus 37

S
Scar
    formation 157
    technique for 151
    tissue 138
Scrunch lines 202
Sebaceous gland activity 263
Serial puncture 75
Simons ratio 58f
Single-point technique 230, 231f
Six horizontal measurements 54f
Skeleton-like look 112
Skin 23f, 80, 82
    atrophy of 99
    blanching of 155f, 156
    discoloration 156, 158
    fascia of 186
    flaccidity and poor quality of 237
    hydrated 160
    necrosis 114f
    on chin, cobblestone appearance of 130f
    roughness 149
Skull 254f
Small gauge needles, use of 105
Smoker's lines 213, 213f
Smooth glabellar area 182
Snap test 248, 265
Soft tissue
    cephalometric points 52, 52f
    layers of 23f
    ptosis of 62
Speech difficulty 264
Standard post botulinum toxin injection 236
Sterile 180
    folliculitis lesions 157
Sternocleidomastoid 250
    test 269
Sternohyoid 236
Strabismus 247, 249
Subcutaneous fat 80, 82, 99
Subcutaneous tissue 253
Sublabial veins 126
Submandibular fat compartments, atrophy of 123
Submental artery 47
Submental fat excess 165
Suborbicularis oculi fat 55, 99, 102f
Suborbital area 99

Superficial fat
    compartment 161
    pads 134
    thin layer of 23f
Superficial filler placement 104
Superficial injection 242
Superficial layer 80
Superficial muscle fibers 260f
Superficial musculoaponeurotic system 36, 81, 86, 112, 123, 126, 136
Superficial temporal
    artery 28f, 29, 152
        frontal branch of 83
    fascia 80, 82
    fat pad 82
Superior labial artery 46, 46f
Superior temporal septum 27
Supraorbital artery 26, 79, 83f
Supraorbital margin 182
Supraorbital notch 24f
Supraorbital vessels 24f
    location of 97f
Supraperiosteal bolus points 88f
Supraperiosteal technique 88
Supratrochlear artery 26, 79
Supratrochlear vessels, location of 97f
Sweat
    and sebum production 260
    glands 172f
Swelling 110, 146
Swift point 89
Synaptosome inhibition assay 269
Syringe, aspiration of 242
Systemic botox exposure 246

T

Tear
    Hirmand's classification of 100t
        trough 20, 21, 34f, 76, 101
            deformity 99
            ligament 30, 31, 98
Teeth 219
    shape of 218
    size of 218
Temple filler injection 88f
Temple hollowness 166
Temporal adhesion 27

Temporal aging, stages of 87t
Temporal area 80, 81
    layers of 80, 82
Temporal bone 80
    zygomatic process of 35
Temporal branch 28f, 39
Temporal ligamentous adhesion 27
Temporal muscle
    atrophy 86
    attaches 133
Temporal region 27
Temporalis fascia 80
Temporalis muscle 28, 80, 82
Temporoparietal fascia 27, 28f
Tenting technique 145
Tissue
    integration 13
    necrosis 156
Tooth and gum tissue complex 218
Tower technique 75
Toxin 147, 270
    higher doses of 236
    injection treatment 173
Transverse nasalis 209
Trigeminal nerve 133
Trough ligament 41
Two-point technique 230, 231f
Tyndall effect 104, 146

U

United States Food and Drug Administration 171
Upper buccal branch 40
Upper eyelids 173
Upper face 166
    concerns 166
    treatment 166, 262
        recommendations for 166
Upper jaw 219
    vertical position of 219
Upper lip 138, 209
    length and degree of movement of 219
    ptosis 247
Upper temporal
    compartment 86f
    region, structures of 80t
Upturned mouth corners 145

V

Valaciclovir 68
Vascular complication 105, 158
Vermillion border 43f, 143
    enhancement, technique for 143f
Vertical fanning 144
Vertical fifths 53, 53f
Vertical maxillary excess 219, 223f
Vibration 74
Viscosity 12
Viscous modulus g 17
Vision, blurred 156
Visual analog scale 174
Visual loss 83, 83f
Vitamin E 136
    supplements 246
Voice, hoarseness of 247
Voluminous lips 137
Volumization 143
V-shaped injection technique 119

W

Western blot assay 269
Wet vermillion 43f
Wrinkle 213
    severity rating scale 118

X

Xeomin 179, 267, 270
Xylocaine, injection of 96f

Y

Yonsei point 220
Youthful jawline 133
Yvoire fillers 19

Z

Zig-zag injection pattern 188f
Zygoma, body of 32f
Zygomatic
    arch 28f, 29, 35, 43, 56f, 103, 241
    branch 39
    eminence 35, 103
    facial vessels 110
    ligament 31, 32f, 41
    region, anterior 99
Zygomaticocutaneous ligament 113, 160
Zygomaticofacial
    nerve 35
    vessels 35
Zygomaticus
    major 36, 46f, 140, 219
    minor 36, 140, 219